ALLE · ZEIT · WACH · 1842

Return to Work
After Coronary Artery Bypass Surgery

Psychosocial and Economic Aspects

Editor: P. J. Walter

With 102 Figures and 204 Tables

Springer-Verlag
Berlin Heidelberg New York Tokyo

Prof. Dr. Paul J. Walter
Department of Cardiovascular Surgery
University Hospital Antwerp
Wilrijkstraat 10, B-2520 Antwerp-Edegem, Belgium

ISBN-13: 978-3-642-69857-6 e-ISBN-13: 978-3-642-69855-2
DOI: 10.1007/978-3-642-69855-2

Library of Congress Cataloging in Publication Data. Main entry under title: Return to work after coronary artery bypass surgery. Proceedings of a symposium held at Herz-Kreislauf-Zentrum Rotenburg/Fulda, May 10–11, 1984. Includes bibliographies and index. 1. Aortocoronary bypass—Patients—Rehabilitation. 2. Aortocoronary bypass—Patients—Employment. 3. Aortocoronary bypass—Patients—Psychology. 4. Aortocoronary bypass—Costs. I. Walter, P. J. (Paul J.), 1935–. [DNLM: 1. Aortocoronary Bypass—rehabilitation—congresses. 2. Employment—congresses. 3. Rehabilitation, Vocational—economics—congresses. 4. Rehabilitation, Vocational—psychology—congresses. WG 169 R439 1984]
RD598.R47 1985 617′.412 85-4620

Softcover reprint of the hardcover 1st edition 1985

2121/3140-543210

Preface

When I gave a presentation on return to work after heart valve replacement at the Tenth Congress of the German Society for Thoracic and Cardiovascular Surgery in 1981, I was surprised by the relatively low level of interest that cardiac surgeons seemed to have in this subject. This stimulated me to intensify my research in this area and to extend it to patients with coronary heart disease.

Obviously, physiological and mechanical aspects of medical treatment are of special interest to the surgeon. For the majority of cardiac surgical patients, that is those with coronary heart disease, the technical problems of the operative procedure have been solved to a great extent. Many studies have demonstrated that, aside from reduction of symptoms, aortocoronary bypass operation can lead to improvement of cardiac performance under stress conditions. However in spite of the technical solutions to hemodynamic problems, it has become very clear that the reintegration of patients into their social sphere has not been accomplished to the extent that might be expected, as exemplified by the relatively low rate of postoperative return to work. Apparently, factors other than hemodynamics and cardiac function impede resumption of the normal lifestyle, enjoyed before the onset of the symptoms of angina pectoris. Return to work after coronary bypass surgery must be seen in a larger psychosocial framework, to understand the deeper reasons for the low incidence. Factors such as the time spent on the waiting list, the role of family and friends, the expectations of the spouse, motivation and guidance from the family doctor, the cardiologist and other hospital staff, and the attitude of employer and colleagues should be studied.

Research should embrace not only, bypass operation, but also percutaneous transluminal coronary angioplasty and conservative treatment.

The great number of coronary operations (about 170000 in the USA in 1983) is a very large burden on the state's social resources. The overall cost to the state could be reduced if it were possible to reintegrate a large number of these patients into working life. The expense of the operation could be recovered within a short time if return to work were increased (higher tax revenue, lower pension and welfare payments).

This book presents the papers from an international symposium which took place on May 10–11, 1984, in the *Herz- und Kreislaufzentrum,* Rotenburg, Federal Republic of Germany, under the patronage of the International Society of Cardiovascular Surgery and the German Society of Thoracic and Cardiovascular Surgery. The scientific committee consisted of H. G. Borst, Hannover; W. D. Johnson, Milwaukee; F. Loogen, Düsseldorf; G. Rodewald, Hamburg; Å. Senning, Zürich; and P. Walter, Antwerp.

For the financial support necessary for the symposium to be held, I would like to thank Pharma Schwarz, Monheim, Federal Republic of Germany, represented by Mr. Gücker. I would like to say a special word of thanks to Mrs. B. Kratzenberg for her excellent organizational support. I am grateful to all the authors for their cooperation, and to Springer-Verlag, represented by Mr. B. Lewerich and his colleagues, for accurate and rapid publication.

Paul J. Walter

Contents

List of Contributors

Almeida, D., Emory University School of Medicine,
69 Butler Street, S. E., Atlanta, GA 30303, USA

Anderson, A. J., Division of Biostatistics, Medical College of Wisconsin, P.O.Box 26509, Milwaukee, WI 53226, USA

Appelbaum, A., Department of Surgery, Hadassah-Hebrew University Hospital, IL-Jerusalem 92-585, Israel

Barboriak, J. J., Department of Pharmacology and Toxicology, Medical College of Wisconsin, Biochemistry Section, Research Service 151 B, Wood, WI, USA

Behrenbeck, D. W., Medizinische Klinik III und Herzchirurgische Klinik der Universität zu Köln, Joseph-Stelzmann-Straße 9, D-5000 Köln 41, FRG

Bentall, H. H., Royal Postgraduate Medical School, Hammersmith Hospital, Du Cane Road, London W12 OHS, GB

Bergmann, G., Medizinische Klinik der Universität, Abteilung Innere Medizin II, Bergheimer Straße 58, D-6900 Heidelberg, FRG

Birck, G., Klinik Roderbirken, D-5653 Leichlingen/Rhld. 1, FRG

Blümchen, G., Klinik Roderbirken, D-5653 Leichlingen/Rhld. 1, FRG

Boll, A., Rehabilitationszentrum Bad Segeberg, Kurpark, D-2360 Bad Segeberg, FRG

Borer, J. S., New York Hospital, Cornell University, New York, NY, USA

Bormann, J., Department of Surgery, Hadassah-Hebrew University Hospital, IL-Jerusalem 92-585, Israel

Boulay, F., Hôpital Central, Centre Hospitalier Régional de Nancy, 29 av de Lattre de Tassigny, F-54500 Vandoeuvre, France

Bourassa, M. G., Institut de Cardiologie de Montréal, 500 E Rue Bélanger, Montréal, Québec, HIT IC8, CDN

Bradford, J. M., Emory University School of Medicine, 69 Butler Street, S. E., Atlanta, GA 30303, USA

Carstens, V., Medizinische Klinik III der Universität zu Köln, Joseph-Stelzmann-Straße 9, D-5000 Köln 41, FRG

Charles, E. D. Jr., School of Public Health, University of Alabama in Birmingham, University Station, Birmingham, AL 35294, USA

Chaves, V., Department de Cardiologie, Université de Genève, CH-1211 Genève, Switzerland

Chiang, J., Department of Surgery, University of Virginia Medical Center, P.O.Box 181, Charlottesville, VA 22908, USA

Clayton, P. D., Department of Thoracic and Cardiovascular Surgery, LDS Hospital, Salt Lake City, UT, and the Department of Medical Biophysics and Computing, University of Utah and LDS Hospital, Salt Lake City, UT, USA

Collins, J. J. Jr., Division of Thoracic and Cardiac Surgery Brigham and Momen's Hospital, 75 Francis Street, Boston, MA 02115, USA

Coustry-Degré, C., Cliniques Universitaire de Bruxelles, Hôpital Academique Erasme, Université Libre de Bruxelles, 808 Route de Lennik, B-1070 Bruxelles, Belgium

Craddock, G. B. Jr., Department of Internal Medicine (Cardiology Division), University of Virginia Medical Center, P.O.Box 181, Charlottesville, VA 22908, USA

Crosby, I. K., Baylor Medical Plaza, 3600 Gaston Ave., 1201 Barnett Tower, Dallas, TX 75246, USA

Dalichau, H., Herzchirurgische Klinik der Universität zu Köln, Joseph-Stelzmann-Straße 9, D-5000 Köln 41, FRG

Danchin, N., Hôpital de Brabois, Centre Hospitalier Régional de Nancy, Route de Neufchateau, F-54500 Vandœvre les Nancy, France

David, P., Institut de Cardiologie de Montréal, 5000 E Rue Bélanger, Montréal, Québec, HIT IC8, CDN

David, P. R., Institut de Cardiologie de Montréal, 5000 E Rue Bélanger, Montréal, Québec, HIT IC8, CDN

Degré, S., Cliniques Universitaires de Bruxelles, Hôpital Academiques Erasme, Université Libre de Bruxelles, 808 Route de Lennik, B-1070 Bruxelles, Belgium

DeRouen, T. A., School of Public Health, University of Washington, Seattle, WA, USA

Dion, W. F., Cardiac Rehabilitation Program, Mount Sinai Medical Center, University of Wisconsin Medical School, 950 N. 12th Street, Milwaukee, WI 53233, USA

Dodge, H. T., University of Washington, Seattle, WA, USA

Domanig, E., II. Chirurgische Universitätsklinik Wien, Spitalgasse 23, A-1090 Wien, Austria

Erdman, R. A. M., Erasmus Universiteit Rotterdam, Fakulteit der Geneeskunde, Thoraxcenter, Postbus 1738, NL-3000 DR Rotterdam, The Netherlands

Faidutti, B., Department de Cardiologie, Université de Genève, CH-1211 Genève, Switzerland

Fentrop. T., Klinik Roderbirken, D-5653 Leichlingen/Rhld. 1, FRG

Fisher, C., Coordinating Center for CASS, University of Washington, Seattle, WA, USA

Flameng, W., Cardiovascular Surgery Department, University Hospital Gasthuisberg, Heretraat, B-3000 Leuven, Belgium

Foster, C., Cardiac Rehabilitation Program, Mount Sinai Medical School, University of Wisconsin Medical School, 950 N. 12th Street, Milwaukee, WI 53233, USA

Frank, K. A., Departments of Psychiatry and Surgery, College of Physicians and Surgeons, Columbia University, New York, NY, USA

Frøysaker, T., Medical Department B, Rikshospitalet, University Hospital, Oslo, Norway

Fuchs, Y., Thoracic and Cardiovascular Surgery Department, Beilinson Medical Center, Tel Aviv University Medical School, IL- Tel Aviv 63474, Israel

Gerhardt, U., Institut für Medizinische Soziologie, Friedrichsstraße 24, D-6300 Giessen, FRG

Gleichmann, U., Gollwitzer-Meier-Institute, D-4970 Bad Oeynhausen, FRG

Glonner, K., Klinik Höhenried für Herz- und Kreislaufkrankheiten, D-8139 Bernried/Obb., FRG

Gotsman, M. S., Department of Cardiology, Hadassah-Hebrew-University Hospital, IL- Jerusalem 92-585, Israel

Gohlke, H., Rehabilitationszentrum für Herz- und Kreislaufkranke, Südring 15, D-7812 Bad Krozingen, FRG

Gottwik, M., Kerckhoffklinik, Benekestraße 2,
D-6350 Bad-Nauheim, FRG

Gould, B., Department of Thoracic and Cardiovascular Surgery, LDS Hospital, Salt Lake City, and the Department of Medical Biophysics and Computing, University of Utah and LDS Hospital, Salt Lake City, UT, USA

Grevenow, P., Cardiac Rehabilitation Program, Mount Sinai Medical Center, University of Wisconsin Medical School, 950 N. 12th Street, P.O.Box 342, Milwaukee, WI 53233, USA

Grodzinski, E., Klinik Roderbirken, D-5653 Leichlingen/Rhld. 1, FRG

Grossmann, P., Medizinische Klinik und Poliklinik B, und Chirurgische Klinik B, Universität Düsseldorf, Moorenstraße 5, D-4000 Düsseldorf, FRG

Guggenmoos-Holzmann, I., Chirurgische Klinik und Institut für medizinische Statistik und Dokumentation der Universität Erlangen-Nürnberg, Maximiliansplatz, D-8520 Erlangen, FRG

Gutmann, M. C., University of Wisconsin Medical School, Milwaukee Clinical Campus, Mount Sinai Medical Center, 950 N. 12th Street, P.O.Box 342, Milwaukee, WI 53201, USA

Hacker, R. W., Herz- und Gefäßklinik, Salzburger Leite 1, D-8740 Bad Neustadt, FRG

Halhuber, M., An der Gotardslust 17, D-5920 Bad Berleburg, FRG

Hammermeister, K. E., Veterans Administration Medical Center, University of Colorado Health Sciences Center, Denver, 1055 Clermont Street, CO, USA

Hahn, K.-J., Abteilung für Herz- und Gefäßchirurgie, Chirurgische Universitätsklinik Hamburg, Martinistraße 52, D-2000 Hamburg 20, FRG

Hanna, S., II. Chirurgische Universitätsklinik Wien, Spitalgasse 23, A-1090 Wien, Austria

Heller, S. S., Departments of Psychiatry and Surgery, College of Physicians and Surgeons, Columbia University, New York, NY, USA

Hoffmann, R. G., Division of Biostatics, Medical College of Wisconsin, P.O.Box 26509, Milwaukee, WI 53226, USA

Hofmann, H., Klinik Höhenried für Herz- und Kreislaufkrankheiten, D-8139 Bernried/Obb., FRG

Hugenholtz, P. G., Erasmus Universiteit Rotterdam, Fakulteit der Geneeskunde, Thoraxcenter, Postbus 1738, NL-3000 DR Rotterdam, The Netherlands

Hurst, J. W., Emory University School of Medicine, 69 Butler Street S.E., Atlanta, GA 30303, USA

Huse-Kleinstoll, G., Universitätskrankenhaus Eppendorf, Abteilung für Herz- und Gefäßchirurgie, Martinistraße 52, D-2000 Hamburg 20, FRG

Hymowitz, Z., Department of Cardiology, Hadassah-Hebrew University Hospital, IL- Jerusalem 92-585, Israel

Ibe, B., Klinik für Herz- und Gefäßchirurgie, Justus-Liebig-Universität, Klinikstr. 29, D-6300 Giessen, FRG

Iberer, F., Universitätsklinik für Chirurgie, Auenbruggerplatz 1, A-8036 Graz, Austria

Jehle, J., Medizinische Klinik B, Universität Düsseldorf, Moorenstraße 5, D-4000 Düsseldorf, FRG

Johnson, W. D., Milwaukee Heart Surgery Associates, S.C., Thoracic and Cardiovascular Surgery, 3112 West Highland Boulevard, Milwaukee, WI 53208, USA

Jones, P. D., Department of Thoracic and Cardiovascular Surgery, LDS Hospital, Salt Lake City, UT, and the Department of Medical Biophysics and Computing, University of Utah and LDS Hospital, Salt Lake City, UT, USA

Jordan, S., Department of Surgery, University of Virginia Medical Center, P.O.Box 181, Charlottesville, VA 22908, USA

Jungmann, H., Curschmann-Klinik, D-2408 Timmendorfer Strand, FRG

Kaiser, D. L., Department of Internal Medicine (Cardiology Division), University of Virginia Medical Center, P.O.Box 181, Charlottesville, VA 22908, USA

Kalmár, P., Abteilung für Herz- und Gefäßchirurgie, Chirurgische Universitätsklinik Hamburg, Martinistraße 52, D-2000 Hamburg 20, FRG

Kaltenbach, M., Johann-Wolfgang-Goethe-Universität, Zentrum Innere Medizin, Abteilung für Kardiologie, Theodor-Stern-Kai, D-6000 Frankfurt/Main, FRG

Kampa, L., Medizinische Klinik und Poliklinik B, und Chirurgische Klinik B, Universität Düsseldorf, Moorenstraße 5, D-4000 Düsseldorf, FRG

Kaplan DeNour, A., Department of Psychiatry, Hadassah-Hebrew University Hospital, IL- Jerusalem 92-585, Israel

Kayser, K. L., 3112 West Highland Boulevard, Milwaukee, WI 53208, USA

Keller, T., Klinik Roderbirken, D-5653 Leichlingen/Rhld. 1, FRG

Keon, University of Ottawa Heart Institute and Faculty of Administration, Program in Health Administration, Civic Hospital, 737, Park Dale Avenue, Ottawa K14148, CDN

King, S. B., Emory University School of Medicine, 69 Butler Street, S. E., Atlanta, GA 30303, USA

Klein, W., Universitätsklinik für Chirurgie, Auenbruggerplatz 1, A-8036 Graz, Austria

Klepetko, W., II. Chirurgische Universitätsklinik Wien, Spitalgasse 23, A-1090 Wien, Austria

Klinner, W., Herzchirurgische Klinik, Klinikum Großhadern, Marchioninistraße 15, D-8000 München 70, FRG

Kloke, M., Medizinische Klinik und Poliklinik B, und Chirurgische Klinik B, Universität Düsseldorf, Moorenstraße 5, D-4000 Düsseldorf, FRG

Knapp, D. N., University of Wisconsin Medical School, Milwaukee Clinical Campus, Mount Sinai Medical Center, Milwaukee, WI 53201, USA

Koch, J., Rehabilitationszentrum Bad Segeberg, Kurpark, D-2360 Bad Segeberg, FRG

Kober, G., Johann-Wolfgang-Goethe-Universität, Zentrum Innere Medizin, Abteilung für Kardiologie, Theodor-Stern-Kai, D-6000 Frankfurt/Main, FRG

Koolen, J. J., Academisch Ziekenhuis, Universiteit van Amsterdam, Meijbergdreef 9, NL-1105 AZ Amsterdam Zuidoost, The Netherlands

Kornfeld, D. S., Presbyterian Hospital, 622 W., 168th Street, New York, NY 10032, USA

Kraft-Kinz, J., Universitätsklinik für Chirurgie, Auenbruggerplatz 1, A-8036 Graz, Austria

Krasemann, E. O., Curschmann-Klinik, D-2408 Timmendorfer Strand, FRG

Krian, A., Medizinische Klinik und Poliklinik B, und Chirurgische Klinik B, Universität Düsseldorf, Moorenstraße 5, D-4000 Düsseldorf, FRG

Kron, I. L., Department of Surgery, University of Virginia Medical Center, P.O.Box 181, Charlottesville, VA 22908, USA

Langbehn, Rehabilitationszentrum Bad Segeberg, Kurpark, D-2360 Bad Segeberg, FRG

Lay, C. M., University of Ottawa Heart Institute and Faculty of Administration, Program in Health Administration, Civic Hospital, 737 Park Dale Avenue, Ottawa K14148, CDN

Leclerc, J. L., Cliniques Universitaire de Bruxelles, Hôpital Academique Erasme, Université Libre de Bruxelles, 808 Route de Lennik, B-1070 Bruxelles, Belgium

Lempp, F., Universitätskrankenhaus Eppendorf, Abteilung für Herz- und Gefäßchirurgie, Martinistraße 52, D-2000 Hamburg, FRG

Lesaffre, E., Medical Informatics Department, University Hospital Gasthuisberg, Herestraat, B-3000 Leuven, Belgium

Levinski, L., Thoracic and Cardiovascular Surgery Department, Beilinson Medical Center, Tel Aviv University Medical School, IL- Tel Aviv 63474, Israel

Levy, M. J., Thoracic and Cardiovascular Surgery Department, Beilinson Medical Center, Tel Aviv University Medical School, IL- Tel Aviv 63474, Israel

Liddle, H. V., Department of Thoracic and Cardiovascular Surgery, LDS Hospital, Salt Lake City, UT, and the Department of Medical Biophysics and Computing, University of Utah and LDS Hospital, Salt Lake City, UT, USA

Loogen, F., Medizinische Klinik und Poliklinik B, Universität Düsseldorf, Moorenstraße 5, D-4000 Düsseldorf, FRG

Magometschnigg, H., II. Chirurgische Universitätsklinik Wien, Spitalgasse 23, A-1090 Wien, Austria

Malm, J. R., Department of Psychiatry and Surgery, College of Physicians and Surgeons, Columbia University, New York, NY, USA

Mannebach, H., Gollwitzer-Meier-Institute, D-4970 Bad Oeynhausen, FRG

Mayer, H. C., Chirurgische Klinik der Universität, Abteilung für Spezielle Thoraxchirurgie, Im Neuenheimer Feld 110, D-6900 Heidelberg, FRG

Meffert, H.-J., Universitätskrankenhaus Eppendorf, Abteilung für Herz- und Gefäßchirurgie, Martinistraße 52, D-2000 Hamburg, FRG

Mehmel, W., Medizinische Klinik der Universität, Abteilung Innere Medizin III, Bergheimer Straße 58, D-6900 Heidelberg, FRG

Meier, B., Centre de Cardiologie, Hôpital Cantonal Universitaire, CH-1211 Genève 4, Switzerland

Mentzer, R. L., Departments of Surgery and University of Virginia Medical Center, P.O.Box 181, Charlottesville, VA 22908, USA

Menzies, S. C., University of Ottawa Heart Institute and Faculty of Administration, Program in Health Administration, Civic Hospital, 737 Park Dale Avenue, Ottawa K14148, CDN

Mibashan, S., Thoracic and Cardiovascular Surgery Department, Beilinson Medical Center, Tel Aviv University Medical School, IL- Tel Aviv 63474, Israel

Moulijn, A. C., Cardiopulmonary Surgery, Akademisch Ziekenhuis, Universiteit van Amsterdam, Meijbergdreef 9, NL-1105 AZ Amsterdam, The Netherlands

Mullen, D. C., Cardiovascular Surgical Associates, 9800 West Bluemound Road, Milwaukee, WI 53226, USA

Neiss, A., Institut für Medizinische Statistik und Epidemiologie, Technische Universität, D-8000 Müchen, FRG

Nitter-Hauge, S., Laboratory of Cardiology, Medical Department B, Rikshospitalet, University Hospital, Oslo, Norway

Oberman, A., Department of Preventive Medicine, University of Alabama in Birmingham, University Station, Birmingham, AL 35294, USA

Pedraza, P. M., Milwaukee Heart Surgery Associates, S. C., Thoracic and Cardiovascular Surgery, 3112 West Highland Boulevard, Milwaukee, WI 53208, USA

Pollock, M. L., Cardiac Rehabilitation Program, Mount Sinai Medical Center, University of Wisconsin Medical School, 950 N. 12th Street, Milwaukee, WI 53233, USA

Polonius, M.-J., Abteilung für Herz- und Gefäßchirurgie, Chirurgische Universitätsklinik Hamburg, Martinistraße 52, D-2000 Hamburg 20, FRG

Rabiner, C. J., Long Island Jewish-Hillside Medical Center, Glen Oaks, New York, NY 11004, USA

Radtke, I., Abteilung für Herz- und Gefäßchirurgie, Chirurgische Universitätsklinik Hamburg, Martinistraße 52, D-2000 Hamburg 20, FRG

Reichart, B., Herzchirurgische Klinik, Klinikum Großhadern, Marchioninistraße 15, D-8000 München 70, FRG

Reifart, N., Johann-Wolfgang-Goethe-Universität, Zentrum für Chirurgie, Abteilung für Thorax-, Herz- und Gefäßchirurgie, Theodor-Stern-Kai, D-6000 Frankfurt/Main, FRG

Riedl, H., Chirurgische Klinik und Institut für medizinische Statistik und Dokumentation der Universität Erlangen-Nürnberg, Maximiliansplatz, D-8520 Erlangen, FRG

Rigler, B., Universitätsklinik für Chirurgie, Auenbruggerplatz 1, A-8010 Graz, Austria

Rodewald, G., Universitätskrankenhaus Eppendorf, Abteilung für Herz- und Gefäßchirurgie, Martinistraße 52, D-2000 Hamburg 20, FRG

Röger, C., Medizinische Klinik III und Herzchirurgische Klinik, Universität zu Köln, Joseph-Stelzmann-Straße 9, D-5000 Köln, FRG

Rosemberg, C., Thoracic and Cardiovascular Surgery Department, Beilinson Medical Center, Tel Aviv University Medical School, IL- Tel Aviv 63474, Israel

Roskamm, H., Rehabilitationszentrum für Herz- und Kreislaufkranke, Südring 15, D-7812 Bad Krozingen, FRG

Rothlin, M. E., Chirurgie A, Universitätsspital, CH-8091 Zürich, Switzerland

Rutishauser, W., Centre de Cardiologie, Hôpital Cantonal Universitaire, CH-1211 Genève 4, Switzerland

Saggau, W., Chirurgische Klinik der Universität, Abteilung für Spezielle Thoraxchirurgie, Im Neuenheimer Feld 110, D-6900 Heidelberg, FRG

Samek, L., Rehabilitationszentrum für Herz- und Kreislaufkranke, Südring 15, D-7812 Bad Krozingen, FRG

Satter, P., Johann-Wolfgang-Goethe-Universität, Zentrum für Chirurgie, Abteilung für Thorax-, Herz- und Gefäßchirurgie, Theodor-Stern-Kai, D-6000 Frankfurt/Main, FRG

Scherer, D., Johann-Wolfgang-Goethe-Universität, Zentrum Innere Medizin, Abteilung für Kardiologie, Theodor-Stern-Kai, D-6000 Frankfurt/Main, FRG

Schmidt, D. H., Cardiac Rehabilitation Program, Mount Sinai Medical Center, University of Wisconsin Medical School, 950 N. 12th Street, Milwaukee, WI 53233, USA

Schmitz, H., Medizinische Klinik III und Herzchirurgische Klinik der Universität zu Köln, Joseph-Stelzmann-Straße 9, D-5000 Köln, FRG

Schmitz, W., Chirurgische Klinik der Universität, Abteilung für Spezielle Thoraxchirurgie, Im Neuenheimer Feld 110, D-6900 Heidelberg, FRG

Schnellbacher, K., Rehabilitationszentrum für Herz- und Kreislaufkranke, Südring 15, D-7812 Bad Krozingen, FRG

Schoop, W., Aggertalklinik, D-5250 Engelskirchen, FRG

Segesser, L. v., Department de Cardiologie, Université de Genève, CH-1211 Genève, Switzerland

Seggewiss, H., Gollwitzer-Meier-Institute, D-4970 Bad Oeynhausen, FRG

Seidel, C., Fachkrankenhaus für Psychosomatik und Durchblutungserkrankungen, Dorfstr. 18, D-8139 Bernried/Starnberger See, FRG

Sennett, S., Cardiac Rehabilitation Program, Mount Sinai Medical Center, University of Wisconsin Medical School, 950 N. 12th Street, Milwaukee, WI 53233, USA

Senning, Å., Universitätsspital, CH-8091 Zürich, Switzerland

Sergeant, P., Cardiovascular Surgery Department, University Hospital Gasthuisberg, Herestraat, B-3000 Leuven, Belgium

Sheikhzadeh, A., Rehabilitationszentrum Bad Segeberg, Kurpark, D-2360 Bad Segeberg, FRG

Sieber, R., Chirurgie A, Universitätsspital, CH-8091 Zürich, Switzerland

Shore, R. T., Milwaukee Heart Surgery Associates S.C., Thoracic and Cardiovascular Surgery, 3112 West Highland Boulevard, Milwaukee, WI 53208, USA

Silomon, H., Schölebergstraße 22/3, D-4500 Osnabrück, FRG

Simonsen, S., Laboratory of Cardiology, Medical Department B, Rikshospitalet, University Hospital, Oslo, Norway

Skupin, M., Johann-Wolfgang-Goethe-Universität, Zentrum für Chirurgie, Abteilung für Thorax-, Herz- und Gefäßchirurgie, Theodor-Stern-Kai, D-6000 Frankfurt/Main, FRG

Stason, W. B., Harward School of Public Health, Center for the Analysis of Health Practices, 677 Huntington Avenue, Boston, MA 02115, USA

Stein, D., Department of Psychiatry, Hadassah-Hebrew University Hospital, IL- Jerusalem 92-585, Israel

Stein, G., Curschmann-Klinik, D-2408 Timmendorfer Strand, FRG

Steinrücken, H., Rehabilitationszentrum für Herz- und Kreislaufkranke, Südring 15, D-7812 Bad Krozingen, FRG

Stocksmeier, U., Institut für Sozialmedizin, Prävention und Rehabilitation e. V., Höhenbergstraße 12, D-8132 Tutzing b. München, FRG

Stoupel, E., Cliniques Universitaires de Bruxelles, Hôpital Académique Erasme, Université Libre de Bruxelles, 808 Route de Lennik, B-1070 Bruxelles, Belgium

Struyven, J., Cliniques Universitaires de Bruxelles, Hôpital Academique Erasme, Université Libre de Bruxelles, 808 Route de Lennik, B-1070 Bruxelles, Belgium

Suy, R., Cardiovascular Surgery Department, University Hospital Gasthuisberg, Herestraat, B-3000 Leuven, Belgium

Thoran, P., Rehabilitationszentrum Bad Segeberg, Kurpark, D-2360 Bad Segeberg, FRG

Torka, M., Chirurgische Klinik und Institut für medizinische Statistik und Dokumentation der Universität Erlangen-Nürnberg, Maximiliansplatz, D-8520 Erlangen, FRG

Tristani, F., Veterans Administration Hospital, Wood, Milwaukee, WI, USA

Troudart, T., Department of Psychiatry, Hadassah-Hebrew University Hospital, IL- Jerusalem 92-585, Israel

Unger, F., I. Universitätsklinik für Chirurgie, Anichstraße 35, A-6020 Innsbruck, Austria

Vallbracht, C., Johann-Wolfgang-Goethe-Universität, Zentrum Innere Medizin, Abteilung für Kardiologie, Theodor-Stern-Kai, D-6000 Frankfurt/Main, FRG

Vandermoten, P., Cliniques Universitaires de Bruxelles,
Hôpital Académique Erasme, Université Libre de Bruxelles,
808 Route de Lennik, B-1070 Bruxelles, Belgium

Vermeulen, A., Akademisch Ziekenhuis, Universiteit van
Amsterdam, Akademisch Medisch Zentrum, Meibergdreef 9,
NL-1105 AZ Amsterdam Zuidoost, The Netherlands

Vetter, H. O., Department of Cardiovascular Surgery,
University of Munich, Klinikum Großhadern, Marchioninistr. 15,
D-8000 München 70, West-Germany

Walker, J. A., Cardiovascular Associates Limited,
2975 S. 29th Street, Suite 300, Milwaukee, WI 53215, USA

Walter, P. J., Cardiovasculaire Heelkunde, Akademisch
Ziekenhuis Antwerpen, Wilrijkstraat 10, B-2520 Edegem,
Belgium

Wegscheider, R., Institut für Sozialmedizin, Prävention und
Rehabilitation e. V., Höhenbergstraße 12,
D-8132 Tutzing b. München, FRG

Welsch, M., Chirurgische Klinik der Universität, Abteilung für
Spezielle Thoraxchirurgie, Im Neuenheimer Feld 110,
D-6900 Heidelberg, FRG

Wenger, N. K., Emory University School of Medicine,
69 Butler Street, S. E., Atlanta, GA 30303, USA

Willner, A. E., Long Island Jewish-Hillside Medical Center,
Glen Oaks, NY, USA

Wilson, S. N., Departments of Psychiatry and Surgery,
College of Physicians and Surgeons, Columbia University,
New York, NY, USA

Zothner, M., Curschmann-Klinik, D-2408 Timmendorfer Strand,
FRG

Return to Work After Coronary Artery Bypass Surgery: Incidence and Main Factors

Age- and Sex-Specific Incidence and Main Factors

A. J. Anderson, J. J. Barboriak, R. G. Hoffmann, D. C. Mullen, and J. A. Walker

Introduction

To facilitate return to gainful employment following coronary artery bypass surgery (CAB), it is necessary to study the factors that affect the decision. Using broad age categories makes it difficult to differentiate the effects of the surgery from retirement. Combining men and women makes the proportions returning to gainful employment dependent on the ratio of men to women in the patient population. Trying to explain return to gainful employment without considering relief of angina following CAB misses the primary risk factor for return to gainful employment. Previous studies, which did not consider all these groups separately, obtained estimates of the proportion employed at 1–2 years after CAB that ranged from 51% to 91% [3, 7, 8, 10, 12, 13, 15–21]. For 3–5 years following CAB the proportion employed ranges from 35% to 72% [1, 2, 4, 5, 9, 11, 14].

In this paper we examine return to gainful employment in 9905 men and 1948 women at 1, 3, 6, and 10 years following CAB. Five age categories for men and three age categories for women are used to separate the effect of natural retirement and disease-related retirement. Angina pectoris following the surgery and patient's employment status prior to the surgery are also used to characterize return to gainful employment.

Methods

The patients in this study had CAB at two Milwaukee area hospitals between 1968 and 1981. The data from the coronary catheterization, surgery, medical history, and life-style factors, including work status, were collected by the Milwaukee Cardiovascular Data Registry. At yearly intervals since 1972 the surviving patients who have not returned the survey within 4 weeks are contacted by telephone. The follow-up rate is better than 95% each year. For the purposes of this study, we utilized the surveys conducted in 1979 through 1983 which contained questions on angina pectoris symptoms and current work status. Although the patients completed surveys throughout the period 1979–1983, they can be included in the analysis for at most two time periods. For example, a patient having CAB in 1976 would have follow-up information only for the 3 and 6 years follow-up. In order to account for this overlap we used maximum-likelihood methods [22] to estimate the probabilities of return to gainful employment.

In order to remove the confounding factor of natural retirement, we have concentrated most of our analysis on patients who would not yet have reached the age of natural retirement (60 or above) at 6 years following CAB. Consequently, retirement will mean disease-related retirement in these patients (age 30–54 years).

Results

Factors Related to Return to Gainful Employment

Table 1 summarizes the number of men and women in each of the five age categories. Seventy percent of the men and 51% of the women were under 60 years of age at the time of the surgery.

The year of surgery and the number of patients included at each of the four follow-up points after CAB are shown in Table 2. The incidence rates of employment following CAB are based on these patient groups.

Table 1. Number of coronary artery bypass patients by age at time of surgery

Age at time of CAB	Men		Women	
	Number	Percent	Number	Percent
30–49	2533	26	274	14
50–54	2039	21	305	16
55–59	2330	23	415	21
60–64	1795	18	469	24
65–79	1208	12	485	25
	9905	100	1848	100

Table 2. Number of patients and range of their year of surgery[a] by years after coronary bypass

Years after CAB	Range of year of surgery	Number surveyed	
		Men	Women
1	1978–1981	4826	1047
3	1976–1981	5540	1212
6	1972–1978	4964	877
10	1968–1974	2601	388

[a] Patient year of surgery; all follow-up studies were in 1979 through 1983

The majority of the men who are working after CAB were employed prior to CAB, as shown in Fig. 1. Fewer than 5% of all the men in each of the age categories became employed following CAB if they were not employed in the 6 months prior to CAB (Employed pre–no, Employed post–yes). The percentage of men deciding to retire after CAB if working prior to CAB increases steadily through age 64. For those aged 60–64 (Fig. 2), 25% were retired prior to CAB and an additional 30% retired immediately after CAB.

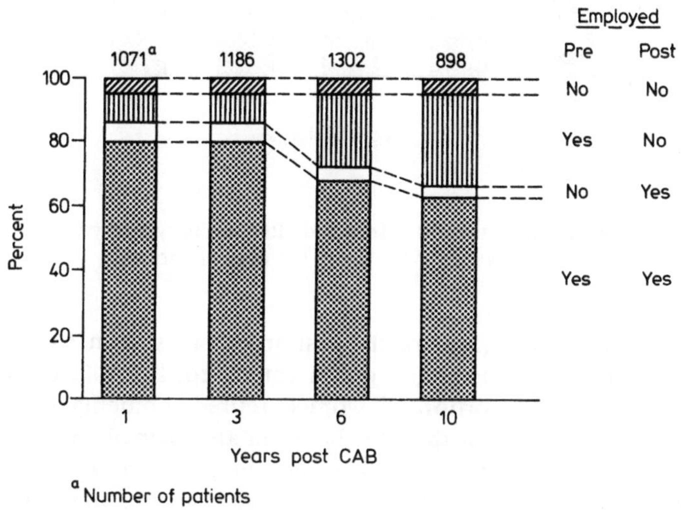

Fig. 1. Employment status before and after coronary artery bypass surgery by years after surgery for males aged 30–49 years at the time of surgery

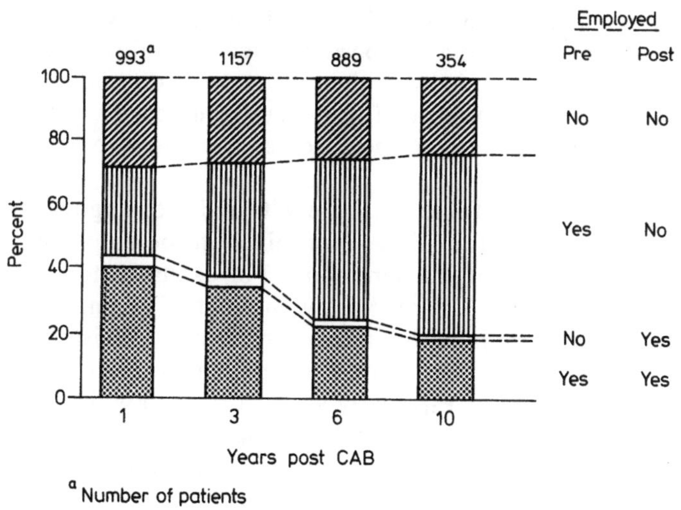

Fig. 2. Employment status before and after coronary artery bypass surgery by years after surgery for males aged 60–64 years at the time of surgery

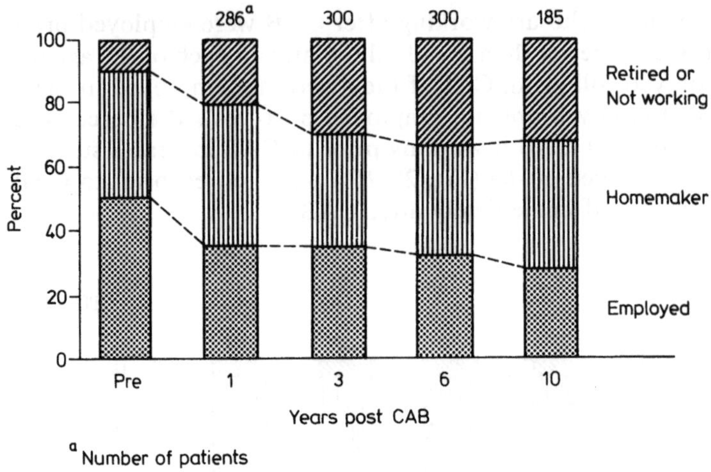

Fig. 3. Employment status before and after coronary artery bypass surgery by years after surgery for females aged 30–54 years at the time of surgery

For women (Fig. 3), the responses are shown to either (1) retired or not working (2) homemaker, or (3) employed, for 1, 3, 6, and 10 years following CAB. The proportion of women retired, homemaker, or employed prior to CAB varies by less than 5% between any year of the surgery. From 1–10 years following CAB, the percent responding homemaker remains consistently near 40% for those less than 55 years of age. The increase in the percent retired from 1 to 10 years following CAB complements the decrease in the percent employed.

Total or partial relief of angina following CAB is a very strong predictor of employment after CAB (Table 3). Ninety percent of the men and 85% of the women had total or partial relief of angina at 6 years following CAB. For men who experience total or partial relief of angina after CAB, the percent employed after CAB is twice that of men who do not experience relief of anginal symptoms. For example, for the age group 55–59, 20% were working six years after CAB when angina persisted as compared to 43% for those with relief of angina.

For women (Table 4), those with relief of angina after CAB are from one and one-half to four times more likely to be employed after CAB than those with persistent angina symptoms. For example, for age 30–54 years and at 6 years after CAB, 35% of those with relief of angina were employed, compared to 22% of those in whom anginal symptoms persisted.

The effect of angina in the few patients who do not experience relief of angina is substantial, especially when combined with employment status prior to CAB. In Table 5 the probability of being employed at 1, 3, and 6 years following CAB is computed separately for men employed prior to surgery and men not employed prior to surgery. Either not working prior to surgery or having persistent angina following surgery reduces the probability of not working following the surgery to 60% or less of that for men who were working prior to

Table 3. Percent of men working by age, years after CAB, and angina pectoris status at year after CAB

a) Men with partial or total relief of angina symptoms

Age at CAB	Pre-CAB	Years post CAB			
		1	3	6	10
30–49	91	88 (978)	86 (1093)	80 (1147)	71 (756)
50–54	90	83 (897)	80 (1147)	70 (947)	46 (538)
55–59	86	73 (1055)	65 (1235)	43 (1156)	26 (552)
60–64	72	42 (941)	33 (1100)	23 (832)	19 (1322)
65–79	38	23 (659)	22 (789)	20 (427)	16 (116)

b) Men with no relief of angina symptoms

Age at CAB	Pre-CAB	Years post CAB			
		1	3	6	10
30–49	87	53 (87)	54 (91)	38 (153)	39 (140)
50–54	84	49 (69)	42 (85)	35 (115)	17 (76)
55–59	81	36 (73)	41 (87)	20 (110)	17 (65)
60–64	69	33 (42)	18 (50)	18 (55)	7 (28)
65–79	32	12 (25)	9 (34)	9 (22)	12 (8)

( ), number of patients

Table 4. Percent of women working by age, years after CAB, and angina pectoris status at year after CAB

a) Women with partial or total relief of angina symptoms

Age at CAB	Pre-CAB	Years post CAB			
		1	3	6	10
30–54	53	41 (237)	41 (259)	35 (256)	31 (156)
55–64	42	27 (440)	24 (502)	15 (365)	8 (149)
65–79	16	8 (271)	9 (336)	12 (137)	17 (29)

b) Women with no relief of angina symptoms

Age at CAB	Pre-CAB	Years post CAB			
		1	3	6	10
30–54	51	7 (28)	15 (39)	22 (41)	11 (28)
55–64	39	13 (45)	8 (50)	8 (52)	12 (24)
65–79	14	8 (26)	14 (26)	4 (26)	(1)

( ), number of patients

Table 5. Probability of gainful employment for males after CAB

Age at CAB	Post-CAB angina	Employed prior to CAB			Not employed prior to CAB		
		1 yr	3 yrs	6 yrs	1 yr	3 yrs	6 yrs
30–49	Relieved	.92	.89	.82	.55	.57	.53
	Persistent	.58	.59	.45	.18	.22	.04
50–54	Relieved	.88	.85	.73	.43	.43	.43
	Persistent	.64	.54	.41	.00	.00	.00

surgery and experienced relief of angina. For the 50–54 year old men, employment status prior to surgery has even more of an effect on the probability of being employed. For both age groups, those who were not employed prior to surgery and experienced persistent angina had the lowest probability of being employed following surgery. The effect of age was a 10% (if employed prior to surgery) or 15% (if not employed prior to surgery) reduction in the probability of employment following CAB.

The effect of not being employed prior to surgery and persistent angina following surgery is shown for women aged 30–54 years old in Table 6. The probability of employment at 3 or 6 years is about one-half if angina is persistent. If the patient is not employed prior to surgery the probability of employment following CAB is less than 0.2.

Table 6. Probability of gainful employment for females after CAB

Age at CAB	Post-CAB angina	Employed prior to CAB			Not employed prior to CAB		
		1 yr	3 yrs	6 yrs	1 yr	3 yrs	6 yrs
30–54	Relieved	.68	.61	.50	.11	.16	.19
	Persistent	.07	.31	.28	.08	.00	.12

In addition to employment prior to CAB and relief of angina following CAB, other factors were significantly related to the decision to be employed following CAB (Table 7). For men less than 65 years of age, those employed in professional (white collar) jobs or with more education return to work at a higher rate than those employed in blue collar jobs or with less education. For males aged 55–64, those categorized as type A prior to surgery or who were self-employed were more likely to be employed after CAB, while poor left ventricular function was related to not being employed following CAB for men under age 55. For women, only education in addition to employment prior to CAB and angina after CAB was predictive of employment following CAB. For both men and women (aged 65 years or more) only working prior to surgery

Table 7. Predictors of employment following CAB

Working prior to CAB
Relief of angina following CAB
Younger age at time of CAB
More education
Professional type employment
Self-employed
Good left ventrical function
Type A behavior

was significantly predictive of working after CAB when all the variables were considered simultaneously.

Reasons for Failure to Return to Gainful Employment

The second part of our study examines reasons for not being employed. These results are based on the 1983 follow-up survey which included a series of questions on why the patients were not employed. Table 8 displays the results of these questions for men aged 30–54 years by anginal status at 3, 6, and 10 years following CAB. Those with persistent angina primarily reported reasons related to their symptoms. A surprising number of men with relief of angina at 3 years after their surgery (25%) indicated that they were able to work but could not because of "lay-offs or plan closings." The decrease in the percentages from 3 to 10 years for those who were able to work but could not because of lay-offs is reflected in an increase in the percentages who were "voluntarily retired" or "retired because of heart problems."

Table 8. Reasons for non-employment in 1983 for males aged 30–54

Reasons for not being employed	Percent of responses					
	Relief of angina at			Persistent angina at		
	3 yrs	6 yrs	10 yrs	3 yrs	6 yrs	10 yrs
1. Heart problems	23	19	17	53	58	51
2. Plant closings or lay-offs	25	17	7	2	1	2
3. Voluntarily retired	15	19	25	2	1	4
4. Retired because of heart problems	22	25	34	19	36	37
5. Other	15	20	17	24	4	6
Number of men not employed	(155)	(255)	(340)	(42)	(81)	(92)

Table 9. Reasons for non-employment in 1983 for females aged 30–54[a]

Reasons for not being employed	Percent of responses Relief of angina at			Persistent angina at		
	3 yrs	6 yrs	10 yrs	3 yrs	6 yrs	10 yrs
1. Heart problems	34	40	19	57	57	64
2. Plant closings or lay-offs	14	4	3	0	0	0
3. Voluntarily retired	31	22	24	0	0	7
4. Retired because of heart problems	7	12	30	28	36	21
5. Other	14	22	24	14	7	7
Number of females not employed	(29)	(50)	(37)	(7)	(14)	(14)

[a] Homemaker not included

Table 9 displays the corresponding results for women aged 30–54 years. Women who had indicated that they were homemakers are not included. Of those with persistent angina, the majority responded that they were not employed because of heart-related problems. For women with relief of angina, 20%–30% "voluntarily retired." The increase in the percentages who responded "retired because of heart problems" is accompanied by a decrease in the percentages who responded "not working because of heart problems."

Summary

The effect of age at the time of CAB on employment following CAB is minimal unless the patients are near retirement age at the time of CAB. Having CAB at age 55 or greater hastens the decision to retire if one was employed prior to the operation.

Patterns of employment following CAB should be studied separately for men and women because of the substantially different rates of gainful employment. Also, additional information is needed to evaluate whether the surgery helped the homemakers to increase their ability to work at home following surgery.

Almost all studies on return to gainful employment are in agreement that working prior to surgery, relief of angina following CAB, higher education level, and occupations requiring less physical demand are predictive of working following CAB. In addition we observed that men aged 55–64 at the time of CAB and who were classified as type A were more likely to be employed at 3 and 6 years following CAB than men classified as type B. Two other studies reported no relation between type A/B personalities and working following CAB [6, 23]. This could be explained by the smaller number of men in the other two studies and the fact that the relation was observed only for men aged 55–64 at the time of CAB in this study.

The probability of being employed following CAB is decreased by 30%–40% if the patient was not employed prior to surgery. Also, the probability of being employed following CAB is decreased by 30%–40% if the patient has persistent angina following CAB. The effect of persistent angina and nonemployment prior to CAB result in an 80% or greater reduction in the probability of being employed following CAB.

The greatest potential for employment following CAB is in patients under age 55 at the time of CAB. At the time of surgery 90% of the men under age 55 were employed, which corresponds to 93% expected from United States Bureau of Labor Statistics figures [24]. At 6 years following surgery 71% of these men were working, while the corresponding figure for the United States is 81% employment. Thus for this age group of men, there is only a potential of an additional 10% who could be employed at 6 years following CAB.

Prior to their CAB, 51% of women aged 30–54 years were employed outside the home. Corresponding figures for the United States show 54% employed. At 6 years following CAB 33% were employed outside the home, while the corresponding United States value is 48%. Thus for women less than 55 years of age at the time of CAB there is a greater potential for return to gainful employment than for men.

Several other studies have detailed reasons for not being employed following CAB [1, 6, 11, 14, 16, 23]. Some of these are adequate savings, disability benefits, and psychological factors. In addition, we have observed that unemployment (lay-offs or plant closings) is a major reason why men under 55 years of age at the time of CAB do not return to gainful employment.

Acknowledgements. The cooperation of St. Luke's Hospital and The Wood Veterans Administration Hospital, both of Milwaukee, Wisconsin and the assistance of The Milwaukee Cardiovascular Data Registry is gratefully acknowledged.

References

1. Almeida D, et al (1983) Return to work after coronary bypass surgery. Circulation 68:205–213
2. Anderson AJ, et al (1980) Retention or resumption of employment after aortocoronary bypass operations. JAMA 243:543–545
3. Barnes et al (1977) Changes in working status of patients following coronary bypass surgery. JAMA 238:12
4. Boulay et al (1982) Strategies for improving the work status of patients after coronary artery bypass surgery. Circulation 66 (III):43–49
5. Danchin et al (1982) Employment following aortocoronary bypass surgery in young patients. Cardiology 69:52–59
6. Dimsdale et al (1982) The association of clinical, psychosocial, and angiographic variables with work status in patients with coronary artery disease. J Psychosom Res 26, 2:215–221
7. Frick et al (1979) Work status after coronary bypass surgery. Acta Med Scand 206:61–64

8. Gutmann et al (1982) Coronary artery bypass patients and work status. Circulation 66
9. Guvendik et al (1982) Symptomatic status and pattern of employment during a five-year period following myocardial revascularization for angina. Ann Thorac Surg 34:4
10. Hammermeister et al (1979) Effect of surgical versus medical therapy on return to work in patients with coronary artery disease. Am J Cardiol 44:105–111
11. Johnson et al (1982) Employment patterns in males before and after myocardial revascularization surgery. Circulation 65, 6:1086–1093
12. Liddle et al (1982) The rehabilitation of coronary surgical patients. Ann Thorac Surg 34
13. Love (1980) Employment status after coronary bypass operations and some cost considerations. J Thorac Cardiovasc Surg 80:68–72
14. Morton; Tolan (1982) Activity level and employment status after coronary bypass surgery. Am J Surg 143:417–420
15. Niles et al (1980) Return to work after coronary artery bypass operation. J Thorac Cardiovasc Surg 79:916–921
16. Oberman et al (1982) Employment status after coronary artery bypass surgery. Circulation 65 (II)
17. Rimm et al (1976) Changes in occupation after aortocoronary vein-bypass operation. JAMA 236:4
18. Smith et al (1982) Employment status after coronary artery bypass surgery. Circulation 65 (II)
19. Symmes et al (1978) Influence of aortocoronary bypass surgery on employment. CMA Journal 118:268–270
20. Wallwork et al (1978) Return to work after coronary artery surgery for angina. Br Med J
21. Westaby et al (1979) Return to work and quality of life after surgery for coronary artery disease. Br Med J 2:1028–1031
22. Zacks (1971) *Theory of statistical inference*. Wiley, New York
23. Zyzanski et al (1982) Employment changes among patients following coronary bypass surgery: social, medical, and psychological correlates. Public Health Rep 97, 6:558–565
24. Handbook of Labor Statistics (1983) US Department of Labor, Bureau of Labor Statistics, December 1983. Bulletin 2175

Psychosocial and Economic Aspects

H. H. Bentall

Patients suffering from coronary artery disease requiring surgery, are generally in the prime of life, and their ability to return to work and to enjoy life is of the utmost importance to the patients themselves and also to the community. It would seem very simple to arrive at figures which answer the kind of questions raised by these statements but in fact there is considerable variation from country to country and the answers are not easy. This variation need not suggest a variation in the quality of surgery nor need it suggest lack of courage or enthusiasm on the part of the patient. There are many factors which affect such patient statistics. In general, reports from the United States, from where the largest numbers of figures originate, show a small reduction in those working at 2 years compared with their preoperative status rather than the benefit which would be expected. However, Liddle and his colleagues (Liddle et al. 1982) from Salt Lake City show a very different picture which they attribute to pre- and post-operative counselling and a more positive approach by the doctor. It is possible, however, that it is the large Mormon population with its strong work ethic which may well be a very important factor in this series. In England the situation is rather different from the common American experience and here I will describe those factors found to be important in the Hammersmith experience and in that of others. In-depth studies of a relatively small number of patients were carried out in 1979 and in 1983.

In the *first study* (Westaby et al. 1979), 156 patients were followed for up to 33 months with a mean of 16.5 months (Table 1). To ensure uniformity, only men were included in the survey and they were classified in a standard way with respect to their employment (Table 2); mean age is not statistically different from group to group and is approximately 52 years for the whole group. Of the *heavy manual workers* (Table 3), none were working without restriction be-

Table 1. The patients

Total		156 patients
Hospital mortality		2 patients
Late mortality		12 patients
Investigated by questionnaire		142 patients
Responded to questionnaire		130 patients
Lost to follow-up		12 patients
Follow-up period	9–33 months	
Mean follow-up	16.5 months	

Table 2. Classification of men in full-time employment

Occupation	No. of pts.	Mean age	Standard deviation
Heavy manual workers	24	50.8	8.9
Skilled workers and tradesmen	41	53.0	7.14
Clerical workers	32	53.1	6.9
Executives and professionals	20	50.9	9.5

Table 3. Heavy manual workers (24 patients)

	Before operation	After operation
Working without restriction		
At original occupation	0	9 } 16 (67%)
At lighter work	0	7 }
Working but restricted by angina	3 (13%)	2 (8%)
Forced to stop work	21 (87%)	5[a] (21%)

[a] 1 patient retired at 65 but was angina free

Table 4. Skilled workers and tradesmen (41 patients)

	Before operation	After operation
Working without restriction		
At original occupation	1 } 2 (5%)	19 } 20 (49%)
At lighter work	1 }	1 }
Working but restricted by angina	15 (37%)	4 (10%)
Forced to stop work	24 (59%)	16[a] (39%)

[a] 1 patient retired at 63 and 1 patient remained redundant; both were angina free

fore operation; three were working but restricted by angina and 87% had been forced to stop work. After operation 75% were working and one patient could have worked but retired at the statutory age of 55. Of the *skilled workers and tradesmen* (Table 4), 59% were forced to stop work but 59% were working after operation; a two further patients who could have worked did not do so for other reasons. Of the *clerical workers* (Table 5), 50% were forced to stop work before operation and 80% were working after the operation. Finally, of the *professionals and executives* (Table 6), 45% were forced to stop work before operation whereas 85% were working after operation. Combining the *whole group* (Table 7), it will be seen that approximately 60% of men were forced to stop work before operation whereas a similar proportion were working without restriction after operation and only 27% were forced to stop work. This result was highly significant, $P < 0.001$.

Table 5. Clerical workers (32 patients)

	Before operation	After operation
Working without restriction		
At original occupation	3 (9%)	18 } 18 (56%)
At lighter work	0	0 }
Working but restricted by angina	13 (40%)	8[a] (25%)
Forced to stop work	16 (50%)	6 (19%)

[a] 2 patients were working part time, having previously been forced to stop

Table 6. Professionals and executives (20 patients)

	Before operation	After operation
Working without restriction		
At original occupation	4 } 4 (20%)	15 } 16 (80%)
At lighter work	0 }	1 }
Working but restricted by angina	7 (35%)	1 (5%)
Forced to stop work	9 (45%)	3 (15%)

Table 7. Work status before and after surgery (117 men)

	Before operation	After operation
Working without restriction		
At original occupation	8 } 9 (8%)	61 } 70 (59%)
At lighter work	1 }	9 }
At work but restricted	38 (32%)	15 (13%)
Forced to stop work	70 (59%)	32[a] (27%)

[a] 2 patients aged 63 and 65 retired after operation but were angina free
1 patient remained redundant but was angina free

We examined the effect of time off work before and after operation related to occupation (Table 8) and it was seen that although there was a wide divergence, the heavy manual workers and the skilled workers and tradesmen had a median time off work before operation of 5 months whereas the clerical and professionals had a very much shorter time. These facts in themselves, however, may also reflect differences in the general practitioners treating the two different groups of patients as well as perhaps a greater determination on the part of the second two groups in getting active treatment for the disablement. As might be expected, the time taken to resume full work was greatest in the heavy manual workers and least with the professionals and executives. When questioning these patients with respect to their employment, we also investigated their *social activities* (Table 9). The four kinds of activity studied are not peculiarly British but perhaps the proportion of those who indulge in gardening would be greater in the South of England, where these figures were gathered,

Table 8. Time off work before and after operation related to occupation (time in months)

	Before operation		After operation		Number of patients retiring
	Range	Median	Range	Median	
Heavy manual workers					
Original work	0–60	5	3–15	5.0	6
Lighter work			3–9	3.0	
Skilled workers and tradesmen	0–180	5	1–12	4.0	17
Clerical workers	0–12	1.5	2–18	4.0	6
Professionals and executives	0–9	2.0	1–6	3.0	2

Table 9. Restriction of social activities (130 patients)

	Before operation	After operation
Hobbies or sports	113 (130)[a]	38/113 (29%)
Gardening	112 (112)	35/112 (31%)
Social activity	116 (130)	30/116 (23%)
Sexual intercourse	99 (103)	29/99 (28%)

[a] Figures in brackets are numbers who indulged in the activity before illness

than in some other parts of the world. Of those who engaged in hobbies or sports before operation, almost all were unable to carry out these activities before operation whereas only 29% were restricted after operation. 100% of gardeners were restricted before operation, whereas only 31% were restricted after operation. Nearly all patients had restriction of other social activities such as Church-going, cinema, clubs etc. before operation whereas only 23% were restricted after operation. Almost all of those who wished to have sexual intercourse before operation were unable, whereas only 28% were still restricted after operation. In general, it is the practice in England to encourage patients to resume all kinds of recreational and social activities after surgery and to encourage their return to work after a convalescent period of 4–6 weeks in sedentary workers and 3 months in manual workers.

In the *second study* from our group (Misra et al. 1984), 120 consecutive patients receiving coronary artery bypass grafting were studied with respect to their employment status in relation to age, preoperative ventricular function, the extent of coronary artery disease, preoperative infarction, and pre- and post-operative angina. These patients were grouped in a similar manner to the previous series and their work status investigated from 6 months to 2 years with a mean of 10 months; we had previously shown that most patients who were going to return to work had done so after 5 months. There was one operative death (0.8%) and one late death. Relief from angina was of the expected pattern, 71% having complete relief requiring no drugs and 22% having relief but requiring drugs. Table 10 shows the ***return to work*** after operation of those working before the onset of angina: 73% returned to work. Of those men who continued to work after the onset of angina, no less than 87% returned to work and of those who were forced to stop work before surgery, 61% returned to work after operation. The *effect of age* on employment is shown in Table 11. It is clearly seen that the younger patients are better able or are more motivated to return to work, but it is also interesting that of those in the decade before normal retirement nearly 60% returned to work. The results found when *occupation groups* were studied (Table 12) show very similar results to those in the earlier studies despite increasing unemployment in the country as a whole; these figures do not quite attain statistical significance at the 5% level.

Table 10. Return to work after CABG

	Percent returning to work after CABG
Men working before onset of angina	73 ($P<0.001$)
Men working after onset of angina	87
Men forced to stop work before surgery	61 ($P<0.05$)

Table 11. Age and return to work

Up to 45	92%	
46–55	76%	
56–65	59%	
		($P<0.05$)

Table 12. Comparison of return to work in different occupational groups

Occupation	Return to work
Manual workers	90%
Skilled workers	60%
Clerical workers	70%
Executive and professionals	71% (NS)

Left Ventricular Function and Extent of Disease. When the preoperative left ventricular function and numbers of coronary arteries involved in the disease were compared with the incidence of return to work, no statistically significant correlation could be found in this series.

Relief of Angina. In both of these series of patients the most significant single factor correlating with return to work was relief of the disabling symptom of angina.

Discussion

Guvendik et al. (1982), also in England, studied 100 men who did not have severe impairment of left ventricular function and whose age range was 30–60 years (mean 49.5 years). These patients were operated on for angina and had the remarkable 1-year employment rate of 91%. They found, however, a progressive decrement over a period of 5 years, down to 73%. They also found that the number and duration of hospital admissions were reduced in patients who had been operated on. Liddle and his colleagues, however, suggest that the low incidence of return to work in some series may be due to medical advice and restriction by the patients' physicians and families.

Liddle and his colleagues give many figures to show that in their series of patients working after operation, the money earned exceeded by a very large factor the total amount of money spent on their illness (up to 7.5 times). Figures like this are not available in England, for the majority of patients are treated within the National Health Service for which no charges are made directly to the patient. If, however, one makes a realistic guess at the real cost of such a treatment it would approximately equal the earnings of the lowest paid worker over a period of 6 months.

It must therefore be true to say that anybody who returns to work for a period exceeding 6 months has a positive benefit to the community quite apart from the relief of suffering in the individual.

References

Bentall HH (1982) Profit and loss in coronary artery surgery. Ann Thorac Surg 34:351–352

Guvendik et al (1982) Symptomatic status and pattern of employment during a five-year period following myocardial revascularization for angina. Ann Thorac Surg 34:383–387

Liddle WV et al (1982) The rehabilitation of coronary surgical patients. Ann Thorac Surg 34:374–382

Misra KK et al (1984) Determinants of work capability and employment after coronary artery surgery. (to be published)

Westaby S et al (1979) Return to work and quality of life after surgery for coronary artery disease. Br Med J 2:1028–1031

The Influence of Economic and Societal Factors

I. K. Crosby, J. Chiang, S. Jordan, R. L. Mentzer Jr., I. L. Kron, D. L. Kaiser, and G. B. Craddock Jr.

Introduction

In the early years after the commencement of coronary bypass surgery in 1968 (Favaloro et al. 1970), patients with multivessel coronary disease were frequently placed on total disability status prior to undergoing coronary artery bypass grafting (CABG). It was the highly motivated or perhaps the self-employed individual who planned to return to work postoperatively. Widespread experience over the last decade (179 000 CABG procedures were performed in the United States in 1983 alone!) with longitudinal follow-up studies has encouraged more aggressive recreational and vocational "mainstreaming" of postoperative patients. Today, CABG, at an expense of $ 15 000 to $ 25 000 per patient, is the single most common surgical procedure performed in the United States. A societal question now arises as to whether the expensive CABG procedure can be offered to all the patients who need it, especially if it does not seem to facilitate a patient's return to professional employment (Crosby and Riddervold 1979; Gutmann et al. 1982; Hammermeister et al. 1979; Weinstein and Stason 1982). With the current economic recession and the escalating cost of health care, it is appropriate to analyze the factors affecting the practicability of professional re-employment for CABG patients.

Previous studies have documented a clear-cut discrepancy between the numbers of postoperative cardiac surgical patients clearly capable of returning to work and the numbers who actually do return to work postoperatively (Crosby et al. 1980; Wellons et al. 1981). The former group includes patients who opted for early retirement and those who had been placed on disability because of their coronary artery disease, and remained so, even though a good postoperative result rendered them capable of working. A symposium was sponsored by the National Center for Health Care Technology in April of 1981, so that lawyers, employers, cardiologists and surgeons, health planners, counselors, consumers, and social workers could provide a multidisciplinary analysis of the factors involved in the postoperative return to work (Eliastam and Gastel 1982).

Because of a changing national economic climate and the need for a clearer delineation of the features that influence a patient's ability, opportunity, and decision to return to work postoperatively, this present study was undertaken.

Materials and Methods

Patients undergoing CABG at the University of Virginia while the national economy was good (1979, 1980) were compared with patients undergoing the same procedure during a bad or "down" economy (1982). Selection criteria were designed so that all patients in the study were of working age, without other major debilitating illnesses, and with a paying job up until the time of their recent cardiac illness. Patients were undergoing their first CABG procedure (not a reoperation) and were less than 63 years old at the time of operation. Patients who died during postoperative follow-up were excluded from the study.

All patients meeting the above criteria were contacted and were surveyed by a detailed questionnaire and by phone conversations with the patient and spouse or with the referring physician. In all, 216 patients were contacted; 62 patients were excluded because (a) they were not gainfully employed prior to operation; (b) they were suffering medical disabilities other than coronary disease; (c) they declined to participate in the detailed financial aspects of the study; or (d) they were not reachable (this was so in five cases). Thus, 154 patients were entered into the study: 81 consecutive patients from the good-economy period (1979–80) and 73 consecutive patients from the bad-economy period in 1982. Patients were also categorized according to the type of work they had performed (Fig. 1). Farmers, factory workers, police officers, and construction workers were all designated as blue-collar workers. Executives, managers, clerks, and professionals were designated as white-collar workers. Postoperatively, each group was divided as to whether the patients were working (W), on disability income (D), or retired/unemployed (R).

	BLUE COLLAR	WHITE COLLAR	TOTAL PATIENTS
GOOD ECONOMY 1979-80	39	42	81
BAD ECONOMY 1982	40	33	73
TOTAL	79	75	154

Fig. 1. Classification of patients

In this study, sources of income were classified under the following headings: wages, union pension, social security disability, unemployment benefits, job benefit plan, social security retirement, and miscellaneous. The annual income for the patient and the family was recorded as being from $ 0 to $ 10000, from $ 10001 to $ 15000, from $ 15001 to $ 20000, from $ 20001 to $ 30000, from $ 30001 to $ 50000, or $ 50001 and over.

The postoperative activity level of the patients was divided into the following categories: I. capable of unlimited activity; II. able to perform most activities; III. limited to mild activities only; and IV. severely limited, confined to bed or chair. These questionnaire categories along with subsequent telephone conversations with the patient, the spouse, and the family doctor enabled us to rank the patients as accurately as possible according to the New York Heart Association Classification.

Results

We were able to follow 97.7% of all the consecutive patients. Figure 2 demonstrates the employment status of white-collar workers during the good and the bad economic periods, showing that 36 of 42 (85.7%) patients returned to work during the good period, and 30 of 33 (90.9%) returned to work during the bad period. There was no significant difference in the employment status of white-collar workers in the two periods. The postoperative blue-collar employment status is outlined in Fig. 3. During the good period, 21 of 39 (53.9%) blue-collar patients returned to work. During the bad period, 30 of 40 (75%) patients returned to work. Thus, there is a statistically significant greater number of blue-collar patients who returned to work after CABG during the bad economic period ($P<0.05$).

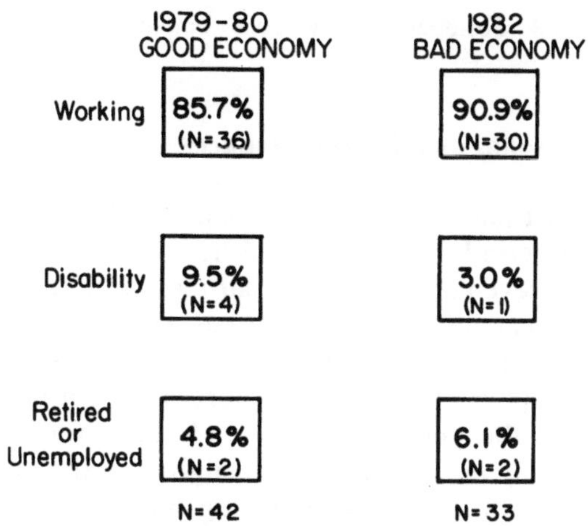

Fig. 2. Postoperative white-collar employment

During the good period, 13 of 39 (33.3%) blue-collar workers were classified postoperatively as disabled; during the bad period, only 6 of 40 (15%) patients were in the disabled category postoperatively. Thus, there was a statistically significant decrease in the number of blue-collar postoperative patients on disability during the bad economic period ($P<0.05$). Despite the fact that the numbers in each group are small, this study shows that a significantly greater number of blue-collar workers were on disability during the good economic period, and that a significantly greater number of blue-collar workers returned to work during the bad economic period. Especially striking is the fact that 31% of the blue-collar workers had a change in jobs during the poor economic period, and some patients' original jobs had been cut entirely.

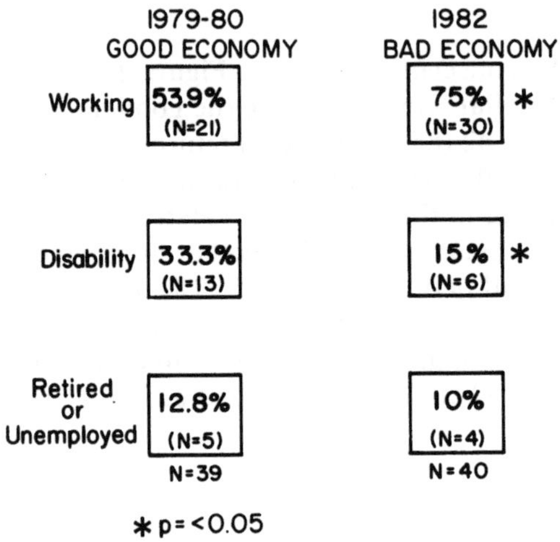

Fig. 3. Postoperative blue-collar employment

Personal and Family Finances

Most patients had incomes derived from several sources. Indeed, in the 1979–80 period, the average white-collar worker had income payments from 1.7 of the seven sources listed earlier, while the average blue-collar worker had payments from 1.3 of the sources. During the 1982 period, the average white-collar worker had payments from 1.2 sources, while the average blue-collar worker had payments from 1.3 sources. In both the good and the bad economic periods, the personal income of the white-collar worker changed little (Fig. 4). Family income decreased slightly in the good economic period, but underwent no significant change during the bad economic period.

There was a sizeable decrease in the average blue-collar postoperative salary during both the good and the bad economic periods. This was largely related to the fact that a much greater percentage of the blue-collar patients did not return to work postoperatively. The total family income did not suffer, however, as the spouses often worked and payments were received from sources other than personal wages. Our interpretation is that society is "looking after" the patient and his or her family when that patient is not working following CABG (Fig. 4).

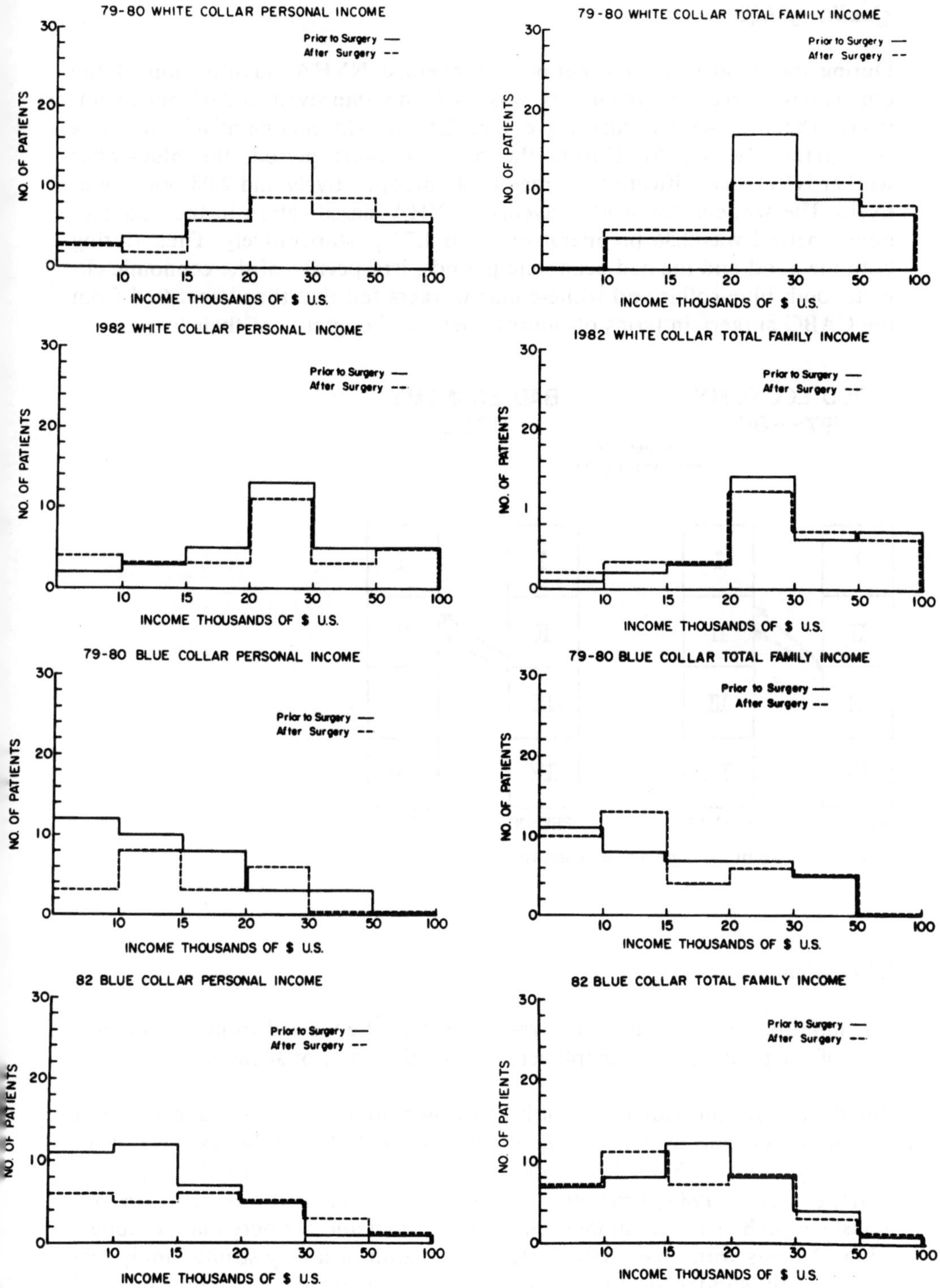

Fig. 4. Personal and total family income (*top,* white-collar; *bottom,* blue-collar)

Quality of Life

During the good economic period, the average NYHA classification of the blue-collar worker before surgery was 2.49; this improved to 2.03 postoperatively. The white-collar worker averaged 2.55 NYHA preoperatively and 1.64 postoperatively (Fig. 5). During the bad economic period, the blue-collar worker NYHA classification averaged 2.49 preoperatively and 2.08 postoperatively. The white-collar worker average NYHA classification in the bad economic period was 2.36 preoperatively and 1.79 postoperatively. Thus, during both the good and the bad economic periods, irrespective of the economic climate, both blue-collar and white-collar workers felt that they benefitted from the CABG surgery in terms of improvement in the quality of their lives.

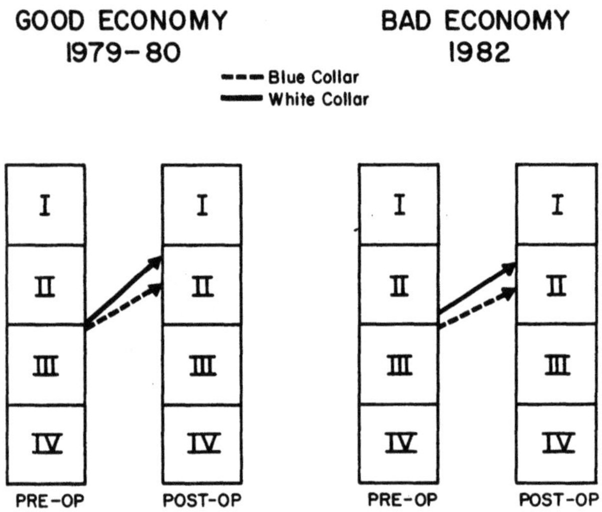

Fig. 5. Change in average NYHA classification

Discussion

It is important that postoperative re-employment be viewed from the perspectives of the patient, of his employer, of his union, and of society.

The Patient. An individual patient is concerned not only with the alleviation of symptoms and improvement in the quality of life, but with the prospect of increased longevity. With CABG patency rates of approximately 50% at 10 years (Campeau et al. 1983; Frick et al. 1983; Seides et al. 1978), patients are obviously apprehensive about their possible life span and the potential or reoperation. Patients with severe ventricular dysfunction or a very strong family history of early sudden death, or patients with associated debilitating medical problems may decide on their own volition never to return to work. Patients may also make that decision based on advice from their family doctor, from their internist, from their cardiologist or surgeon, or from family members.

The Employer. While many employers are sensitive to the medical needs of their faithful employees, in this litigious era they have to be concerned with and protected against the possibility that a particular job or work activity could bring on or worsen the symptoms of cardiovascular disease. For example, if a person lifting heavy objects at work experiences severe chest pain or sustains a myocardial infarction, he is probably entitled to Workers' Compensation benefits (R. W. Galiher Jr, panelist in discussion of Boulay et al. 1982 at the National Center for Health Care Technology's assessment forum on Coronary Artery Bypass Surgery: Economic, Ethical and Social Issues, April 1981, in Washington, DC.). Many employers have little interest in trying to support a patient through periods of reduced productivity because of cardiac disease, and, at the same time, they are vulnerable to lawsuits related to injuries sustained by employees while in the job. Thus patients are coerced into retirement or disability. Some employers (e.g., the automobile industry) simply refuse to re-employ CABG patients (T. S. Turner, panelist in discussion of Boulay et al. 1982).

The Union. Guidelines concerning retirement and disability vary from union to union. Although these guidelines are generally beneficial to the union member with a medical problem, they sometimes benefit the union membership at large, rather than the individual worker. At the 1981 Washington Symposium, the president of the Detroit AFL-CIO admitted that there was considerable discrimination against CABG patients by their fellow workers (T. J. Turner, panelist in discussion of Boulay et al. 1982). This hostile attitude is an unpleasant fact of life and is probably fueled by the high unemployment rate in the auto industry. After a CABG patient returns to work, he and his physician might, at least initially, desire a lighter job for him, but such jobs are reserved for people with considerable seniority in the employee hierarchy, and the senior workers generally resent these jobs being given to patients who have recently undergone cardiac surgery. They also resent CABG patients being supported at a lower productivity rate, while there are perfectly healthy union members unable to get a job (T. J. Turner, panelist in discussion of Boulay et al. 1982). They would prefer the CABG patients to take their total disability pension.

The Teamsters Union has a different approach; it evidently contracts with an employer to provide a definite number of healthy union members to work for that employer (E. F. Walsh, panelist in discussion of Boulay et al. 1982). If a worker gets a cardiac illness, they promptly replace him with another healthy employee, and the afflicted employee is placed on medical retirement. He has no choice in the matter (E. F. Walsh, panelist in discussion of Boulay et al. 1982). Although this works out well from the employer's point of view and from the union's point of view, it may be quite frustrating to the individual patient.

Sometimes there is a financial disincentive to returning to work. With a monthly check from Workers' Compensation (as his disease was aggravated by his job!), plus a union disability check, plus a social security check, plus more more favorable federal income tax considerations of these checks, the CABG patient may be financially more secure if he stops working than if he returns to work full-time and pays his taxes (R. W. Galiher, panelist in discussion of Boulay et al. 1982).

Society. The explosion of medical science in terms of sophisticated diagnostic and therapeutic procedures has left behind some of society's traditional concepts of retirement and disability. Society has been slow to accept that approximately 50% of the nation's deaths in any year will come from heart disease; at the same time, it is struggling with the ramifications of improved longevity. Thus, industry and society generally are making attempts to medify the criteria for medical disability and the guidelines for early retirement. The commercial airline pilot who has CABG surgery can now return to his former occupation 2 years after surgery, if he has an angiogram that demonstrates patent grafts and undergoes a yearly stress test demonstrating no symptoms or EKG abnormalities.

Such national and international tendencies as higher employment rates, shorter average working weeks, and the idea of employees taking early retirement in order to enjoy it in good health also influence a patient's decision and ability to return to work after CABG.

Work Capability Postoperatively. From a series of patients with ventricular aneurysms operated on between 1973 and 1978, there was a clear distinction between postoperative capability and actual employment. Figures 6 and 7 outline the striking differences: although 82% of the patients themselves felt that

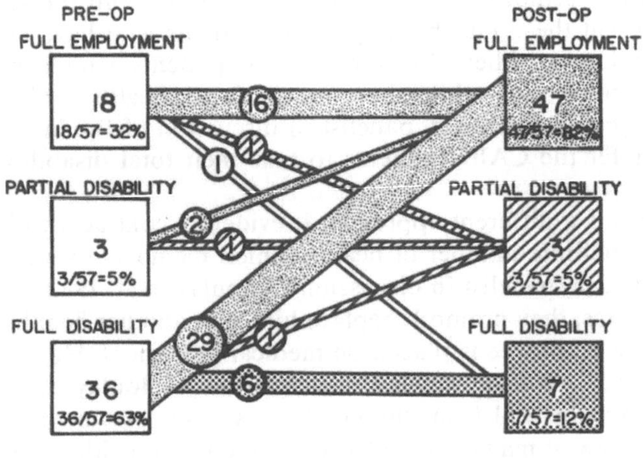

Fig. 6. Work capability

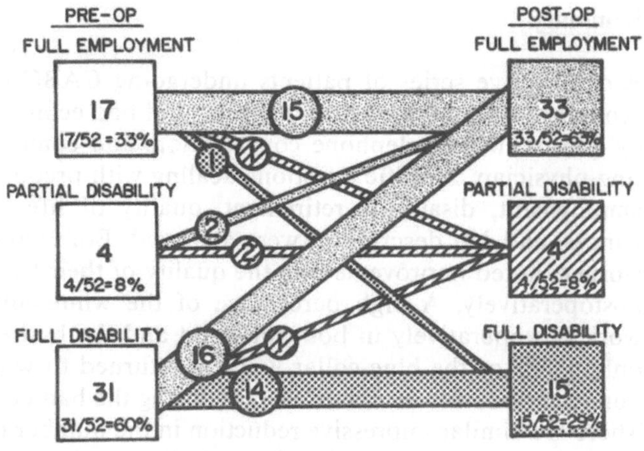

Fig. 7. Actual employment status

they were capable of full-time work postoperatively, only 63% were so employed. Only 12% of the patients felt they were totally disabled postoperatively; however, from society's perspective, because some patients were retired and some had been placed on total disability prior to surgery, 29% were still classified as totally disabled (Crosby and Riddervold 1979; Wellons et al. 1981).

The design of this present study excludes people who had retired preoperatively, who were unemployed preoperatively, who are of retirement age (more than 63 years old), and who have major associated medical disabilities. Thus, there is a clearer delineation of the factors influencing postoperative re-employment in the work-able patients. It is encouraging to note such a high percentage of patients returning to work postoperatively. Although only 54% of the blue-collar workers returned to work after CABG during the period of good economy, there was a significant increase (up to 75%) in the number of blue-collar workers employed after CABG during the period of bad economy. White-collar workers (85.7% during the good economic period and 90.9% during the bad economic period) enjoyed a high rate of return to work after CABG, irrespective of the economic times. The decrease in the number of patients on disability among blue-collar workers from 33.3% to 15% during the bad economic period may reflect changes in society allowing these patients to be re-employed after CABG, or more stringent criteria for disability. There is an enormous challenge to society in changing its attitudes about rehiring healthy postoperative workers (Boulay et al. 1982) and about finding alternative types of employment for workers with restricted physical capabilities postoperatively.

Generalizations from this study must be made very cautiously due to the small sample numbers and the potential ambiguities in the sample population. Patients in this study all live in the western half on the state of Virginia and the eastern part of West Virginia. This is, therefore, an area study, and the results cannot be interpreted as a national trend.

Summary

A consecutive series of patients undergoing CABG during a period of good economy (1979–80) and during a period of bad economy (1982) were contacted by questionnaire, telephone conversation, and communication with the referring physician. Specific questions dealing with preoperative and postoperative employment, disability, retirement, quality of life, personal and family finances, and job description were analyzed. Both white-collar and blue-collar workers noted improvement in the quality of their lives (NYHA classification) postoperatively. A high percentage of the white-collar workers returned to work postoperatively in both the good and the bad economic periods. While only 53.9% of the blue-collar workers returned to work during the good economic period, this increased to 75% during the bad economic period ($P<0.05$). There is a similar impressive reduction in the number of blue-collar workers on disability, from 33.3% during the period of good economy down to 15% during that of bad economy ($P<0.05$). The average personal and family income of the white-collar workers did not change much during the good or the bad economic periods, although the average personal income of the blue-collar worker in both the good and the bad economic times was decreased after CABG (fewer of them returned to work). Yet, because of spouse and other family member employment and income from other sources, the total family income of the blue-collar patient did not suffer.

References

Boulay FM, David PP, Bourassa MG (1982) Strategies for improving the work status of patients after coronary artery bypass surgery. Circulation [Suppl III] 66:43–49

Campeau L, Enjalbert M, Lesperance J, Vaislic C, Grondin CM, Bourassa MG (1983) Atherosclerosis and late closure of aortocoronary saphenous vein grafts: Sequential angiographic studies at 2 weeks, 1 year, 5 to 7 years, and 10 to 12 years after surgery. Circulation [Suppl III] 68:II-1

Crosby IK, Riddervold HO (1979) Coronary artery bypass surgery: Who needs it and who pays for it? Nord Med 94:188–189

Crosby IK, Wellons HA, Martin RP, Schuch D, Muller WH (1980) Employability: A new indication for aneurysmectomy and coronary revascularization. Circulation [Suppl I] 62:I-79–I-83

Eliastam M, Gastel B (eds) (1982) Technology assessment forum on coronary artery bypass surgery: Economic, ethical, and social issues. American Heart Association Monograph #92: Circulation (Part II) 66. American Heart Association, Dallas, TX

Favaloro RG, Effler DB, Groves LK, et al (1970) Direct myocardial revascularization by saphenous vein graft: Present operative technique and indications. Ann Thorac Surg 10:97–111

Frick MH, Valle M, Pekka-Tapani H (1983) Progression of coronary artery disease in randomized medical and surgical patients over a five-year angiographic follow-up. Am J Cardiol 52:681–685

Gutmann MC, Knapp DN, Pollock ML, Schmidt DH, Simon K, Walcott G (1982) Coronary artery bypass patients and work status. Circulation [Suppl III] 66:33–42

Hammermeister KE, DeRouen TA, English MT, Dodge HT (1979) Effect of surgical versus medical therapy on return to work in patients with coronary artery disease. Am J Cardiol 44:105–111

Seides SF, Borer JS, Kent KM, Rosing DR, McIntosh CL, Epstein SE (1978) Long-term anatomic fate of coronary artery bypass grafts and functional status of patients five years after operation. N Engl J Med 298:1213–1218
Weinstein MC, Stason WB (1982) Cost-effectiveness of coronary artery bypass surgery. Circulation [Suppl III] 66:56–66
Wellons HA, Bodily SE, Martin RP, Crosby IK (1981) Combined aneurysmectomy and coronary revascularization: A critical assessment of financial, survival rate and quality of life results. Primary Cardiol 7:65–72

Employment Status: Pre- and Postoperative Characteristics

H. O. Vetter, H. Hofmann, K. Glonner, A. Neiss, B. Reichart, and W. Klinner

Introduction

Within the last 5 years the number of patients undergoing coronary artery bypass grafting (CABG) has significantly increased in Germany. Coronary bypass surgery is carried out to relieve anginal pain, to prevent myocardial infarction, and to improve functional capacity in patients with coronary artery disease (CAD). Contrary to expectations, only 50%–75% of patients who recover from CABG are reported to return to work postoperatively (Oberman and Kouchoukos 1979; Gutmann et al. 1982; Boulay et al. 1982; Gohlke et al. 1982; Smith et al. 1982; Almeida et al. 1983).

In the evaluation of CABG patients this study was designed to correlate preoperative variables with a set of postoperative characteristics influencing the rate of return to work.

Patients and Methods

Patients operated on for CAD in the University Clinic of Cardiovascular Surgery at Munich between January 1979 and December 1980 were included in this study. Patients who needed reoperation because of graft occlusion and patients with additional surgical procedures in conjunction with CABG were excluded from the investigation. The remaining 865 patients were sent a questionnaire in September 1982, aimed at collecting the following data: work status [present occupation, return to employment (including change of work), and interest in a retraining program for another job], self-assessment of quality of life, existence of anginal pain after surgery, frequency of preoperative recreational physical activities, and postoperative participation in a rehabilitation program. There were 800 patients who responded. Sixty-two patients (7.8%) died during the follow-up period. In addition, for the final analysis 162 patients who had retired prior to CABG as well as 25 housewives were excluded. The remaining 551 patients, 522 males and 29 females, were divided into six groups according to their occupation. White-collar workers comprised 68 patients in group I (managers, officials) and 184 patients in group II (public employees). There were 173 patients in group III (skilled blue-collar workers) and 75 patients in group IV (unskilled blue-collar workers). Group V consisted of 51 self-employed persons, while group VI was made up of the 25 housewives who were not included in our investigation.

Table 1. Preoperative Characteristics

Characteristic	No.	%
Sex:		
male	522/551	94.7
female	29/551	5.3
Prior myocardial infarction:		
1	337/551	61.2
2 or more	50/551	9.1
Coronary artery disease:		
single vessel	62/551	11.3
double vessel	128/551	23.2
triple vessel	361/551	65.5
left main	91/551	16.5
Ejection fraction (%):		
less than 50	75/551	13.6
more than 50	476/551	86.4
Recreational activity:		
frequent	117/551	21.2
occasional	213/551	38.7
none	221/551	40.1

The average duration of follow-up was 33 months (21–45 months). The age of the investigated population ranged from 28 to 65 years (mean age 51.3 ± 6.1 years). All preoperative characteristics are shown in Table 1. 61.2% of the patients had at least one myocardial infarction before CABG. 13.6% had an ejection fraction below 50%. 59.9% stated in the questionnaire that they had been involved in frequent or occasional recreational physical activities.

Obstruction in coronary arteries with a reduction in luminal diameter of 50% or more was considered significant. According to this evaluation a single vessel disease was found in 11.3%, a double in 23.2%, and triple in 65.5%. In 16.5% the left main stem was significantly narrowed.

Statistical differences were determined by chi-square or Student's *t*-test, as appropriate.

Results

All essential postoperative data obtained by the questionnaire are listed in Table 2. When the postoperative work status of the 551 patients was analyzed, 314 patients (58.1%) had returned to work, and 264 (48.9%) were still working at the time of the follow-up survey. 230 patients (42.6%) had retired after CABG, 38 (7.0%) were still disabled, and 8 (1.5%) were unemployed.

Figure 1 shows the differences in work status between white-collar workers and self-employed persons in comparison to the blue-collar workers. Only

Table 2. Postoperative Characteristics

Characteristic	No.	%
Chest pain at follow-up:		
same or less	304/544	55.9
none	240/544	44.1
Quality of life:		
improved	434/546	79.5
unchanged	81/546	14.8
worse	31/546	5.7
Return to work	314/540	58.1
Working at follow-up	264/540	48.9
Retired after surgery	230/540	42.6
Disability	38/540	7.0
Unemployment	8/540	1.5
Rehabilitation program:		
yes	419/551	76.0
no	132/551	24.0
Influence of rehab. program:		
improved	208/419	49.6
unchanged	186/419	44.4
worse	25/419	6.0

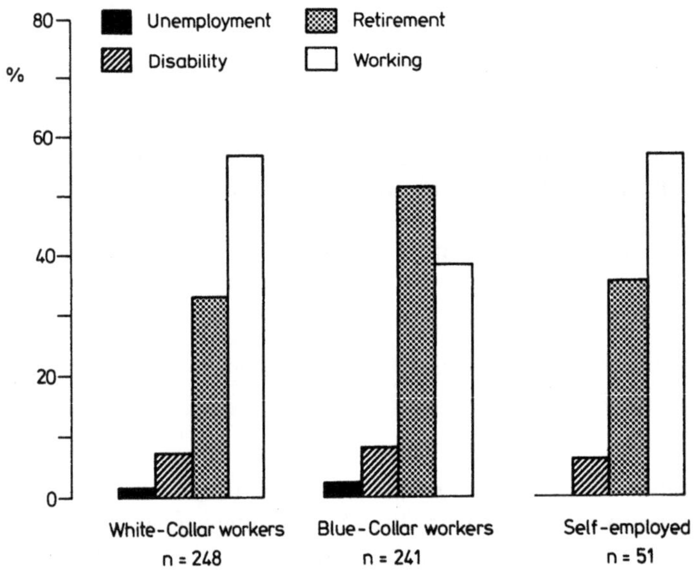

Fig. 1. Work status of the patients in different occupational groups 33 months after CABG. Retirement after surgery was remarkably high among blue-collar workers; therefore the percentage of working patients at the time of follow-up in this group was significantly lower than that in the white-collar and self-employed groups

among the white- and blue-collar workers were a few patients unemployed. Disability amounted to 5.9%–7.3% in all groups. Retirement after surgery was 33.5% for the white-collar workers, 53.1% for the blue-collar workers, and 37.2% for the self-employed group. Therefore, the percentage working at the time of follow-up was 58.1% for the white-collar workers, 37.8% for the blue-collar workers, and 56.9% for the self-employed group.

Of the patients who returned to work, 5.2% changed employers, 19.9% moved to a less physically demanding job with the same employer, and 74.9% kept their previous job. Only six patients participated in a retraining program for another occupation during the follow-up period.

Most patients (45%) were out of work for 4–6 months; in 10.0% of cases the time between surgery and return to work was more than 12 months. In Fig. 2 the average time between surgery and return to work is shown for the different occupational groups. A significant difference was found between group I (white-collar workers) and group IV (blue-collar workers); the former were out of work for an average of 5.6 ± 2.6 months, while the latter averaged 7.8 ± 2.9 months ($P < 0.05$). In fact, the self-employed persons were out of work only for an average of 5.3 ± 3.0 months ($P < 0.01$).

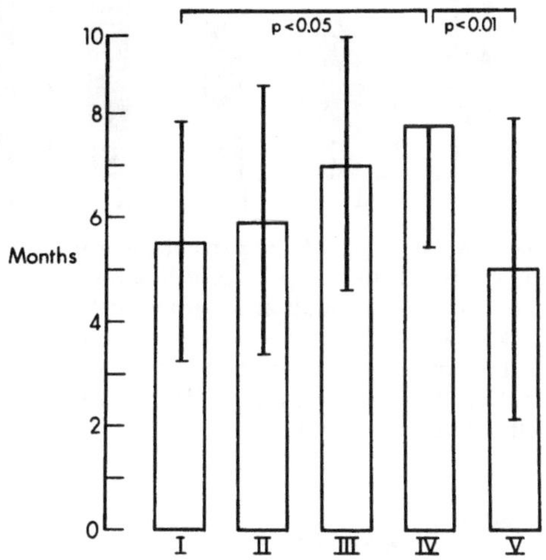

Fig. 2. Average time between surgery and return to work after CABG. Among the different occupational groups the unskilled blue-collar workers (IV) were out of work for the longest period. The shortest time was found for the self-employed persons (V). *I and II,* white-collar workers; *III,* skilled blue-collar workers. Means ± SD

The number of patients participating in a rehabilitation program was lower in group I than in group IV. The percentage of participation was as follows: 69% in group I, 77% in group II, 77% in group III, 85% in group IV, and 59% in group V. In groups I to IV a higher percentage of patients participating in a rehabilitation program postoperatively were working at the time of follow-up (Fig. 3); only group V, the self-employed patients, showed a somewhat lower percentage in that respect.

Freedom from postoperative anginal pain after surgery was reported by 44% of the surviving patients. 59% of these patients were working at the time of the investigation. However, only 41% of those still complaining about angina

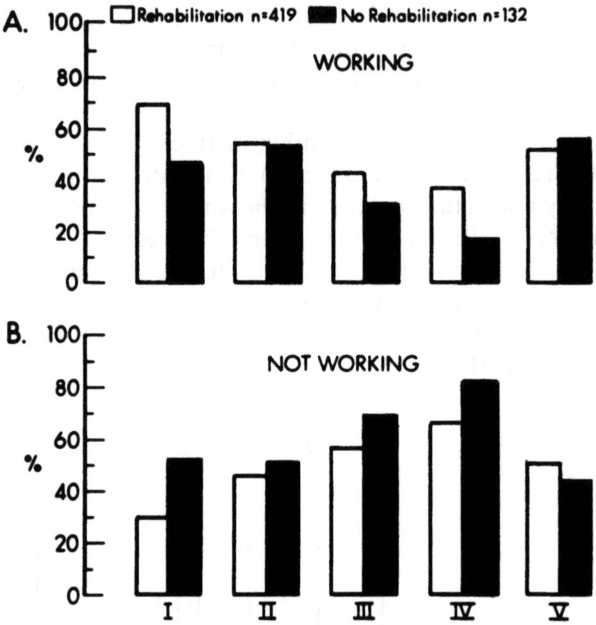

Fig. 3. A, B. In part A the percentage of patients working at the time of follow-up after CABG is shown. In all subgroups except V, a higher percentage of patients was employed after participation in a rehabilitation program postoperatively. Part B shows the patients who did not go back to work after surgery. In correspondence with the aforementioned findings, a higher percentage of patients in groups I to IV was not involved in a rehabilitation program. *I and II,* white-collar workers; *III,* skilled blue-collar workers; *IV,* unskilled blue-collar workers; *V,* self-employed persons

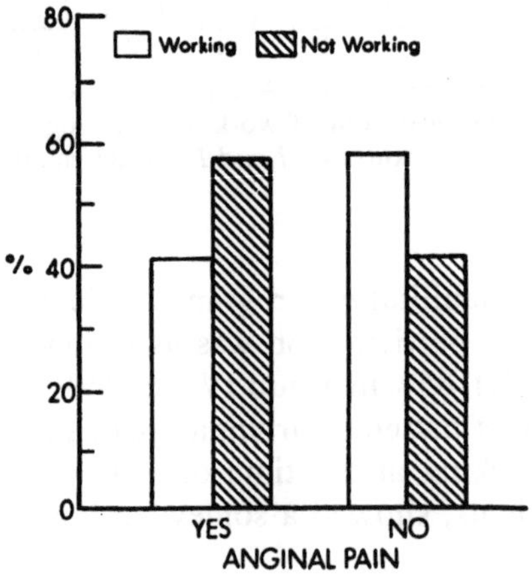

Fig. 4. Work status of patients after CABG in relation to postoperative anginal pain. At the time of follow-up 58.5% of the patients free of postoperative anginal pain had returned to work, whereas almost the same proportion (58.7%) who still had angina pectoris no longer worked

pectoris after surgery returned to work (Fig. 4). In contrast to these data, the majority of patients (80%) experienced an improvement in their quality of life (Table 2).

The mean age of the employed patients (49.5±6.6 years) was approximately 3–7 years lower in all occupational groups than the mean age of the nonworking patients (52.2±5.8 years). One exception existed within group IV (unskilled blue-collar workers), in which there was no significant difference between the mean age of the working and the nonworking persons at the time of the survey (Fig. 5).

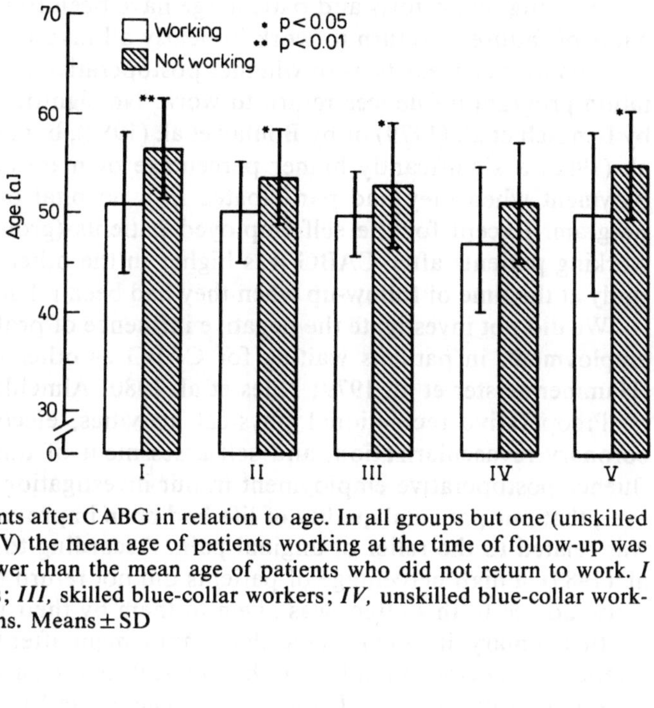

Fig. 5. Work status of patients after CABG in relation to age. In all groups but one (unskilled blue-collar workers, group IV) the mean age of patients working at the time of follow-up was approximately 3–7 years lower than the mean age of patients who did not return to work. *I and II,* white-collar workers; *III,* skilled blue-collar workers; *IV,* unskilled blue-collar workers; *V,* self-employed persons. Means ± SD

Discussion

The results regarding return to work were comparable to those of other European investigations (Wallwork et al. 1978; Frick et al. 1979; Nitter-Hauge 1981). Studies from Germany have been somewhat different, as rates of return to work after CABG have been reported as considerably lower, amounting to 50%–55% 1–4 years after surgery (Gohlke et al. 1982). Lower rates of return to work were also reported by Bluemchen et al. (1979), but the follow-up of their investigation was only 19 months; therefore the work status of a higher percentage of patients was still undecided, and 66% of their population were blue-collar workers. The results reported by Benesch et al. (1979) regarding postoperative employment for white-collar workers and self-employed persons were similar to those in our investigation. Studies from the United States of America report higher rates of return to work (Rimm et al. 1976; Barnes et al. 1977;

David 1979; Gutmann et al. 1982; Almeida et al. 1983). This may be due to the differences in the health care systems of the two countries, and to the shorter preoperative waiting period in the U.S.A. for patients undergoing CABG (Hacker et al. 1983).

According to the answers in our questionnaire, the rate of return to work was influenced by age, existence of anginal pain, and postoperative participation in a rehabilitation program. 44% of our patients were free of anginal pain after surgery, and 59% of this group returned to work. Of the symptomatic patients only 41%, however, were working at the time of follow-up. This result was confirmed by the patients of Gutmann et al. (1982). Postoperative existence of angina pectoris and patient age have been found to be major determinants of failure to return to work in nearly all investigations.

A controversy exists as to whether postoperative participation in a rehabilitation program influences return to work. No significant influence was found by Benesch et al. (1979) or by Boulay et al. (1982), but according to Gutmann et al. (1982) a significantly higher percentage of male patients returned to employment when they had participated in a hospital out-patient rehabilitation program. Except for the self-employed patients (group V) the percentage of working patients after CABG was higher in the other groups (I to IV) of our study at the time of follow-up when they had been rehabilitated postoperatively.

We did not investigate the negative influence of prolonged preoperative unemployment, in patients waiting for CABG as other investigators have done (Hammermeister et al. 1979; Niles et al. 1980; Almeida et al. 1983).

Preoperative recreational physical activities, ejection fraction, degree of coronary revascularization, and self-assessment of quality of life did not influence postoperative employment in our investigation. It can be added, however, that our patients' quality of life had been improved by 80%, which mostly was related to the relief of anginal pain. According to a report by Almeida et al. (1983), a high percentage of patients did not return to work after CABG because advice to this effect was given to them by their physicians.

In summary, it can be stated that employment after CABG is more often influenced by socioeconomic than by medical factors, and that this is even more accentuated in patients of lower social classes and performing physically demanding jobs.

References

Almeida D, Bradford JM, Wenger NK, King SB, Hurst JW (1983) Return to work after coronary bypass surgery. Circulation [Suppl II] 68:205–213

Barnes GK, Ray MJ, Oberman A, Kouchoukos NT (1977) Changes in working status of patients following coronary bypass surgery. JAMA 238:1259–1262

Benesch L, Neuhaus KL, Rivas-Martin J, Loogen F (1979) Clinical results and return to work after coronary heart surgery. In: Roskamm H, Schmuziger M (eds) Coronary heart surgery. Springer, Berlin Heidelberg New York, pp 379–384

Blümchen G, Scharf-Bornhofen E, Brandt D, van den Bergh C, Bierck G (1979) Clinical results and social implications in patients after coronary bypass surgery. In: Roskamm H, Schmuziger M (eds) Coronary heart surgery. Springer, Berlin Heidelberg New York, pp 375–378

Boulay FM, David PP, Bourassa MG (1982) Strategies for improving the work status of patients after coronary artery surgery. Circulation [Suppl III] 66:43-49

Danchin N, David P, Robert P, Bourassa MG (1982) Return to work after coronary surgery: Is there a need for a comprehensive rehabilitation program? In: Mathes P, Halhuber MJ (eds) Controversies in cardiac rehabilitation. Springer, Berlin Heidelberg New York, pp 81-83

David P (1979) Contribution factors preventing return to work of cardiac surgery patients. In: Roskamm H, Schmuziger M (eds) Coronary heart surgery. Springer, Berlin Heidelberg New York, pp 370-374

Frick MH, Harjola PT, Valle M (1979) Work status after coronary bypass surgery. Acta Med Scand 206:61-64

Gohlke H, Gohlke-Baerwolf C, Schnellbacher K, Heidecker K, Samek L, Goernandt L, Stuerzenhofecker P, Roskamm H (1982) Long-term effects of aortocoronary bypass surgery of exercise tolerance and vocational rehabilitation. In: Mathes P, Halhuber MJ (eds) Controversies in cardiac rehabilitation. Springer, Berlin Heidelberg New York, pp 71-80

Gutmann MC, Knapp DN, Pollock ML, Schmidt DH, Simon K, Walcott G (1982) Coronary artery bypass patients and work status. Circulation [Suppl III] 66:33-42

Hacker RW, Schuck R, Torka M (1983) Tod auf der herzchirurgischen Warteliste. Dtsch Med Wochenschr 108:1786-1789

Hammermeister KE, DeRouen TA, English MT, Dodge HT (1979) Effect of surgical versus medical therapy on return to work in patients with coronary artery disease. Am J Cardiol 44:105-111

Niles NW, van der Salm TJ, Cutler BS (1980) Return to work after coronary artery bypass operation. J Thorac Cardiovasc Surg 79:916-921

Nitter-Hauge S (1981) Correlation studies between employability, left ventricular hemodynamics and exercise ECG before and after aortocoronary bypass surgery. Acta Med Scand [Suppl] 645:1-7

Oberman A, Kouchoukos NT (1979) Working status of patients following coronary bypass surgery. Am Heart J 98:132-134

Rimm AA, Barboriak JJ, Anderson AJ, Simon JS (1976) Changes in occupation after aortocoronary vein-bypass operation. JAMA 236:361-364

Smith HC, Hammes LN, Gupta S, Vliestra RE, Elveback L (1982) Employment status after coronary artery bypass surgery. Circulation [Suppl II] 65:120-125

Wallwork J, Potter B, Caves PK (1978) Return to work after coronary surgery for angina. Br Med J 2:1680-1681

Employment Status of Patients After Coronary Artery Bypass Surgery

R. W. Hacker, H. Riedl, I. Guggenmoos-Holzmann, and M. Torka

Despite a definite improvement in the symptomatic status of patients after coronary artery bypass grafting (CABG), the socioeconomic consequences of this operation are rather limited. The finding that medical parameters do not seem to play a decisive role in return to work after surgery [11, 16] is confirmed by the fact that the return-to-work rate differs widely among countries with different social systems [1, 2, 7, 8, 12, 14]. The following data illustrate the situation in the Federal Republik of Germany.

Materials and Methods

Out of 2700 patients with CABG, operated on between 1974 and 1981 at the Chirurgische Universitätsklinik Erlangen, Federal Republik of Germany, there were 1486 surviving males under the age of 60 at the time of follow-up. Pre-, intra-, and early postoperative data, as gathered from the hospital charts, are not complete for all parameters (Tables 1, 2). Follow-up data were obtained by telephone interviews with patients and physicians. Information concerning occupational status is available for 1484 (99.9%) of 1486 patients. The follow-up period ranged from less than 1 year to 9 years postoperatively, with a mean of 4.0 (SE = 2.2) years.

The majority of patients did not work prior to surgery. Most of them had been declared disabled by the time of coronary angiography, at a mean of 3.9 (SE = 3.0) months before surgery.

The various parameters analyzed for their possible influence on postoperative work status are shown in Tables 1 and 2. Preoperative blood pressure was measured in the ascending aorta during cardiac catheterization. Relative body weight was calculated according to the BROCA formula [10]. The time interval between coronary angiography and surgery was taken as an approximate measure of the duration of preoperative disability, since most of the patients had been declared disabled at the time of coronary angiography. Left ventricular function was determined by single plane ventriculography in the RAO projection. Obstructions in coronary arteries with a reduction in luminal diameter of 50% or more were regarded as significant.

Patients were considered completely revascularized if all major coronary arteries with a 50% or greater reduction in luminal diameter had received at least one bypass graft. Secondary branches (e. g., left diagonal or posterolateral circumflex) were grafted only if they supplied large areas of myocardium.

Table 1. Preoperative variables tested for their influence on postoperative work status: Univariate analysis

Independent variables analyzed	No. of patients	Working (%)	Unlimited working ability (%)
Age			
≦40 years	34	76.5[c]	58.8[c]
41–50 years	271	62.8[c]	47.4[c]
51–59 years	1079	41.7[c]	34.0[c]
Occupation			
Blue-collar workers	547	34.4[c]	25.3[c]
White-collar workers	646	59.4[c]	48.1[c]
Self-employed	157	63.7[c]	49.0[c]
Myocardial infarction			
Yes	835	46.9	36.7
No	638	48.7	39.5
Blood pressure			
≦160/95 mmHg	891	47.8	38.1
>160/95 mmHg	243	42.0	35.0
Body weight			
≦BROCA+10%	1109	49.8	39.1
>BROCA+10%	356	44.4	34.2
Time interval between angiography and operation			
≦3 months	731	51.0[a]	42.0[b]
>3 months	714	44.4[a]	34.1[b]
Left ventricular function			
Normal	681	47.9	36.4
Hypokinetic segments	513	49.3	40.5
A-/dyskinetic segments	256	43.0	35.9
Left ventricular enddiastolic pressure			
≦12 mmHg	563	46.4	36.5
>12 mmHg	610	47.9	40.8
No. of obstructed vessels			
1	335	52.2	40.6
2	455	45.9	34.1
3	572	47.6	38.7
Left main stenosis	124	43.6	40.3

[a] $P<0.05$
[b] $P<0.01$
[c] $P<0.001$

Early postoperative complications include all types of complications during the hospital of patients following CABG.

Postoperative coronary arteriography with assessment of graft patency was performed in 414 (27.9%) patients at a mean time of 1 year after surgery. The overall graft occlusion rate was 8.9%.

The symptomatic status of patients (functional class) was categorized according to the classification of the New York Heart Association [9].

Table 2. Intra-/postoperative variables tested for their influence on postoperative work status: Univariate analysis

Independent variables analyzed	No. of Patients	Working (%)	Unlimited working ability (%)
No. of coronary anastomoses			
1	511	48.1	36.3[a]
2	629	46.4	35.3[a]
3	298	48.3	43.8[a]
>3	48	58.3	52.1[a]
Revascularization			
Complete	920	49.2	40.7[a]
Incomplete	564	45.4	33.4[a]
Early complications			
Yes	49	40.8	39.6
No	1435	48.0	37.8
Wound infection			
Yes	177	41.8	32.2[b]
No	1307	48.6	38.7[b]
Myocardial infarction			
Yes	74	21.6[c]	6.8[c]
No	1410	49.2[c]	39.5[c]
Graft patency			
All open	355	49.9	38.2[c]
Not all open	57	42.1	21.1[c]
Functional class (NYHA)			
I	788	62.2[c]	60.1[c]
II	406	37.2[c]	18.2[c]
III	208	21.6[c]	3.9[c]
IV	82	28.1[c]	7.3[c]
Subjective working ability			
Unlimited	563	84.9[c]	
Limited	725	30.6[c]	
Nonexistent	196	4.6[c]	

[a] $P<0.05$
[b] $P<0.01$
[c] $P<0.001$

The subjective working ability reflects the patient's own estimate. Possible limitations are not necessarily restricted to symptoms caused by coronary heart disease.

The statistical analysis consisted of Pearson's chi-square test to analyze the dependency of working status on each explanatory variable. Interrelations between factors with a significant effect ($P<0.05$) were accounted for by a multivariate logistic regression analysis. In a stepwise procedure those factors were selected which significantly increased the predictive power. The statistical criterion used was a likelihood ratio test [4].

Results and Discussion

Seven hundred and nine (47.8%) patients had returned to work at the time of follow-up. This percentage barely changed within the 9-year follow-up period, although the percentage of patients with subjectively unlimited working ability declined slightly during the same period of time (Fig. 1).

Of all the factors which by univariate statistical analysis had shown an influence on the likelihood of going back to work (Tables 1, 2), only three remained after applying a multivariate analysis (Table 3): the subjective ability to work, the type of occupation, and the patients' age at the time of follow-up.

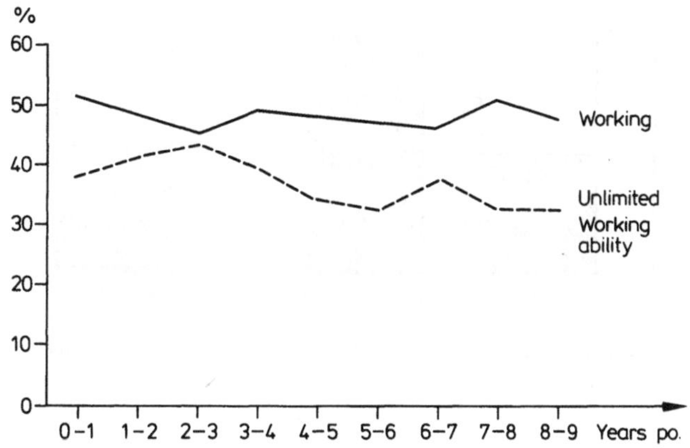

Fig. 1. Work status and working ability vs length of follow-up after CABG

Table 3. Variables tested for their influence on postoperative work status: Multivariate analysis

Independent variables analyzed	LR-chi square	*DF*	*P*
Subjective working ability postoperatively	567.91	2	<0.001
Age	60.84	2	<0.001
Occupation	43.40	4	<0.001
Myocardial infarction postoperatively	1.40	1	NS
Time interval between angiography and operation	2.25	2	NS
Functional class (NYHA)	3.19	3	NS

Symptoms

Functional class, in contrast to working ability, achieved statistical significance by univariate analysis only. It is obvious that the absence of angina pectoris does not necessarily imply unlimited working ability: Although 788 (53.1%) patients fell into functional class I, only 563 (37.9%) considered themselves completely fit for work.

In the working group the percentage of patients either in functional class I or without limitations was about equal, at 69.1% and 67.4%, respectively (Fig. 2). In the nonworking group, however, the respective figures were different, at 38.5% and 11.0%, indicating that at least some of these patients – although without angina – fail to return to work for medical reasons other than symptoms of coronary heart disease [2, 3, 5].

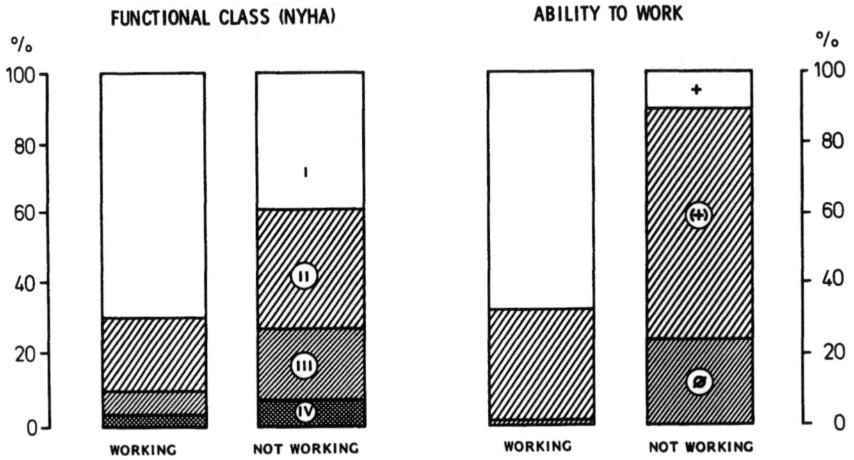

Fig. 2. Functional class and working ability vs work status

Age

Advanced age had a negative influence on work status: The closer the retirement age, the less likely it was that the patient would return to work. The difference between the percentage of patients working and the percentage of patients with unlimited working ability decreased from 17.7% for patients under age 40 to 7.7% for patients over age 50. This shows that the older the patients were, the less they tended to go back to work when subjective limitations of their working ability persisted.

Occupation

There was no appreciable difference in work status between employers and employees, as long as employees were white-collar workers. How much of the less favorable situation for blue-collar workers is due to the physical demands of their job and how much to a different attitude toward their work remains unknown from our data. The finding that the ability to work was lowest among blue-collar workers can be interpreted in both ways. It seems to be of interest, however, that the difference between the percentage of working people and the percentage of people with unlimited working ability decreased from 14.7% for self-employed to 9.1% for blue-collar workers.

Medical and Surgical Treatment

To examine the question of whether there is a difference in work status after medical and surgical treatment of coronary heart disease, we compared our data with the data of 483 medically treated patients, as published by Weiss [15]. These patients took part in a rehabilitation program after having had a myocardial infarction before age 60. 53% of them were back at work 18 months later.

If we apply the same selection criteria, that is an age below 60 and previous myocardial infarction, to our surgically treated patients, we end up with 765 patients, 49% of whom were back to work 4 years postoperatively.

In different subgroups, adjusted for age and occupation, the percentage of working patients was essentially the same following medical and surgical treatment (Fig. 3).

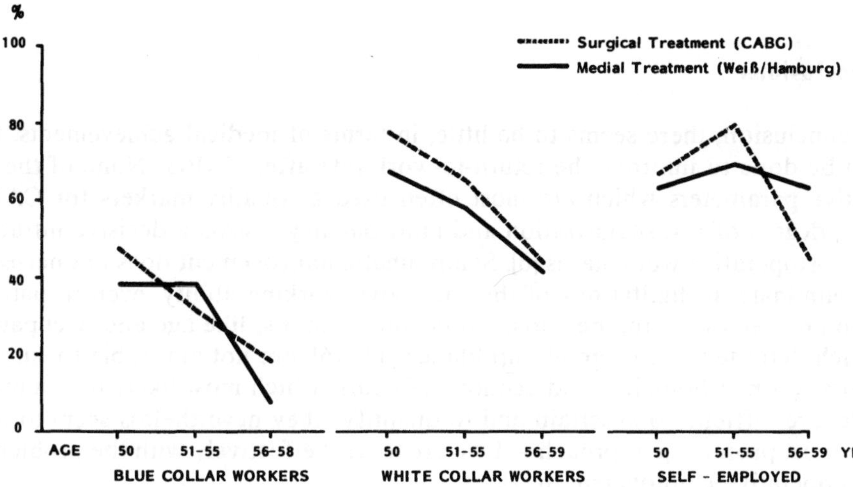

Fig. 3. Return-to-work rate by age and occupation: surgical vs medical treatment of patients with myocardial infarction

General Employment Rate

Compared to the employment rate of the general male population in the Federal Republik of Germany [13], the postoperative employment rate of our patients was considerably lower (Fig. 4). The difference increased with age from 25% for patients in their early forties to 48% for patients in their late fifties. This could, at least in part, be due to the multimorbidity of older patients, who are free of angina pectoris nearly as often as the younger ones, but nevertheless remain unfit for the demands of their job due to ailments caused by diseases other than coronary heart disease [2, 3, 5].

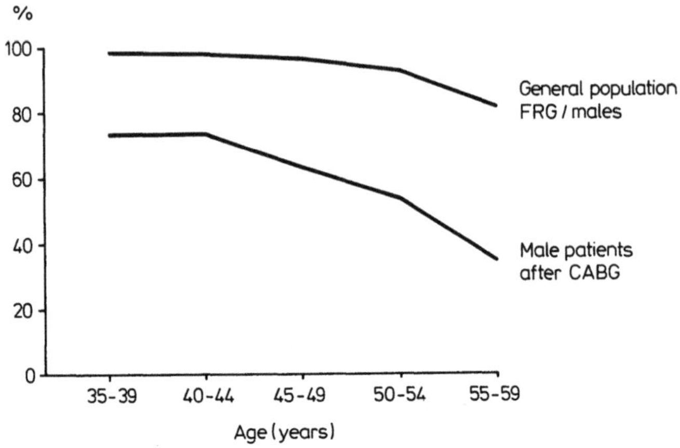

Fig. 4. Employment rate by age: Male population of Federal Republik of Germany vs male patients after CABG

Conclusions

In conclusion, there seems to be little, in terms of medical achievements, that can be done to improve the return-to-work rate after CABG. None of the objective parameters which are most often used as quality markers for CABG, e.g., degree of revascularization and graft patency, shows a decisive influence on postoperative work status [6]. Symptomatic improvement does not necessarily eliminate all limitations of the subjective working ability, even in patients who are free of angina pectoris. Nonmedical factors, like age and occupation, which definitely are of great importance [11, 16], are not amenable to surgery. Moreover psychological and economic factors, which most likely play a major role, are difficult to ascertain and to quantify; they nevertheless seem to offer the most promising approach – if we are to deal effectively with the problem of postoperative employment [6, 7].

References

1. Almeida D, Bradford JM, Wenger NK, King SB, Hurst JW (1983) Return to work after coronary bypass surgery. Circulation 68:II-205
2. Boulay FM, David PP, Borussa MG (1982) Strategies for improving the work status of patients after coronary artery bypass surgery. Circulation 66:III-43
3. Danchin N, David PP, Bourassa MG, Robert P, Chaitman BR (1983) Factors predicting working status after aortocoronary bypass surgery. Can Med Assoc J 126:255
4. Fienberg SE (1980) The analysis of cross-classified data. MIT Press, Cambridge Mass
5. Gutmann MC, Knapp DN, Pollock ML, Schmidt DH, Simon K, Walcott G (1982) Coronary artery bypass patients and work status. Circulation 66:III-33
6. Jensen RL, Clayton PD, Liddle HV (1982) Relationship between graft patency, postoperative work status, and symptomatic relief. J Thorac Cardiovasc Surg 83:503
7. Johnson WD, Kayser KL, Pedraza PM, Shore RT (1982) Employment patterns in males before and after myocardial revascularization surgery. Circulation 65:1086

8. Liddle HV, Jensen RL, Clayton PD (1981) The rehabilitation of coronary surgical patients. Ann Thorac Surg 34:374
9. New York Heart Association, Criteria Committee (1964) Disease of the heart and blood vessels. Little Brown, Boston
10. Ries W (1970) Fettsucht. Barth, Leipzig
11. Smith HC, Hammes LN, Gupta S, Vlietstra RE, Elveback L (1983) Employment status after coronary artery bypass surgery. Circulation 65:120
12. Speiser K, Pfluger N, Rothlin M (1982) Die berufliche Rehabilitation nach aorto-koronarer Bypassoperation, Schweiz Med Wochenschr 112:1095
13. Statistisches Jahrbuch für die Bundesrepublik Deutschland (1982) Kohlhammer, Stuttgart
14. Walter P, Thies B, Gerhardt U (1983) Wie viele Patienten nehmen nach einer Koronaroperation ihre Arbeit wieder auf? Med Klin 78:276
15. Weiss B (1983) Wiederaufnahme der Arbeit nach erstem Herzinfarkt. Dtsch Med Wochenschr 108:1872
16. Zyzanski SJ, Rouse BA, Stanton BA, Jenkins CD (1982) Employment changes among patients following coronary bypass surgery: Social, medical, and psychological correlates. Public Health Rep 97:558

Can Aortocoronary Bypass Surgery Improve Return to Work?

M. E. Rothlin, R. Sieber, and Å. Senning

Numerous reports on employment status after coronary artery bypass grafting (CABG) have been published from the United States, Canada, and European countries. Oberman et al. [8] found no net gain in the return to work after CABG for the studies carried out in the United States [1, 2, 4, 5, 7]. On the other hand several reports from Canadian and European centers have shown a moderate positive effect of CABG on the postoperative employment status as compared to the preoperative status [6, 9, 10, 11] or to a comparative control group of patients treated medically [3]. It is of interest that, on average postoperative employment status was the same in the American, Canadian, and European reports, namely about 61%. However, preoperatively 68% of the patients operated on in the United States were employed but only 43% of those operated on in Canada or European countries. In a study reported from this institution [9], the rate of vocational rehabilitation observed in the first postoperative year was higher that reported by other authors [2–7, 10, 11]; we therefore restudied the same problem in a defined population of 238 male patients after an average postoperative observation time of 3.7 ± 0.7 years.

Patients and Methods

Two hundred and thirty-eight patients with CABG performed between January 1979 and August 1981 enrolled in a prospective study including angiographic control of bypass patency 3 months postoperatively. Only male patients having chronic angina were included. Patients requiring an intervention for valvular disease or left ventricular aneurysm and patients presenting for a reintervention or an emergency operation were not included. Preoperative characteristics of the 238 patients enrolled are listed in Table 1. Postoperative data of the presented population are shown in Table 2. All patients came for a first postoperative examination 6 weeks after the intervention and for postoperative angiography 3 months after operation. Thereafter they were followed by their private physicians. All patients received a questionnaire regarding their health and vocational status at the beginning of 1984. Out of the 238 patients, 4, who all had left this country after early postoperative reexamination, could not be traced, corresponding to a follow-up of 98.3%.

A patient was defined to be working if he had full-time employment or if he was able to perform more than 50% of his job, i. e., he was not receiving a pension. A patient doing 50% or less of his job is eligible for a pension in this

Table 1. Preoperative characteristics of the 238 patients

Age (years)		53.3 ± 7.4
Duration of symptoms (months)		36.6 ± 40.8
Angina (NYHA)		2.5 ± 0.7
Stress test (% of predicted)		61.0 ± 26.0
Previous infarction	0	43%
	1	49%
	>1	8%
Main vessels involved	1	13%
	2	32%
	3	55%
Ejection fraction		0.59 ± 0.09
LVEDP (mmHg)		13.1 ± 5.7

Table 2. Postoperative characteristics of the 238 patients

Angina (NYHA)	1.5 ± 0.6
Stress test (% of predicted)	84.0 ± 23.1
Number of distal anastomoses per patient	3.2 ± 1.1
Patent distal anastomoses per patient	2.6 ± 1.2
Ejection fraction	0.59 ± 0.10
LVEDP (mmHg)	11.6 ± 5.0

country and was therefore defined to be "not working". For statistical analysis of the data, chi-square and student's *t*-test were used, as convenient.

Results

Out of the 238 patients traced, 7 had died during an average postoperative follow-up of 3.7 ± 0.7 years, corresponding to a yearly mortality of 0.8%. Eight patients were receiving a pension because their age was above 65 years before the operation. The remaining 219 patients were studied for their vocational status 3.7 ± 0.7 years after CABG.

As may be seen from Fig. 1, nine patients not working preoperatively and five patients working preoperatively had reached the age of pension. One-half of the unemployed patients remained so at the late postoperative follow-up, while 43% had resumed vocational activity. Out of the 105 patients working before CABG, 18% were unemployed and 77% were working at late postoperative follow-up. Of the patients below the age of 65 years at late follow-up there were 100 working before operation and 130 working 3.5 years after operation, corresponding to a net gain of 30%. The corresponding figures of unemployed patients were 105 before operation and 75 at late follow-up.

Table 3 illustrates several variables that may influence the return to work after CABG. It may be seen that the age of patients and the severity of angina were significantly lower and the duration of preoperative unemployment sig-

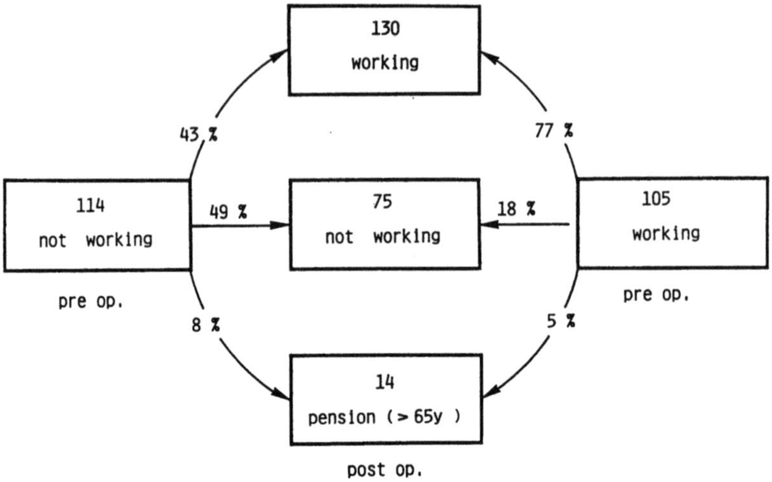

Fig. 1. Return to work after CABG

Table 3. Factors influencing return to work after CABG

		Working patients	nonworking patients	*P*
Age (years)		51.2± 6.6	53.9± 6.5	<0.01
Bypass patency (%)		84.4±23.8	80.4±28.1	NS
Ejection fraction (%)		60.9±11.2	59.9± 9.8	NS
Angina (NYHA)		1.3± 0.5	2.1± 0.9	<0.001
Preoperative duration "off work"		2.4± 3.6	7.2± 7.3	<0.001
Blue-collar		45%	55%	<0.001
White-collar		78%	22%	
Postoperative	Yes	72%	28%	<0.001
rehabilitation program	No	51%	49%	

nificantly shorter in patients resuming longlasting vocational activity. Bypass patency was also better in patients resuming their work, but this difference did not reach statistical significance. Return to work was significantly higher in white-collar or self-employed patients than in professions requiring more severe physical activity. Patients who attended a formal 3-week rehabilitation program at a specialized institution presented with a significantly higher rate of vocational rehabilitation.

Discussion

The presented data confirm the previously reported observation of a net gain in return to work after CABG [6, 9, 10, 11]. About one-half of patients not working preoperatively resumed their vocational activity for over 3 years after

CABG; this is less than what was found when vocational status was assessed within the first postoperative year [9]. In confirmation of previously reported findings [4, 6, 8, 9, 10], several factors were significantly related to return to work; these were age of the patient, duration of preoperative unemployment, presence and severity of postoperative angina, motivation of the patient to resume work, and physical stress involved with professional activity. It is of particular interest that a formal rehabilitation program is a factor with a beneficial effect on return to work, if tested by univariate analysis. Multivariate analysis is required in order to prove that rehabilitation program is an independent variable.

It is well known to any physician regularly involved with postoperative check-up of patients with CABG that a number of factors not directly related to coronary artery disease may be decisive for the postoperative employment status. These include the attitudes of private physicians, employers, and relatives toward the patient, and the socioeconomic conditions and welfare status of the patient himself and of the community he is living in. These factors are very subjective and of marked complexity. The person most likely to influence actively the nonmedical factors which influence return to work ist the private physician attending the patient before operation and during the first postoperative months. For this duty the private physician needs proper information on his patient from the heart surgical center and clear explanations on the expected capacity of the patient to resume his work. Moreover it is desirable that patients continue their professional activity as long as is possible before operation.

References

1. Anderson AJ, Barboriak JJ, Hoffmann RG (1980) Retention or resumption of employment after aortocoronary bypass operations. JAMA 243:543
2. Barnes GK, Ray MJ, Oberman A, et al (1977) Changes in working status of patients following coronary bypass surgery. JAMA 238:1259
3. Frick MH, Harjola PT, Valle M (1979) Work status after coronary bypass surgery. Acta Med Scand 206:61
4. Hammermeister KE, DeRouen TA, English MT (1979) Effect of surgical versus medical therapy on return to work in patients with coronary artery disease. Am J Cardiol 44:105
5. Love JW (1980) Employment status after coronary bypass operations and some cost considerations. J Thorac Cardiovasc Surg 80:68
6. Neuhaus KL, Benesch L (1978) Probleme der Arbeitsaufnahme nach koronarchirurgischen Eingriffen. Med Welt 29:478
7. Niles NW, Vander Salm TJ, Cutler BS (1980) Return to work after coronary artery bypass operation. J Thorac Cardiovasc Surg 79:916
8. Oberman A, Wayne JB, Kouchoukos NT et al (1982) Employment status after coronary artery bypass surgery. Circulation [Suppl II] 65:115
9. Speiser K, Pfluger N, Rothlin M (1982) Die berufliche Rehabilitation nach aortokoronarer Bypassoperation. Schweiz Med Wochenschr 112:1095
10. Symmes JC, Lenkei SCM, Berman ND (1978) Influence of aorto-coronary bypass surgery on employment. Can Med Assoc J 118:268
11. Wallwork J, Potter B, Caves BK (1978) Return to work after coronary artery surgery for angina. Br Med J 2:1680

Factors Contributing to Resumption of Work*

M. Welsch, G. Bergmann, D. Mayer, H. C. Mehmel, W. Saggau, and W. Schmitz

Introduction

Within the last 17 years aortocoronary bypass surgery (ACBS) as an essential basic principle of therapy for atherosclerotic coronary artery disease (CAD) has gained an important standing. Venous aortocoronary bypass graft (ACBG) for eliminating relevant coronary artery stenosis was introduced by Rene Favaloro in 1967 [6].

In most cases vena saphena magna has been used for ACBG, and complete revascularization has become the main object at ACBS [14].

The aims of ACBS consist in improvement of life expectancy and quality of life. The life expectancy of surgically treated patients is approaching that of the average population. The prognosis of patients with multiple vessel disease and main stem stenosis undoubtedly has improved [5, 11–13, 15, 16]. Improvement of the quality of life by virtue of a drastic reduction in anginal complaints has been achieved in 85%–90% of patients, while complete removal of angina pectoris can be registered in 60%–75% of all patients [13, 17]. It is true that based on the progress of the primary disease, the extent of the symptomatic recovery gradually decreases on a scale of 3%–4% per year [9], but in the majority of the patients such a decrease does not occur for some years. The symptomatic improvement normally makes possible professional rehabilitation [1, 2, 4, 7, 8, 16–18]. In view of these positive results of ACBS regarding symptoms and signs as well as prognosis of CAD for all involved in health care, the proportion of patients resuming work after ACBS in West Germany and the resulting social and economic effect is disappointing [9, 17]. While according to relevant studies the probability of professional reintegration in West Germany ranges between 20% and 57%, in the USA 63%–80% resume work postoperatively, without essential differences with respect to the result of the operation, individual exercise tolerance, and professional demand [1, 2, 4, 7, 9, 10, 16–18].

Patients and Methods

To assess the postoperative clinical and occupational status of patients with CAD who underwent ACBS we analyzed the data of 121 patients (90% male)

* Dedicated to Prof. Dr. Dr. H. C. W. Schmitz on occasion of his 60th birthday

Table 1. Further clinical characteristics (121 patients)

Myocardial infarction	72	(59.5%)
- anterior localization	39	
- posterior localization	33	
Coronary artery disease	2.2 ± 0.8	(1-3)
- single CAD	30	(24.8%)
- double CAD	36	(29.7%)
- triple CAD	55	(45.5%)
- left main included in 1-3 CAD	22	(18.2%)
Ejection fraction (%)	54.1 ± 9.0	(23-68)

with an average age of 47.9 ± 5.5 years (range, 30–55 years) at the time of surgery; all of these patients had been working up to this event. The average severity of preoperative angina pectoris judged by the criteria of the Canadian Cardiovascular Society was 3.5 ± 0.6, with a range of 1–4. Further preoperative clinical characteristics are shown in Table 1 and 3.

These patients were taken from a total number of 521 patients who underwent ACBS between April 1981 and May 1983 at the Department of Cardiac Surgery at the University Clinic of Heidelberg.

The data of the Federal Agency for Statistics show that the average frequency of early retirement in Germany in 1982 was 17.5% at the age of 58 years and 21.5% at 59 years. Furthermore the Agency came to the conclusion that 25% of all males had prematurely left employment before reaching the age of 60. These facts led us to fix the upper age limit for inclusion in the study at 55 years at the time of surgery. Preoperative retirement or application for this and a second disease influencing the capability to work were further exclusion criteria.

The surgical procedure was performed with aid of pulsatile cardiopulmonary bypass at moderate whole systemic hypothermia (25°–28°C). The cardiac arrest was induced by continuous aortic cross-clamping with profound topical cardiac cooling (10°–15°C) and infusion of cardioplegic Bretschneider solution (4°C).

For the direct myocardial revascularization, vena saphena magna grafts were used exclusively. The proximal anastomoses were performed with a partial occlusion clamp after completion of distal anastomoses. Figure 1 depicts the frequency and extent of the inserted grafts.

In order to determine early graft patency, coronary angiographic restudy was done in each patient using the Sones or Judkins technique in the Heart Catheter Laboratory of the Department for Cardiology, on average 1.6 ± 0.5 (range 1–3) months after ACBS. These second angiographic study reports were reviewed to obtain the following parameters:

1. Number of diseased vessels with stenosis of cross-sectional diameter greater than 50%
2. Condition of inserted grafts
3. Measurement of biplane left ventricular ejection fraction

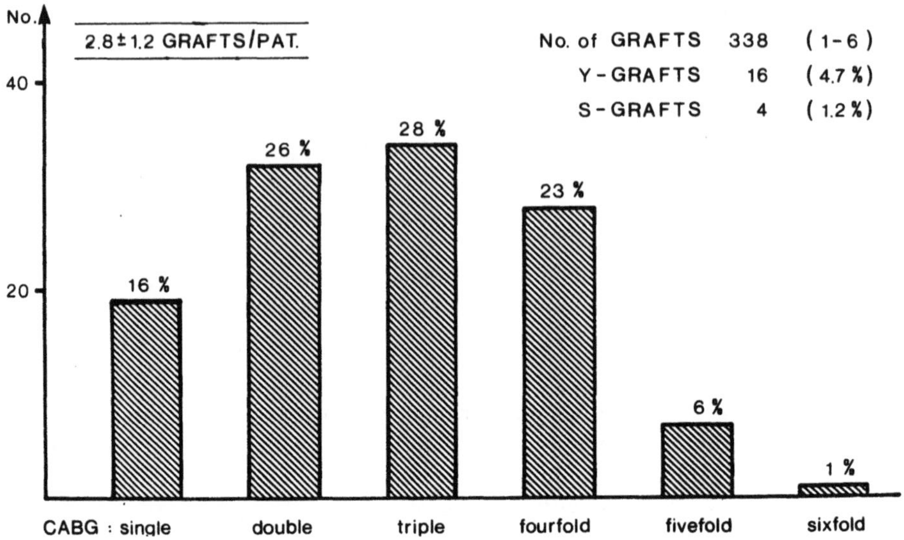

Fig. 1. Frequency and extent of the inserted coronary artery bypass grafts (CABG)

Besides using the patency rate to assess revascularization, a scale for angiographic qualitative determination of revascularization developed by Roskamm et al. [13] was modified by adding one further grade.

The severity of angina pectoris was classified using the criteria of the Canadian Cardiovascular Society [3]. The clinical data include information obtained from pre- and postoperative selective coronary arteriography and left ventriculography at 30° right anterior oblique and 60° left anterior oblique projections with a cineradiographic film; also included is information from the surgical procedure and data on the pre- as well as the postoperative symptomatology. The demographic and relevant historical facts contained information concerning the work status before and after surgery, the reason for failure to return to work, and patients' satisfaction with the outcome of the operation; this information was collected by the same person using a standardized questionnaire at the last reexamination, which on average was performed 22 ± 16.9 months after surgery, with a range of 9–34 months. The symptomatic relief and rehabilitation was determined for each patient at the same time.

A computerized data base containing the mentioned clinical and demographic information for each of the 121 patients was constructed and analyzed via the HADES basis and SAS statistical system of the University Calculating Centre. All data were then correlated with the patients' postoperative work status.

Results

Patency Rate

At the coronary angiographic restudy, performed on average 1.6 months after ACBS, 310 of 338 inserted grafts were open. The corresponding early mean patency rate was 91.7%. With a patency rate of 96%, 112 grafts were connected with the left anterior descending artery (LAD); there were 68 grafts to the diagonalis artery (DIAG) and 67 grafts to the right coronary artery (RCA), each with a patency rate of 91%. The patency rate of 46 grafts to the posterior lateral artery (RPL) was 94%. The lowest patency rate was found in 45 grafts to the obtuse marginal artery (ROM), with 80% (Fig. 2).

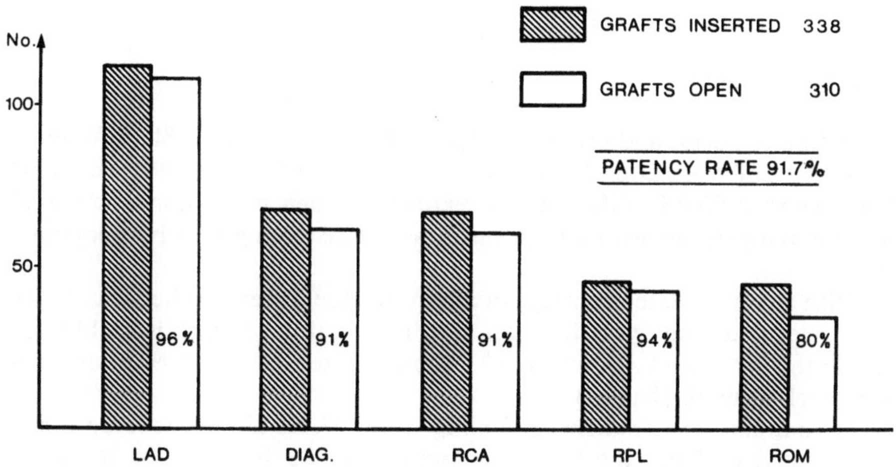

Fig. 2. Localization of the inserted grafts and the corresponding patency rate (for abbreviations, see text)

Grade of Revascularization

A differentiated analysis of the operative results is possible with the division of the angiographic data into five grades of revascularization. This takes into consideration the extent of stenosis, the angiographic condition of the grafts, and the different value of the varying vascular regions.

Complete revascularization – all vessels with a significant stenosis (greater than 50%) were provided with an open graft – was achieved in 62.8% of all cases. Incomplete revascularization – all main branches with a significant stenosis were provided with an open graft – was found in 10.7% of the patients. In 15.8% we observed a sufficient revascularization – all main branches with a significant stenosis were provided with an open graft but at least one graft had a significant stenosis –, while an insufficient revascularization was registered in 9.9% – all main branches with a significant stenosis were grafted but at least

Table 2. Grade of revascularization

	Localization – stenosis >50%	Condition of inserted grafts	n	%
I – Complete	All vessels	Open	76	(62.8)
II – Incomplete	Main branches	Open	13	(10.7)
III – Sufficient	Main branches	With signif. stenosis	19	(15.8)
IV – Insufficient	Main branches	At least one occluded	12	(9.9)
V – Miscarried	All vessels	Occluded	1	(0.8)

one graft was occluded. In one patient the revascularization miscarried – all grafts were occluded (Table 2).

Employment Status

According to social and economic status, there are considerable differences in resumption of work after ACBS: Of the blue-collar workers, 39% went back to work, whereas 88.9% of the employees resumed their professional activity. 75% of the employers carried on their business, while among the civil servants 50% retired.

With a comparable mean age in all groups the difference between blue-collar worker and employees in relation to resumption of work is highly significant at the 0.1% level. On average 3.3 months after ACBS 52.9% of all patients were back at work (Table 3).

In contrast to the patients resuming work, 47.1% did not take up a professional activity within the follow-up period of 22±16.9 months (range, 9–34 months).

Table 3. Resumption of work in relation to type of employment

Employment status	No./total pat.	%	Mean age
Blue-collar	32/82[a]	(39.0)	46.0±5.2
Employees	24/27[a]	(88.9)	47.0±6.7
Employers	6/8	(75.0)	45.9±5.5
Civil servants	2/4	(50.0)	46.5±2.1
	64/121	(52.9)	46.4±5.7

[a] $P<0.001$

Factors Without a Visible Influence

Relevant factors without a visible influence on resumption of work are the extent of CAD, with an identical average vascular involvement of 2.2±0.8 in the "worker" and "nonworker" groups, and prior myocardial infarction, which was similar in both groups (35 vs 37 respectively). The number of inserted grafts per patient was nearly identical in the two groups, at 2.8±1.1 compared with 2.8±1.2. The grade of revascularization in the "worker" group (1.8±1.1) was comparable with that in the "nonworker" group (1.7±1.1). The mean patency rate, at 92.7%±0.15% and 91.6%±0.17%, was not essentially different. The time lapse between the first symptoms and coronary angiography (15.4±24.3 vs 16.8±22.7 months) exerted no visible influence on resumption of work. The "waiting time" between coronary angiography and ACBS was 4.0±3.1 months in the "worker" group as against 3.9±2.5 months in the "nonworker" group, and without visible influence. Participation in ambulant coronary training groups (5 in the "worker" group vs 2 in the "nonworker" group) was amazingly low.

Factors with a Significant Influence

Some influencing factors of varying statistical significance were found.

The 64 workers were significantly younger (average age, 46.3±5.7 years) than the 57 nonworkers (average age, 49±4.7 years) ($P<0.001$). As to the rate of resumption of work, the lack of physical stress at work showed a highly significant influence. Whereas out of 39 white-collar workers (27 employees, 8 employers, and 4 civil servants) 82.1% continued working after ACBS, out of 82 blue-collar workers only 39% resumed their professional activity ($P<0.001$). Based on the comparable initial degree (3.4±0.7 vs 3.5±0.3), the extent of the angina symptoms after ACBS averaged 1.2±0.5 in the "worker" and 1.5±0.8 in the "nonworker" group, the difference being significant at the 1% level.

The participation in the rehabilitation program, with 40 patients in the "worker" and 22 patients in the "nonworker" group was significantly different at the 1% level. Whereas preoperatively both groups showed a similar value of left ventricular ejection fraction (54.6% vs 53.8%), the mean postoperative value, at 60.1%±5.3% in the "worker" and with 57.4%±8.5% in the "nonworker" group, was significantly different at the 5% level (Table 4).

Table 4. Significant differences between patients retiring (57) or working (64) after surgery

	"Worker"	"Nonworker"
Age	46.3±5.7	49.7±4.7[c]
White-/blue-collar	32/32	7/50[c]
Angina pectoris	1.2±0.5	1.5±0.8[b]
Ejection fraction	60.1±5.3	57.4±8.5[a]
Participation in rehabilitation program	40	22[b]

[a] $P<0.05$
[b] $P<0.01$
[c] $P<0.001$

Discussion and Conclusion

The aim of ACBS consists in improving life expectancy and quality of life [4, 5, 11–13, 15]. The improvement in quality of life through the drastic reduction or complete removal of angina pectoris was achieved in a large proportion of patients [7, 13, 16, 17]. Symptomatic improvement normally allows occupational rehabilitation [7, 16]. A study comparing medical and surgical treatment of CAD found no difference between the two for patients returning to work [10]. Despite comparable surgical results with respect to the grade of myocardial revascularization, individual exercise tolerance, and professional demand, many studies show that the extent of resumption of work in other countries is significantly higher than in West Germany [1, 2, 7–10, 16–18]. Visible differences are based on a different social system with less chance of calculating the pension that will be received, on a significantly shorter morbidity – pre- and postoperatively – and on a considerably shorter waiting time for preoperative filtering diagnosis as well as ACBS. The variables which influenced the postoperative resumption of professional activity after ACBS were, in order of importance: age, type of physical activity in preoperative occupation, anginal class, participation in rehabilitation program, and left ventricular function.

Compared to the retired patients, patients resuming work:

- Are younger at the time of surgery,
- belong to occupational groups with a lack of physical stress at work,
- have a good or improved left ventricular function,
- and participate more frequently in a rehabilitation program.

We conclude that a strategy for improving resumption of work is to decrease the considerable waiting time for preoperative filtering diagnosis and surgery. Moreover, with five objective predictive factors it is possible to discern patients with the poorest resumption of work prognosis and to submit them to an individualized postoperative rehabilitation program.

References

1. Anderson AJ, Barborjak JJ, Hoffmann RG, Mullen DC (1980) Retention or resumption of employment after aortocoronary bypass operations. JAMA 243:543
2. Benesch L, Neuhaus KL, Rivas-Martin J, Loogen F (1979) Clinical results and return to work after coronary heart surgery. In: Roskamm H, Schmuziger M (eds) Coronary heart surgery. Springer, Berlin Heidelberg New York
3. Campeau L (1976) Grading of angina pectoris. Circulation 54:522
4. Denolin H (1981) Rehabilitation bei Herzkranken. In: Krayenbühl HP, Kübler W (eds) Kardiologie in Klinik und Praxis. Thieme, Stuttgart, pp 71–71.10
5. Detre K, Peduzzi P, Murphy M, Hultgren H, Thomson J, Obermann A, Takaro T (1981) Effect of bypass surgery on survival in patients in low- and high-risk subgroups delineated by the use of simple clinical variables. Circulation 63:1329–1338
6. Favaloro, RG (1969) Saphenous vein graft in the surgical treatment of coronary artery disease. Operative technique. J Thorac Cardiovasc Surg 58:178
7. Gehring J, Koenig W, Wrana N, Mathes P (1984) Aortocoronare Bypass-Operation: Welche Faktoren beeinflussen die Arbeitswiederaufnahme? Herz/Gefäße 4:205–223

8. Gohlke H, Gohlke-Bärwolf C, Samek L, Stürzenhofecker P, Schmuziger M, Roskamm H (1982) Verbesserte anginafreie Arbeitstoleranz bis zu 6 Jahren nach der Bypass-Operation in Abhängigkeit vom Revaskularisationsgrad. Schweiz Med Wochenschr 112:1616-1618
9. Hacker RW, Torka M, v d Emde J (1982) Revaskularisation des Myokards durch aortocoronaren Bypass. Dtsch Ärzteblatt 47:23-28
10. Hammermeister KE, De Rouen TA, English MT, Dodge HT (1979) Effect of surgical versus medical therapy on return to work in patients with coronary artery disease. Am J Cardiol 44:105
11. Lichtlen PR (1978) Natural history of coronary artery disease based on coronary angiography. Cleve Clin Q 45:153
12. Marthur VS, Hall RJ, Gracia E, de Castro CM, Cooley DA (1980) Prolonging life with coronary bypass surgery in patients with three-vessel disease. Circulation [Suppl I] 62:90-98
13. Roskamm H, Schmuziger M et al (1981) Bestimmt die Vollständigkeit der Revaskularisation die funktionelle Verbesserung und die Überlebensdaten koronaroperierter Patienten? Z Kardiol 70:590-599
14. Schmuziger M (1982) Herzchirurgie. In: Roskamm H, Reindell H (eds) Herzkrankheiten. Springer, Berlin Heidelberg New York, pp 802
15. Suter B, Hirzel HO, Fischer M, Turina M, Senning A, Krayenbühl HP (1982) Bringt die aortocoronare Bypass-Operation einen Nutzen bei Patienten mit fortgeschrittener Koronarsklerose und schlechter Ventrikelfunktion? Schweiz Med Wochenschr 112:1688-1694
16. Symmes JC, Lenkei SCM, Bermann ND (1978) Influence of aortocoronary bypass surgery on employment. Can Med Assoc J 118:268-270
17. Walter P, Thies B, Gerhardt U (1983) Wie viele Patienten nehmen nach einer Koronaroperation ihre Arbeit wieder auf? Med Klin 78:276-280
18. Wenger NK (1982) Coronary bypass surgery as a rehabilitative procedure. Adv Cardiol 31:80-85

Summary of the Discussion

A. Oberman

Generally, the presenters this morning focused on four basic factors impacting on return to work - the relief of angina, age, prior occupation, and the duration of time not working prior to surgery. Dr. Anderson also brought out the importance of considering females separately and alluded to important psychological factors, especially type A, as being related to work rehabilitation. Unfortunately, he did not have time to elaborate on the possible implications.

Dr. Crosby mentioned many of the extraneous complicating factors, such as the state of the economy. The discussion afterwards concerned both the commonalities and unique problems among different societies. Differences between the U.S. and Europe in terms of work rehabilitation programs and socio-economic processes relating to return to work were brought out. But the consensus on determinants of return to work among the presenters was quite striking compared to any differences. The rates of return to work postoperatively were similar, even though, as pointed out by Dr. Bentall and others, the percentage of those working prior to surgery was much lower in Europe than in the U.S. Return to work was found to be greater in patients who had not been forced to give up work immediately after surgery. Dr. Bentall stated unequivocally that relief of angina was the main determinant in return to work after coronary artery bypass grafting. Several speakers stressed the importance of rehabilitation, although they were unable to define those components of the rehabilitation process that might lead to return to work. Dr. Vetter pointed out the disappointing percentage of patients working in view of the good left ventricular function and improvement in self-assessment for quality of life found afterwards. He also noted the exceptionally high retirement rates. Dr. Hacker discussed the importance of the period of unemployment prior to surgery. He described a previously reported finding, that perhaps it is not so much one's disability, but one's perception of disability and subjective estimate of problems that is paramount. Unfortunately, physicians' attitudes sometimes contribute to retirement. In Dr. Hacker's study, according to estimates by physicians, more than one-third of patients prematurely retired were free of angina pectoris. Dr. Rothlin discussed the increasing rates of return to work and related the trends to rehabilitative efforts. He noted that local unemployment rates and welfare attitudes were important considerations. There appeared to be some lack of agreement among the presenters on the relative value of medical as opposed to nonmedical determinants. Dr. Welsch stressed the roles of revascularization and good left ventricular function in permitting a higher percentage of patients to return to work. He also attributed improvements in resumption of work to special rehabilitation programs.

In summing up this morning's session, there is remarkable agreement in terms of the disappointing rates of return to work and those factors identified as being associated with failure to return to work. Despite the emphasis on the relief of angina as a determinant in resuming gainful employment, the view that nonmedical factors contributed in large part to rehabilitative efforts was inescapable.

Employment Patterns in Males Before and After Myocardial Revascularization Surgery: A Study of 2229 Consecutive Patients Followed for as Long as 10 Years*

W. D. Johnson, K. L. Kayser, P. M. Pedraza, and R. T. Shore

Introduction

Loss of productivity is the dominant economic factor associated with coronary artery disease. For the typical male with coronary artery disease, 1 year's earnings frequently exceed the direct cost of revascularization surgery. We have investigated the work status of all 2812 males who underwent coronary artery surgery from January 1968 through March 1978. No patient has been excluded. The purpose of the study is to compare the pre- and postoperative employment characteristics of our entire male patient population with the employment characteristics of a sampling of the United States population compiled by the United States Bureau of Labor Statistics (USBLS). We have not compared our patients with a similarly diseased population that underwent a different form of treatment. Rather, we compared our entire surgical experience with a standard - the U.S. population.

Methods

In November 1978, all living patients operated on for coronary artery disease by the surgeon authors were mailed a questionnaire. They were asked to describe their work status as: working normally with little or no limitation, working but with some limitations, or not working or retired. They were asked to describe their work status both before their heart surgery and on the date of the survey. We also asked, "If you are not now working full time at the job of your choice please indicate the main reason why." In January 1979, nonresponders were sent a follow-up questionnaire. Nonresponders to the second questionnaire were then contacted by telephone during February through April 1979. In May 1979, the survey was terminated.

This report does not include the data on women because: (1) Their age distribution and work patterns are so different from those of men that they would have to be handled separately. (2) They constitute only 16% of our entire patient population. (3) The USBLS counts only employment for pay, which excludes homemaking. This further reduces the number of usable women sub-

* First published in Circulation 65:6 (1982) and reprinted here by permission of the American Heart Association, Inc.

jects to the point where the group and subgroup sizes would be too small for analysis.

The USBLS data used for comparison are those for white males because our surgical population contains far fewer nonwhites than the general U.S. population. Figure 1 shows the effect of age and time on participation in the U.S. labor force as reported by USBLS. (Participation in the U.S. labor force is defined as persons employed plus those classified as unemployed expressed as a percent of all persons in the sample. A more precise and detailed explanation is given in the Handbook of Labor Statistics [1].) In general, participation in the labor force represents the percentage of employed and employable persons. The percentage of persons working is obtained by multiplying the participation in the labor force by the employment rate. The employment rate for white males older than age 40 years is higher than the entire U.S. population and varies from 96% to 98.5% for the period of this study. Because of this high employment rate, the distrinction between "participation in the labor force" and "persons working" need only be made for precise comparisons. Where the distinction is appropriate, we make it; where it is not, we ignore it. Figure 1 demonstrates the slight falloff in employment for the 40- and early-50-year-old age groups and the very sharp dropoff in the late 50- and 60-year-old age groups. White males leave the labor force at a very slow rate before age 55 years and much more rapidly thereafter. Surprisingly, these patterns changed from 1968 to 1978. In 1978, many more white males were leaving the work force at age 50 years and older than were in 1968. This migration from the work force has been investigated [2–4] and is attributed mainly to early voluntary retirement.

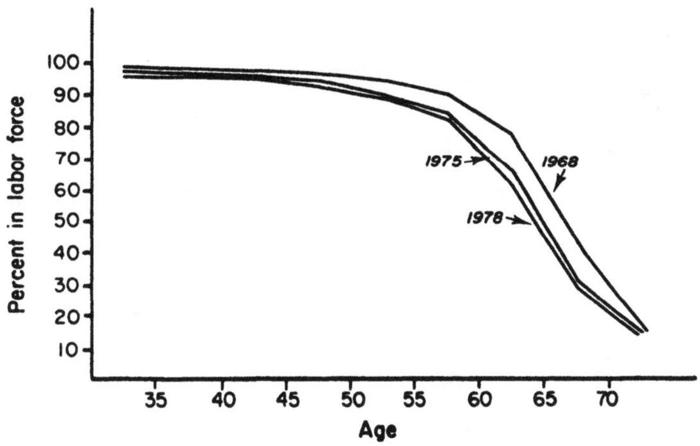

Fig. 1. U.S. Bureau of Labor Statistics: Participation in civilian labor force – white males

Clinical Material

The study group consisted of 2812 male patients operated January 1968 through March 1978; 456 (16.2%) were known to be dead in early 1979, leaving

2354 potential survivors. Of these, 127 (5.4%) were either lost or refused to answer questions, leaving 2229 responders, the subjects of this report. The study series was then divided into groups and subgroups by age and date of surgery (Table 1). For brevity and clarity, we present all other data by percentages only, but the number of subjects in any group can be determined by referring to Table 1. In our terminology, a group contains subjects classified by age or date of surgery. A subgroup contains subjects classified by age and date of surgery. Table 2 shows the percent follow-up for all groups, which is uniformly good throughout the years of surgery. Only the youngest age groups show a slightly lower follow-up, probably because of higher mobility.

Table 1. Number of subjects in each group and subgroup

	Year of surgery									
	1968		1969		1970		1971		1972	
Age (years)	1	2	1	2	1	2	1	2	1	2
0–44	5	0	15	5	23	5	25	6	18	4
45–49	3	5	17	4	31	10	24	9	33	9
50–54	12	0	19	7	34	16	30	21	29	32
55–59	5	3	12	18	21	34	22	25	41	25
60–64	1	12	4	18	18	32	18	32	20	38
65–69	0	5	0	12	6	19	3	19	7	29
70+	0	1	0	3	0	17	1	11	0	11
Total	26	26	67	67	133	133	123	123	148	148

	Year of surgery											
	1973		1974		1975		1976		1977–1978		Total	
Age (years)	1	2	1	2	1	2	1	2	1	2	1	2
0–44	23	8	39	15	41	16	47	31	52	43	288	133
45–49	35	15	58	27	51	39	59	47	72	60	383	225
50–54	55	34	43	56	80	60	89	67	101	88	492	381
55–59	60	51	58	47	87	80	89	97	138	124	533	504
60–64	28	57	38	54	45	84	73	85	114	137	359	549
65–69	8	34	11	38	23	38	31	48	52	69	141	311
70+	4	14	1	11	3	13	7	20	17	25	33	126
Total	213	213	248	248	330	330	395	395	546	546	2229	2229

1, age at surgery; *2*, age at survey

Table 2. Percent follow-up

Age (years) at surgery	0–44	45–54	55–59	60–64	65+	Total	
	90.3%	94.3%	95.7%	96.8%	96.7%	94.6%	
Year of surgery	1968–70	1971–72	1973	1974	1975	1976	1977–78
	95.0%	92.8%	95.1%	94.3%	95.1%	96.6%	93.8%

Results

Work Status Before Operation and at Survey Date Compared with USBLS Data

Because of the marked effect of age on employment status, we made all comparisons on an age-for-age basis. Preoperative data are grouped by age at surgery, and postoperative data by age at survey. Our subject subgroup sizes are too small to be analyzed separately; therefore, we have regrouped them by age and date of surgery. For each age group and each date-of-surgery group, we calculated a USBLS weighted average as follows: The number of subjects in each subgroup was multiplied by the USBLS percent of white males working for that age and year using the data in Fig. 1. These "expected workers" were then summed within the group and divided by the total number of subjects in the group to give a weighted average. Figure 2 shows the comparison broken down by age. If disability is defined as the difference between our subjects and the USBLS weighted average, the younger groups have the highest preoperative disability, and there is little change postoperatively. For the 60–64-year-old group, there was no disability preoperatively and moderate disability at the survey date. The 65–69-year-old group contained far more subjects who were working preoperatively than USBLS, but at the survey date, the percentage was about the same as that from the USBLS. The patients who were 70 years of age or older had a much higher employment rate both pre- and postoperatively than the USBLS rate, but this is at least partly because particularly preopera-

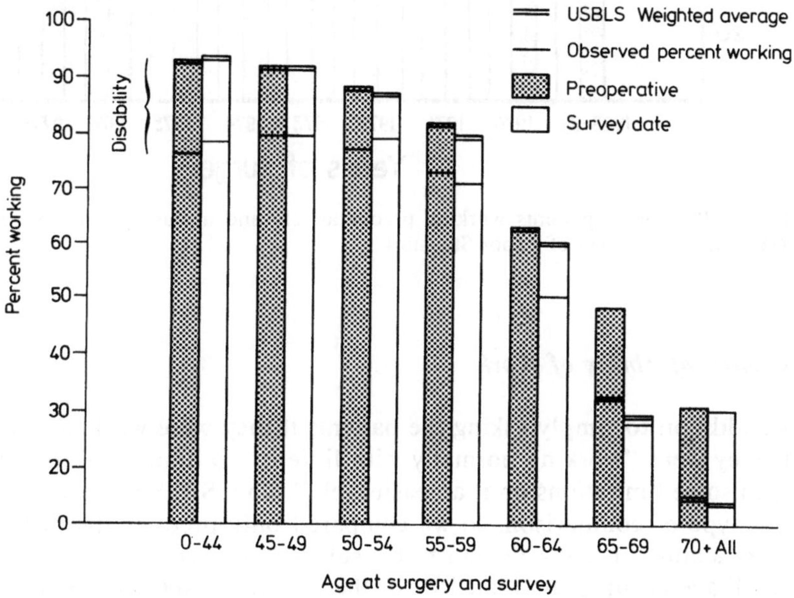

Fig. 2. Percent of patients working preoperatively and at survey date by age (years). *USBLS*, U.S. Bureau of Labor Statistics

tively, they have a lower median age than the USBLS subjects older than 70 years.

Figure 3 shows the same data broken down by year of surgery. The amount of preoperative disability as defined above decreased markedly from 1968 to 1978. The improvement in disability shows no trends. The best years were 1968–1969 and 1971. The poorest years were 1970 and 1975. These data show no recognizable trends that indicate that the effects of surgery deteriorate with time, except the effect of aging.

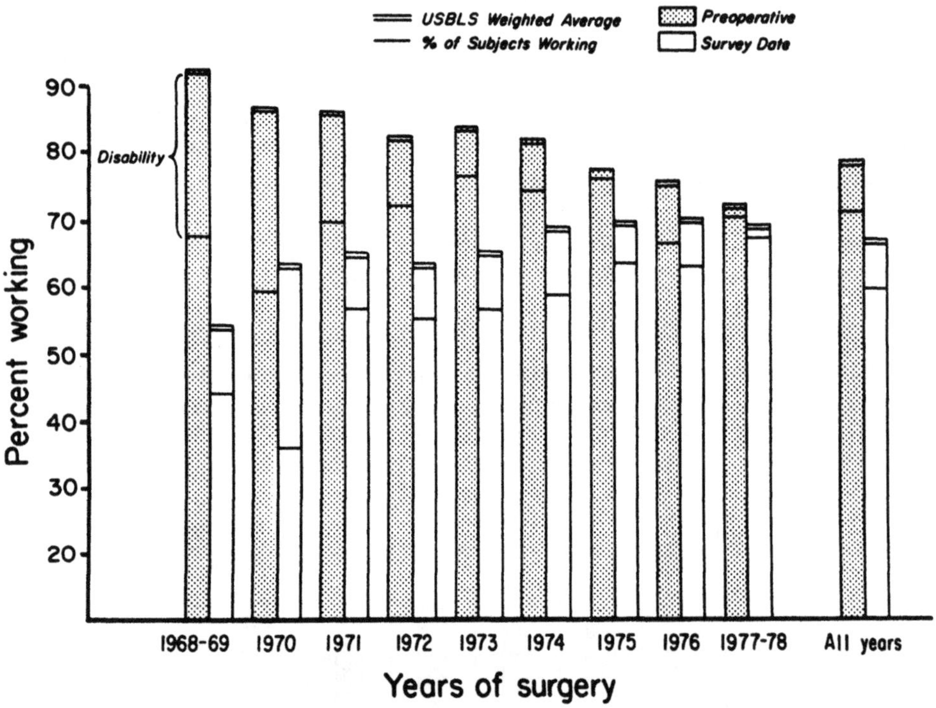

Fig. 3. Percent of patients working preoperatively and at survey date by year of surgery. *USBLS*, U.S. Bureau of Labor Statistics

Quality of Ability of Work

In addition to simply asking the patients if they were working, we asked them if they were "working normally with little or no limitation" or "working, but with some limitations or at an easier job." No USBLS figures are available for this type of comparison, so we compared only preoperative with survey date work status. Figure 4 demonstrates substantial preoperative partial disability: In all age groups, less than 50% of the patients described themselves as working without limitations. Postoperatively, the younger patients demonstrated remarkable improvement; the older patients remained about the same. This is a somewhat subjective judgment on the part of the patient, but shows a remarkable improvement in the patient's judgment of his ability to work.

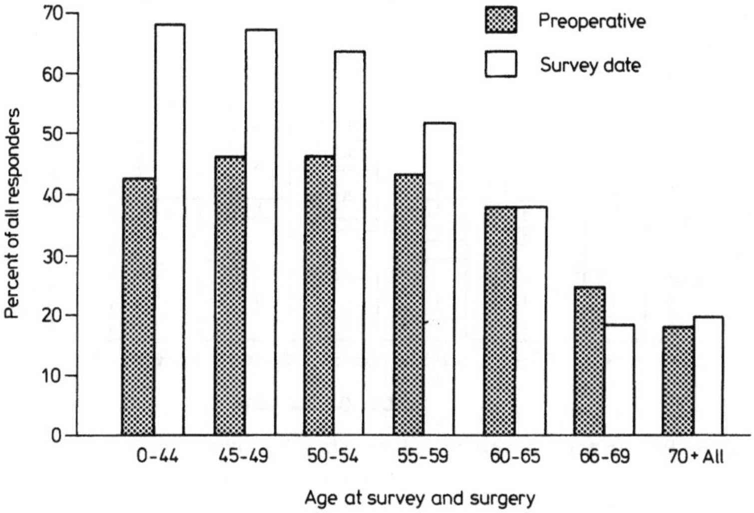

Fig. 4. Percent of patients working normally with little or no limitations preoperatively and at survey date by age

Reason for Not Working

We asked patients, "If you are not now working full time at the job of your choice, please indicate the main reason why." Figure 5 shows the results by age at survey. In all groups younger than age 65 years, physical disability was the reason cited most often. "Company policy" was an insignificant factor in all age groups, accounting for only 2.6% overall. Doctor's advice was an important factor in the 55–59- and 60–64-year-old groups, cited by 8%–12% of patients. After age 65 years, the "desire to relax and enjoy life" became the dominant reason. Up to age 65 years, the three factors not under the patient's control – physical disability, company policy, and doctor's advice – steadily increase with age, but after age 65 years, the desire to enjoy life is the dominant reason.

Figure 6 shows the same data broken down by year of surgery. There is only one clear pattern: "Physically not able" increases markedly as time from surgery increases. None of the other answers have a pattern. We might dismiss this observation as due to aging, but this is not the case. Only 2 years of age at survey separate patients operated early vs those operated in later years. This is because the median age at surgery in the early years was 51 years and had increased to 55 years in the later years. Therefore, this effect must be attributed to a deterioration of the effects of surgery, progression of disease, or improvement in the quality of surgery, or probably a combination of all three.

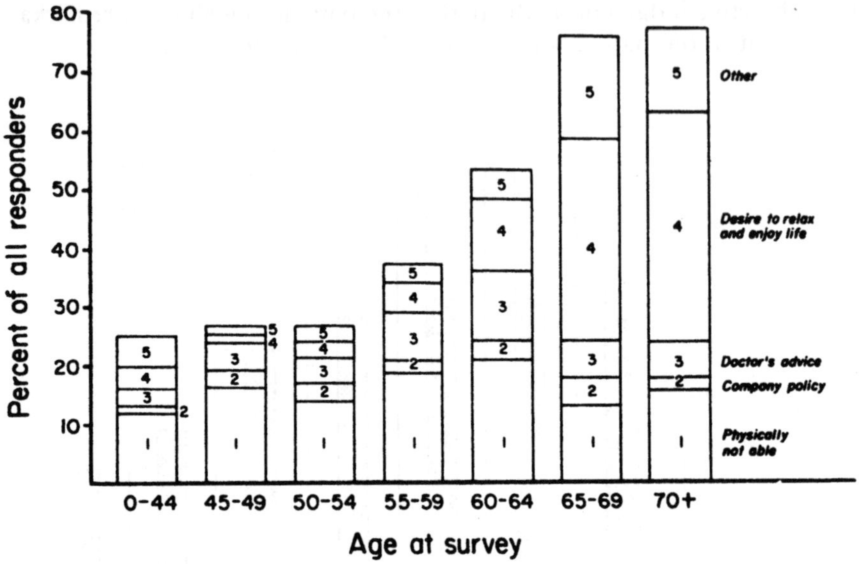

Fig. 5. Reason for not working full time at job of choice by age at survey

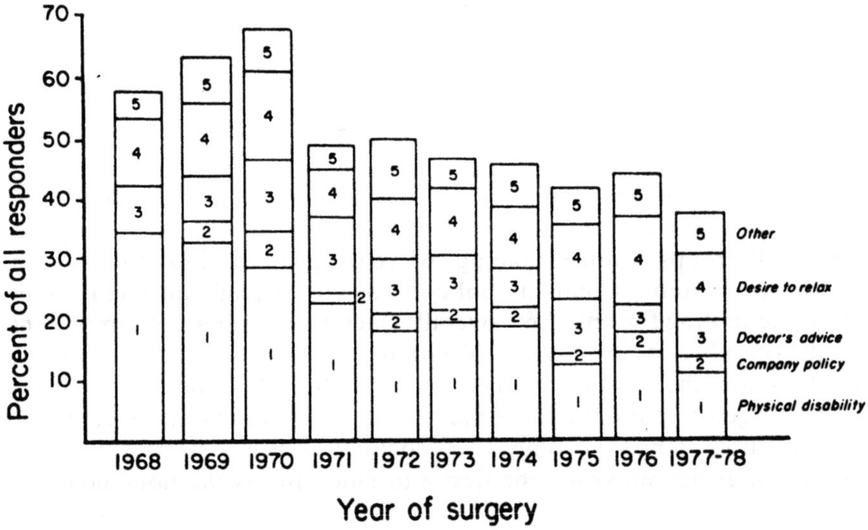

Fig. 6. Reason for not working full time at job of choice by year of surgery

The Effect of Preoperative Resting Left Ventricular Function on Work Status

Our data bank contains left ventricular function (LVF) data on patients operated on after January 1972. Therefore, all data in this section refer to male patients operated on since 1 January 1972. We have divided these patients into two categories of LVF: good ventricles (GV) and bad ventricles (BV). A GV has, at most, one major area (e.g., anterior wall or inferior wall) of distinct hypokinesis or akinesis, or two major areas of moderate or slight hypokinesis. The ejection fraction of a GV is generally greater than 0.35, measured in the right anterior oblique view, at rest, by the method of Dodge. A BV has at least one major area of dyskinesis, two or more areas of distinct hypokinesis or akinesis, or requires resection of at least 6 cm of scar. The ejection fraction is generally less than 0.35 Tables 3 and 4 describe the study group. The BV group contained a larger proportion of nonresponders; we do not know why. Follow-up of the BV group is still more than 91%, compared with more than 95% in the GV group. Other than the difference in follow-up, the only notable difference is that mortality in the GV group is almost six times higher than that in the BV group. Tables 5 and 6 show the comparison of preoperative and survey employment broken down by age, date of surgery, and LVF. In the BV group, preoperative employment was lower except among those 65–69 years old. The change in employment with surgery was similar in BV and GV groups and generally followed the pattern of the 1968–1978 group: little or no change for the younger patients and a loss for the older ones. The overall amount of change was almost identical in BV and GV groups.

Table 3. The study group classified by ventricular function

	Good ventricle	Bad ventricle
Total patients	1636	478
Known dead	73 (4.5%)	125 (26.2%)
Nonresponders	67 (4.3%)[a]	31 (8.8%)[a]
Responders	1496	322
Median age (years) at surgery	55	55
Median age (years) at survey	58	58

[a] $\chi^2 = 11.08$; $P < 0.001$

Table 4. Number of subjects in the good ventricle and bad ventricle groups

				At surgery		At survey	
Year of surgery	GV	BV	Age (years)	GV	BV	GV	BV
1972	68	16	0–44	178	33	100	16
1973	178	35	45–49	249	44	166	27
1974	201	48	50–54	311	72	265	54
1975	251	80	55–59	369	88	331	84
1976	338	57	60–64	263	49	364	77
1977–1978	460	86	65–69	101	29	201	41
			70+	25	7	69	23
All years	1496	322	All ages	1496	322	1496	322

Abbreviations: *GV* = good ventricle; *BV* = bad ventricle

Table 5. Work status by left ventricular function and age - 1880 male responders who had surgery between January 1972 and March 1978

	Percent working					
	Good ventricle			Bad ventricle		
Age[a] (years)	Preop	Postop	Δ%	Preop	Postop	Δ%
0–44	78.7	81.0	+2.3	67.0	68.8	+1.8
45–49	83.9	83.1	+0.8	72.7	70.4	−2.3
50–54	73.0	81.1	+8.1	76.4	79.6	+3.2
55–59	80.5	76.4	+4.1	56.9	60.7	+3.8
60–64	66.5	56.9	−9.4	53.1	37.7	−15.4
65–69	46.5	27.4	−19.1	51.7	31.7	−20.0
70+	36.0	37.7	+1.7	14.3	26.1	+11.8
All years	75.1	65.2	−9.9	62.4	53.5	−8.9

[a] Age at surgery = preop; age at survey = postop

Table 6. Work status by left ventricular function and date of surgery - 1880 male responders who had surgery between January 1972 and March 1978

	Percent working					
	Good ventricle			Bad ventricle		
Year of surgery	Preop	Postop	Δ%	Preop	Postop	Δ%
1972	72	56	−18	69	44	−25
1973	82	61	−21	51	37	−14
1974	76	61	−15	73	50	−23
1975	80	67	−13	74	54	−20
1976	70	65	−5	49	68	+19
1977–78	74	69	−5	59	61	+2
All years	75.1	65.2	−9.9	62.4	53.5	−8.9

There appears to be a deterioration with time after surgery in excess of that attributable to aging alone. In all age groups, there was a general trend of fewer persons working as the time since surgery increased.

Tables 7 and 8 show the percentage of patients working "full time with little or not limitation" broken down by age, date of surgery and LVF. Significantly fewer BV patients were in this category preoperatively and at the survey, but the improvement after surgery was about the same in both groups. There does appear to be a trend of fewer patients working with little or no limitation as the time from surgery increases.

The "main reason for not working full time at job choice" is shown in Table 9, broken down by LVF. The BV group has a higher total percentage and this higher total percentage is accounted for by "physically not able" and "doctor's advice." Both of these reasons were cited about twice as often by patients in the BV group as by those in the GV group.

Table 7. Working with little or no limitation by left ventricular function and age – 1880 male responders who had surgery between January 1972 and March 1978

	Percent working with little or no limitations					
	Good ventricle			Bad ventricle		
Age[a] (years)	Preop	Postop	Δ%	Preop	Postop	Δ%
0–44	44.9	71.0	+26.1	33.3	62.5	+29.2
45–49	49.8	71.7	+21.9	38.6	55.6	+17.0
50–54	48.9	63.8	+14.9	50.0	64.8	+14.8
55–59	49.9	55.6	+5.7	33.0	45.2	+12.2
60–64	40.7	44.2	+3.5	28.6	29.9	+1.3
65–69	25.7	19.9	−5.8	24.1	14.6	−9.5
70+	20.0	29.0	+9.0	14.3	8.7	−5.6
All ages	45.3	51.1	+5.8	35.7	40.1	+4.4

[a] Preop = age at surgery; postop = age at survey

Table 8. Working with little or no limitation by left ventricular function and year of surgery – 1880 male responders who had surgery between January 1972 and March 1978

	Percent working with little or no limitations					
	Good ventricle			Bad ventricle		
Year of surgery	Preop	Postop	Δ%	Preop	Postop	Δ%
1972	41.2	41.2	0	43.8	25.6	−8.2
1973	46.6	43.3	−3.3	25.7	20.0	−5.7
1974	43.3	49.8	+6.5	47.9	41.7	−6.2
1975	53.4	53.4	0	42.5	43.8	+1.3
1976	41.4	48.8	+7.4	28.1	43.9	+15.8
1977–78	44.8	56.5	+11.7	30.2	44.2	+14.0
All years	45.3	51.1	+5.8	35.7	40.1	+4.4

Table 9. Reason for not working full-time at job of choice – good ventricles vs bad ventricles

	Good ventricle (%)	Bad ventricle (%)
Physically not able	13.4	23.3
Company policy	2.7	1.6
Doctor's advice	5.8	11.2
Desire to relax	12.7	9.3
Other reasons	5.9	7.1
Total	40.5	52.5

Shifts in Employment Patterns

Figure 1 shows a fairly sharp "knee" around age 55 years. Portions of the curves up to the age 55 years and over age 55 years are reasonably linear. Before age 55 years, attrition rate from the labor force is about 0.5% per year. After age 55 years, it is about 5.0% per year. If we choose a subgroup younger than age 55 years throughout the study period and assume a constant 0.5% per year attrition rate, analysis becomes greatly simplified. Similarly, we separated those older than 55 years throughout the study period and assumed a constant 5.0% per year attrition rate. Figure 7 shows how 738 male patients younger than 55 years at the survey date changed their employment status over the period of surgery to survey (average 3.8 years). There was essentially no change in total employment; 10.6% of patients not working preoperatively were working postoperatively, but this was balanced by 10.3% of patients going the other way. A significant gain was made, however, when 20.7% of patients moved from limited to unlimited ability to work against only 5.3% in the opposite direction; 7.9% went from no work at all to unlimited employment against only

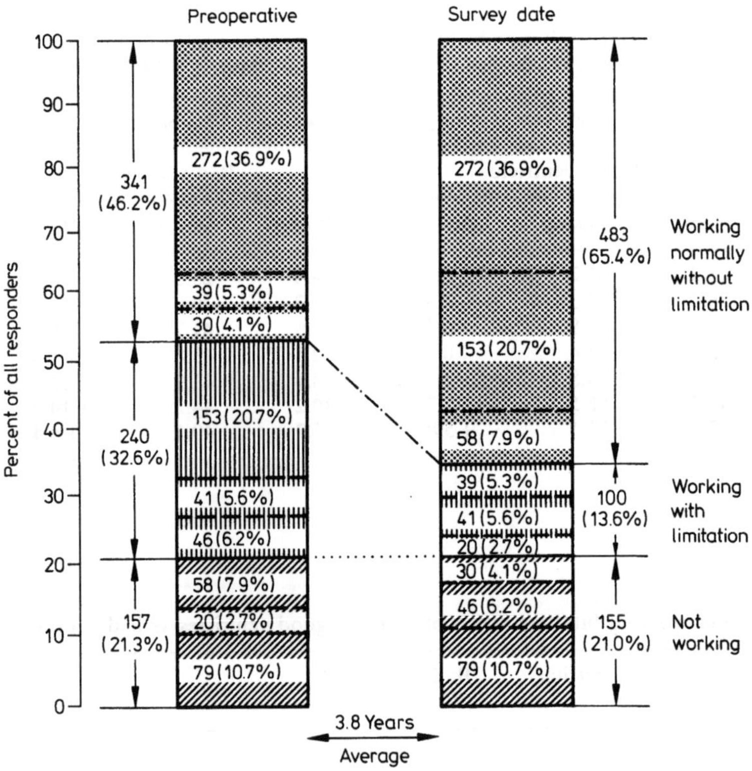

Fig. 7. Preoperative to postoperative shifts in employment; 738 male patients younger than age 55 years throughout the study period. The best way to determine where a subgroup shifted is to identify the subgroup by its exact size; e. g., the second subgroup from the top in the left column consists of 39 patients. This group can be found in the right column as the fourth subgroup (the top subgroup of the second group)

4.1% in the opposite direction. Thirty-one percent of patients improved their work status; 53.2% remain unchanged and 15.5% showed a decline. Using the data in Fig. 1, we would have an expected attrition of 0.5% per year or about 2% over the study period; we observed no change.

The group of 1065 patients older than 55 years at surgery (Fig. 8) show an entirely different and almost opposite picture; 24.2% went from working to nonworking, but only 5.7% went in the other direction, for an overall loss of 18.5% over the average 3.5 years from surgery to survey. A loss of 14.0% from unlimited work status to no work was balanced by only 3.4% in the other direction. Only 16.1% of patients improved their status; 55.8% remained the same; and 28.0% dropped. During the 3½ years from surgery to survey, we would have an expected loss of about 5.0% per year or 17.5%, according to Fig. 1; we observed a loss of 18.5%.

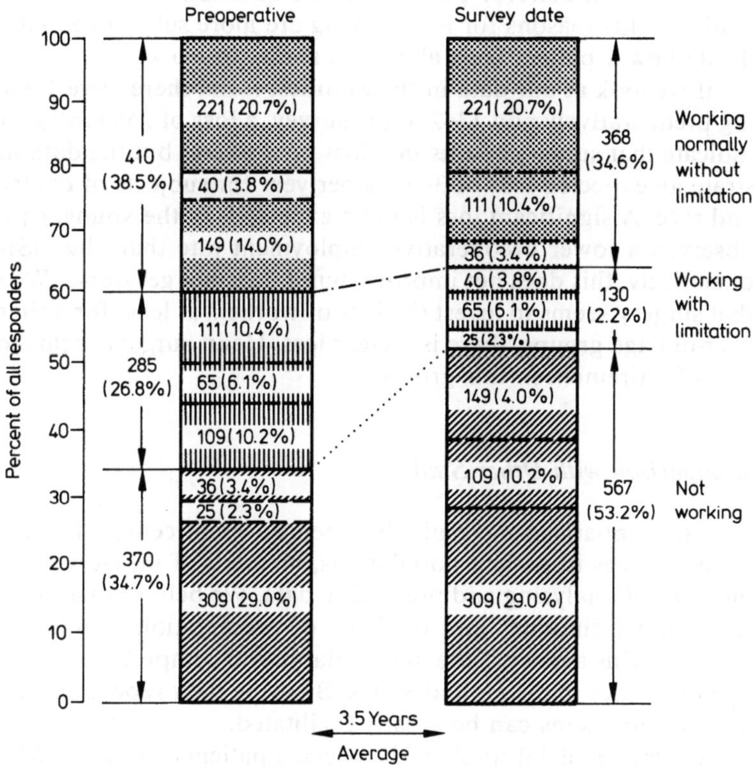

Fig. 8. Preoperative to postoperative shifts in employment, 1065 male respondents older than age 55 years throughout the study period

Discussion

The primary purpose of this study is to compare the work status of our entire population of heart surgery patients with the United States population as published by the USBLS. We have included all of our myocardial revascularization patients. In order to get a high follow-up on all patients, we had to keep the questionnaire short and simple. We never exceed one page typed double-spaced. Because of these limitations, we can examine only very superficially the motivation and reasons for working or not working. This approach has obvious limitations, but eliminates errors produced by any type of sampling. We have no sampling error because we did not sample. Our errors are caused by subjects answering questions incorrectly and the fact that the 6% lost to follow-up may not be typical of the responders. We would expect that the questions concerning whether or not the patient is working are straightforward, purely objective, and, therefore, accurate. The questions on how well the patient can work and his reasons for not working are more subjective, but at least they indicate how a patient feels about his ability to work.

If we look at our data in their crudest form, there were 1598 patients working preoperatively and 1342 at the survey, a loss of 256 (16%). This alone might indicate that surgery results in a loss of workers; but the data in Fig. 1 demonstrate an expected loss of 3%–5% per year for subjects of comparable age, sex, and race. A significant loss is to be expected. In the younger patients, we have observed a lower preoperative employment rate than the USBLS data. Postoperatively, this does not improve, but it does not get worse. We might conclude that surgery seems to arrest the loss of workers at least for a time. In the 60–70-year-old age groups, there is a clear loss. Heart surgery seems to accelerate the rate of retirement in this group.

Comparison with Other Studies

Precise comparison of results between different centers is impossible because of differences in patient populations, methods of measuring employment, and methods of analyzing and presenting data. We believe that investigators should try to use techniques and methods of presentation similar to USBLS where possible. This agency is the most reliable and comprehensive source of employment statistics in the United States. By using their reports as models and standards, comparisons can be greatly facilitated.

Symmes et al. [5] studied 329 selected patients. Overall, 56.8% were working preoperatively and 70.5% postoperatively, an impressive gain. However, they used an unusual definition of preoperative employment: A patient was considered employed only if his salary had been totally unaffected by his heart disease. This resulted in a very low preoperative employment rate. The postoperative employment rate in this study was unremarkable. Patients were followed for 2–60 months (mean 23 months).

Russell et al. [6] studied 67 surgical patients randomized into the National Cooperative Unstable Angina Study. Among these patients, 85% were working preoperatively and only 45% 1½ years later. This is by far the largest decrease after surgery we have seen. We see no reason for this large decrease except, perhaps, that the very small group size contains, by chance, a high proportion of poor results.

Crosby et al. [7] reported 52 patients who underwent aneurysmectomy and coronary artery bypass grafting. Over the 11-month follow-up, employment increased from 40% preoperatively to 71% postoperatively.

Hammermeister et al. [8] reported on 1198 somewhat selected patients surveyed 3–8 years postoperatively. Employment dropped from 77.8% preoperatively to 68.2% postoperatively.

Barnes et al. [9] reported that 350 of 909 patients who "attended a special follow up clinic" had not "retired" before surgery. Follow-up averaged 12.2 months. Preoperatively, 73% were working; postoperatively 74%.

In the report by Anderson et al. [10], 564 male patients were surveyed 1 and 4 years postoperatively. The method of selection of this group is unclear, but it is drawn from a much larger cohort of patients operated during the stated time, 1969 through 1974. In a subgroup of 315 patients younger than 55 years at surgery, 95.9% were working preoperatively. One year later, only 89.8% were working, and 4 years after surgery, 88.9% were working. This group showed a higher preoperative employment rate than the national age-, sex- and race-adjusted average. The attrition rate at 4 years is about what one would expect (Fig. 1).

Niles et al. [11] reported a net increase of 10% in 105 patients followed an average of 20 months. In this group, the preoperative employment rate was only 50%, which is very low. No other data presented explain this. The postoperative employment rate of 60% is a good increase, but still low compared with other studies.

Love [12] reported on 100 patients followed 6 months to 2 years. Preoperatively, 64% were working; postoperatively, 54%.

Many of these reports investigated factors associated with not working postoperatively. Factors mentioned were age, work status preoperatively, left ventricular function, length of preoperative disability, graft patency, symptom relief, and education.

An annotation by Oberman and Kouchoukos [13] mentioned "doctor's advice" and "company policies" as reasons for not working. Although data are scanty, they reported that many patients may not be working because of medical advice and the reluctance of companies to hire patients back after surgery. Our data tend to discount employers as a significant factor in not returning to work. Only 2.6% of the patients cited this as the primary reason for not working. Doctor's advice, however, was cited by 7.6% of patients as the main reason for not working, and one may assume that it may be an important secondary factory in many other patients' reason for not working. If all physicians advising patients not to work would reverse their advice, many patients might return to work, but mortality might also rise. The advice not to work may, in many cases, be good advice. In patients with good ventricular function and successful bypass surgery, however, this should never be a patient's main reason for not working.

Summary

Loss of productivity is a major concern among patients with heart disease. To assess the effect of surgery on this factor, we surveyed every living male patient of the surgeon authors operated on from January 1968 through March 1978 (96% follow-up) and compared their pre- and postoperative work status with the U.S. population as reported by the U.S. Bureau of Labor Statistics (USBLS). Comparisons were made on an age-for-age basis and adjustments were made for changes in national employment patterns from 1968–1978.

Preoperatively, our younger patients had a 10% lower employment rate than the U.S. male population at large according to the USBLS. Postoperatively, many returned to work, but an equal number who worked preoperatively did not postoperatively. The ability to work full time with little or no limitation increased 20% after operation. The main reason for not working was physical disability, with doctor's advice a distant second. Older patients showed a trend of accelerated retirement after surgery. A few returned to work, but many more retired. The ability to work full-time without limitation increased 4%. Thirty percent of all older subjects cited a desire to relax as their main reason for not working. Compared with the early years of surgery, patients in later years were older and did not show as much preoperative disability. There was some evidence of a deterioration of the effects of surgery. Patients with severely impaired left ventricular function fared worse both pre- and postoperatively, but the improvement was the same as for patients with normal or moderately impaired left ventricular function.

References

1. US Dept of Labor Bureau of Labor Statistics (1979) Handbook of Labor Statistics, 1978. US Govt Print Off, Washington, DC, pp 1–4, tables IV and LX
2. Rones PL (1979) Older men – the choice between work and retirement. Monthly Labor Review, November 1978, p 3
3. Rosenfeld C, Brown SC (1979) The labor force status of older workers. Monthly Labor Review, November 1979, p 12
4. Deutermann WV (1977) Another look at working-age men who are not in the labor force. Monthly Labor Review, June 1977, p 9
5. Symmes JC, Lenkei SCM, Berman ND (1978) Influence of aortocoronary bypass surgery on employment. Can Med Assoc J 118:268
6. Russell RO Jr, Wayne JB, Kronenfeld J, Charles ED, Oberman A, Kouchoukos NT, White C, Rogers W, Mantle JA, Rackley CE (1980) Surgical versus medical therapy for treatment of unstable angina: changes in work status and family income. Am J Cardiol 45:134
7. Crosby IK, Wellons HA, Martin RP, Schuch D, Muller WH (1980) Employability – a new indication for aneurysmectomy and coronary revascularization. Circulation [Suppl I] 62:I-79
8. Hammermeister KE, DeRouen TA, English MT, Dodge HT (1979) Effect of surgical versus medical therapy on return to work in patients with coronary artery disease. Am J Cardiol 44:105
9. Barnes GK, Ray MJ, Oberman A, Kouchoukos NT (1977) Changes in working status of patients following coronary bypass surgery. JAMA 238:1259
10. Anderson AJ, Barboriak JJ, Hoffman RG, Mullen DC (1980) Retention or resumption of employment after aortocoronary bypass operations. JAMA 243:543

11. Niles NW, Vander Slam TJ, Cutler BS (1980) Return to work after coronary artery bypass operation. J Thorac Cardiovasc Surg 79:916
12. Love JW (1979) Employment status after coronary bypass operations and some cost considerations. J Thorac Cardiovasc Surg 80:68
13. Oberman A, Kouchoukos NT (1979) Working status of patients following coronary bypass surgery. Am Heart J 98:132

Reemployment Related to Functional and Hemodynamic Changes

S. Nitter-Hauge, T. Frøysaker, and S. Simonsen

Patients and Methods

The present study includes available follow-up data in a total of 70 male survivors of aortocoronary bypass surgery. In these patients the employment status has been related to objective criteria of haemodynamic improvement, such as number of grafts implanted, graft flow, graft patency, left ventricular function and results of exercise tolerance testing using a bicycle ergometer. The mean age at the time of surgery was 52 years, with a range of 30–65 years. Longstanding angina pectoris with or without myocardial infarction together with the demonstration of critical coronary arterial stenosis (75% or greater reduction in lumen diameter) in one or more of the major vessels, and a left ventricular ejection fraction above 0.50 were the usual prerequisites for referral to surgery. The mean interval between operation and the time of the restudy was 14 months, with a range of 8–33 months. According to their working status at follow-up, the patients were divided into two subgroups:

1. *Actually working,* i.e. all patients who at the time of restudy were working more than 4 h, a day
2. *Non-working,* i.e. all patients who at the time of restudy were not working (temporary or permanent disability)

Operative Procedure

Operative technique included extracorporeal circulation with general cooling of the patients to 28 °C in those undergoing double/triple bypass surgery. During single bypass operations the cooling of the patients was stopped at 32°–30°C. The nonhemic priming volume caused a moderate haemodilution, with reduction of the hematocrit to approximately 25%–30%. The flow rate in the heart-lung machine was kept at a level of 2–3 l/m^2 body surface. The left ventricle was routinely vented through the apex cordis, except in patients undergoing single vein bypass to LAD, when no vent was applied. The hearts were electrically fibrillated before incision of the coronary arteries. Aortic cross-clamping was used in distal anastomoses to LAD and the circumflex artery, while anastomoses to the distal right artery and the posterior descending artery were performed using Silastic tapes as snares. After the rewarming of the patient was started, the heart was defibrillated. The vein grafts were thereafter anastomosed proximally to the aorta. As soon as the patients had been rewarmed, the heart-lung machine was disconnected and the completion of the proximal anastomoses was eventually done on a beating heart.

Catheterization Technique

Before operation and at the restudy, all patients underwent left heart catheterization with coronary angiography including graft angiography. The contrast material used was Isopaque Coronar [metrizoate meglumine/Na/Ca (58/9/1) 370 mg I/ml]. Left ventricular pressures were measured before and 2 min after left ventriculography. Pressures were recorded with Elema Schönander equipment (Transducer EMT 35 and Mingograf 81). The baseline was the 4th intercostal space in the anterior axillary line. The end-diastolic pressure was measured at the intercept between the "a" wave and the rapid ventricular upstroke. The ejection fraction was measured by outlining the internal contour of the left ventricle in systole and diastole; the formula given by Arbogast et al. (1973) was used.

Exercise Tests

Exercise testing was performed with the patient sitting on an electrically braked Elema bicycle. ECG was monitored on an oscilloscope and recorded on a six-channel ink jet ECG recorder (Mingograf 61, Siemens-Elema, Stockholm) at a paper-speed of 50 mm/s. Before the exercise test, a 12-lead ECG was taken with the patient recumbent. Subsequently, with the patient seated on the bicycle, bipolar chest-head connections CH_1-CH_7 were made with the indifferent electrode attached to the forehead. The initial work load was 300 kpm ($\sim$50 W), increasing by 300 kpm ($\sim$50 W) every 6 min. ECGs were taken at 2-min intervals during exercise, at the end of the exercise period, and subsequently at 2-min intervals until return to baseline, as well as at any time during the tests when significant changes were noted on the oscilloscope. The patients were exercised to symptomatic endpoints; moderately severe angina/dyspnea, or exhaustion. ST-segment depression of 2 mm or more, lasting at least 0.08 s from the J-point regardless of slope of the ST-segment, during maximal exercise or recovery was interpreted as positive. A test was considered negative if no significant ST-segment changes occurred. If ST-depressions were present in the resting state, additional changes of the same magnitude as referred to above had to be present for an ECG to be labelled positive. ST-changes of the vasoregulatory type have been disregarded. The results from the exercise ECG were expressed as the cumulative work performed in each case, determined by adding the work performed on each load. None of the patients were taking digitalis, diuretics or other drugs known to produce false-positive tests.

Statistics

The statistical data are presented as mean ±1 standard deviation from the mean (SD). The statistical significance of the difference between two variables was analysed using Student's *t*-test. *P* values above 0.05 were not considered to be significant.

Results

Of a total of 70 men included in this study, 31 (44%) were recorded as working while 39 (56%) were recorded as temporarily sick or permanently disabled at follow-up. In this series of men under 65 years, age per se apparently was not related to working status, and there was no significant correlation between working status and duration of symptoms. However, our data indicate a relationship between working status and (a) type of preoperative employment and the physical strain associated with it, as well as (b) the preoperative working status (Fig. 1). There were relatively more "blue-collar" than "white-collar" workers among the unemployed patients than among those who were employed at the time of restudy. Return to work was much more common among those working up to the time of operation than among those who were temporarily or permanently disabled before operation.

Analysis of data obtained from the operating theatre showed that the number of grafts per patient as well as graft flow was nearly the same in the nonworking group and in the working group. Follow-up arteriography showed that graft patency rate also was very similar, with an average of 1.3 grafts/patient in the employed group vs. 1.2 grafts/patient in the non-working group (Fig. 2).

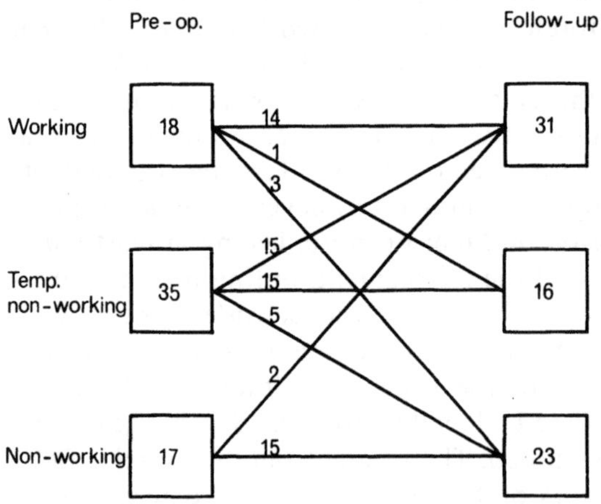

Fig. 1. Employment status in 70 men examined before aortocoronary bypass surgery and at follow-up

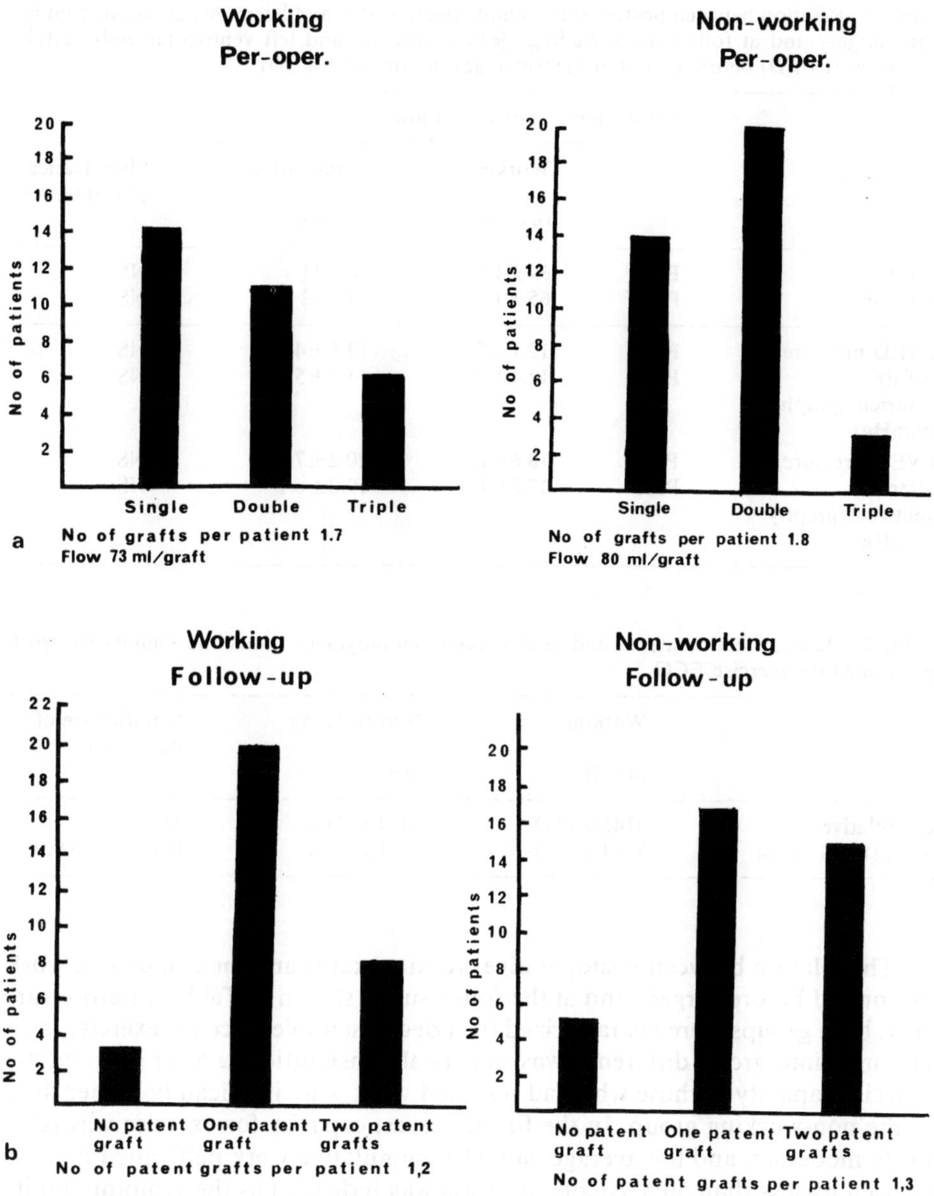

Fig. 2. **a** Number of grafts implanted, and **b** number of grafts patent at follow-up in working and non-working patients

Analysis of the haemodynamic pattern showed that the ejection fraction and the left ventricular end-diastolic pressures measured before and after left ventriculography were the same when working and non-working patients were compared (Table 1).

Table 1. Relation between postoperative employment status and haemodynamic function before surgery and at follow-up, including ejection fraction and left ventricular end-diastolic pressures *(LVED)* before and after ventriculography (mean ± 1 SD)

		Employment status at follow-up		
		Working (*n* = 31)	Non-working (*n* = 39)	Significance of difference
Ejection fraction (%)	Pre	69 ± 11	68 ± 11	NS
	Post	65 ± 15	64 ± 12	NS
LVED pressure before ventriculography (mmHg)	Pre	12.1 ± 5.5	12.5 ± 4.8	NS
	Post	12.4 ± 7.0	14.2 ± 5.2	NS
LVED pressure after ventriculography (mmHg)	Pre	18.6 ± 8.1	20.2 ± 7.9	NS
	Post	17.2 ± 6.9	19.8 ± 6.1	NS

Table 2. Relation between pre- and postoperative employment status and cumulative work performed on exercise ECG

		Working (*n* = 31)	Non-working (*n* = 39)	Significance of difference
Cumulative work (kpm)	Pre	3142 ± 1992	3494 ± 2764	NS
	Post	7644 ± 2952	5151 ± 3383	$0.01 > P > 0.001$

The relation between postoperative working status and the cumulative work performed before surgery and at the follow-up is shown in Table 2. Before surgery, both groups were characterized by a decreased tolerance for exercise, and the small intergroup difference was statistically insignificant. After surgery, the exercise capacity in those who had resumed work was significantly higher than in the non-working group. In the former cases, capacity for exercise was relatively moderate, and the average value for cumulative work performed had increased by less than 50%. Angina pectoris was indicated as the symptom limiting muscular performance at the end of exercise in approximately 20% of the patients at the follow-up study, while exhaustion was the limiting symptom in the remaining patients. In this respect, there was no difference between the working and the non-working group.

Figure 3 shows the data for the maximal exercise capacity (cumulative work performed) in each patient for whom pre- and postoperative values were available. The patients are divided according to their preoperative and follow-up employment status. Of seven patients who were actually working before and after surgery, all but one had increased their exercise tolerance to normal val-

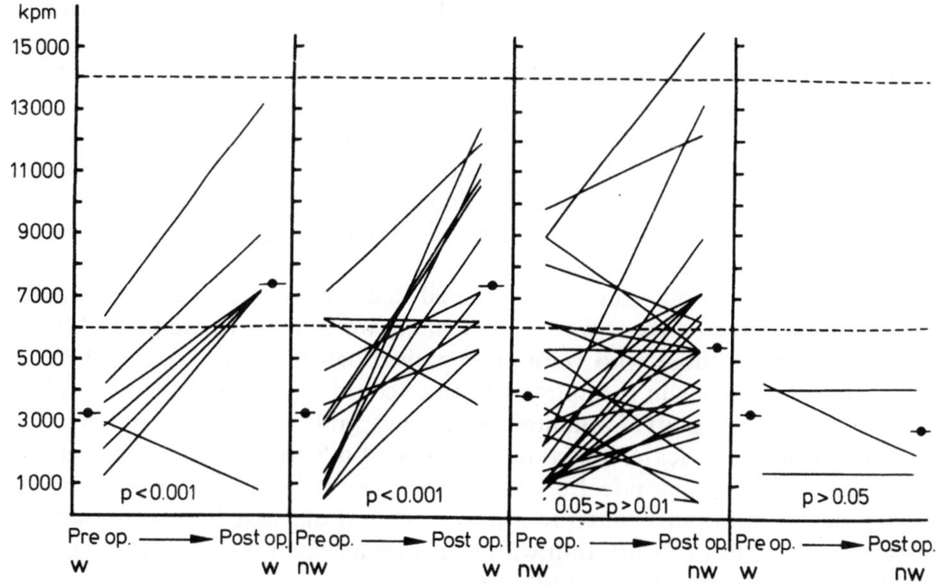

Fig. 3. Maximal exercise capacity (cumulative work performed) before operation and at follow-up in working and non-working patients. The patients are divided into subgroups according to their working status. *w*, working; *nw*, non-working. -•-, mean value. *Interrupted lines* mark upper and lower limits of normal range according to Erikssen et al. (1977)

ues. Of 13 patients who were not working before operation and working at follow-up, all but two had improved their tolerance for exercise up to normal or to subnormal values. A total of 29 patients were working neither before nor after the operation. In this subset of patients, the improvement in physical tolerance for exercise was less significant, and only one-third had exercise capacity within normal range. Finally, a small group of patients (three) who were working before operation but not afterwards had an unchanged and very low exercise capacity.

Discussion

Several studies have evaluated the effect of coronary bypass surgery on work status. Cannom et al. (1974) reported that 63% of middle-aged men went back to work within 1 year after operation. Rimm et al. (1976) found that 83% were back to work within 14 months after operation. The same percentage of reemployment was also reported in a study from Norway by Hoel et al. (1975). Other investigators, however, correlating work status after surgery with the preoperative work status, have given a more differentiated view on the possibility for reemployment in operated patients. English et al. (1975) concluded that 71% of patients employed within 3 months before surgery returned to work, whereas of those not employed preoperatively only 18% returned to work. In their study educational level or manual labour did not influence return to employment, Barnes et al. (1975) stated that only 10% of those who were not working before operation returned to work after operation, while in the group working full-time before surgery, no overall changes were noted. According to Logue et al. (1976), patients who were strongly motivated because of economic considerations usually did go back to work, whereas those with a generous disability programme often retired after surgery. Although 90% of their patients had symptomatic improvement and relief of angina, only 50% returned to work, which is close to our finding.

The results from our study also showed that the postsurgical employment rate was higher among those who were actually working up to the time of operation than among those who were unemployed before the operation (45% vs. 13%). The discrepancy in reemployment rates could not be explained by differences in number of grafts implanted, graft flow, graft patency or objective parameters of left ventricular function such as end-diastolic pressure or ejection fraction. Thus, the anatomical outcome of the operation did not appear to be of significant importance when return to work was discussed. Previous studies of the rate of return to work following valve replacement surgery have yielded similar results (Nitter-Hauge et al. 1976).

An important factor in the present study is the observation that the physical capacity measured by ECG exercise tests was reduced in those who felt unable to work compared with the group who were working. Among patients who returned to work we found a significant and rather uniform improvement in exercise tolerance. A majority of patients in this subgroup performed more than 100 W for 6 min, which is normal for healthy men of the same age (Erikssen et al. 1977). This contrasts with the observations made in the non-working patients. In this subgroup about two-thirds of the patients performed less than 100 W for 6 min and had a maximal physical capacity less than that which would be expected in normals.

A number of studies (Bartel et al. 1973; Lapin et al. 1973; Rimm et al. 1976) have found a significant improvement in exercise tolerance after bypass surgery. It appears from the present study that the individual tolerance for exercise after operation not only can be related to the preoperative capacity, but to a large extent to the postoperative employment status. Patients going back to work in general had improved their physical capacity more than those who felt unable to work. Whether this means that those who resumed work also more quickly had improved their physical performance than non-workers, or indicates a permanent situation of reduced physical capacity in the latter group, is difficult to say. It might be that in non-working patients return to work is hampered by a reduced physical capacity demonstrable more than a year after operation. A analogous situation has previously been observed in correlation studies between employment status and physical capacity in patients with sustained myocardial infarction (Benestad 1968). It is likely that the differences between the two series of patients reflect a lack of training effect in the non-working group. To what extent a proper rehabilitation program can normalize the exercise tolerance in patients who feel unable to resume work after bypass surgery remains an open question in the absence of experimental data, but should be of considerable interest when discussing the role of bypass surgery for the rehabilitation of these patients.

Summary

The occupational status of a group of 70 male patients, 30–65 years of age, operated on with aortocoronary bypass surgery, was studied and related to left ventricular function, number of patent grafts, and exercise ECG. The patients were divided into two groups; one ($n=39$) consisted of subjects unable to work ("non-working" group), while the other ($n=31$) consisted of subjects working up to the time of examination ("working" group). The non-working group had a higher percentage of men in manual occupations (77 vs. 48%), and more of them had been temporarily or permanently disabled before operation compared with the working group (87 vs. 55%). There was no correlation between employability and (a) objective parameters of left ventricular function such as left ventricular end-diastolic pressure before and after angiography and ejection fraction or (b) number of patent grafts per patient. The working group had in general increased their tolerance for exercise and had a higher exercise capacity than the non-working group. In the working group, all but three patients had a normal exercise tolerance. The increase in exercise tolerance in the non-working group was more modest, only one-third of the patients having a normal exercise capacity. Exhaustion and angina pectoris were the two principal limits upon exercise.

References

Arbogast R, Solignac A, Bourassa MG (1973) Influence of aorto-coronary saphenous vein bypass surgery on left ventricular volumes and ejection fraction. Comparison before and one year after surgery in 51 patients. Am J Med 54:290–296

Barnes GK, Oberman A, Kouchoukos NT, et al. (1975) Changes in working status of patients undergoing saphenous vein bypass surgery (SVBS). Circulation [Suppl 2] 51–52:118

Bartel AG, Behar VS, Peter RH, et al. (1973) Exercise stress testing in evaluation of aorto-coronary bypass surgery, report of 123 patients. Circulation 48:141–148

Benestad AM (1968) Determination of physical work capacity and exercise tolerance in cardiac patients. Acta Med Scand 183:521–529

Cannom DS, Miller DG, Shumway NE (1974) The longterm follow-up of patients undergoing saphenous vein bypass surgery. Circulation 49:77–85

English MT, Logan GA, Eyer KM, et al. (1975) Employment following coronary artery bypass graft surgery. Circulation [Suppl 2] 144:51–52

Erikssen J, Rasmussen K, Forfang K, Storstein O (1977) Exercise ECG and cas history in the diagnosis of latent coronary heart disease among presumably healthy middle-aged men. Eur J Cardiol 5, 6:463–476

Hoel B, Eie H, Semb G, Sivertsen E (1975) Aortocoronary vein bypass in patients with angina pectoris. Acta Med Scand 197:383–390

Lapin ES, Murray JA, Bruce RA, Winterscheid L (1973) Changes in maximal exercise performance in the evaluation of saphenous vein bypass surgery. Circulation 47:1164–1173

Logue B, King SB, Douglas JS Jr (1976) A practical approach to coronary artery disease with special reference to coronary artery bypass surgery. Curr Probl Cardiol 1

Nitter-Hauge S, Frøysaker T, Hall KV (1976) Reemployment related to functional and haemodynamic changes after aortic valve replacement. Ann Chir Gynaecol Fenniae 65:124–131
Rimm AA, Barboriak JJ, Anderson AJ, Simon JS (1976) Changes in occupation after aortocoronary vein bypass operation. JAMA 236:361–364

Determinants of Vocational Rehabilitation

V. Carstens, C. Röger, H. Schmitz, D. W. Behrenbeck, and H. Dalichau

In patients with coronary artery disease and angina pectoris, aortocoronary bypass surgery has gained widespread acceptance due to the dramatic relief of pain experienced by most patients [4, 5, 10]. Theoretically this improvement in pain should have a positive impact on employment. However, despite relief of symptoms, patients who have undergone coronary artery bypass grafting generally have an overall reduction in employment from preoperative levels [4, 6, 8, 11, 14, 16].

The purpose of our study was to identify those factors that influence the return to work after surgery and to examine if there is a relation between resumption of work postoperatively and the functional result of the intervention expressed by exercise capacity. In a second investigation we tried to identify those variables that influence working status in patients with angiographically proved coronary artery disease, who are not operated on.

Methods

The study consisted of two groups. Group A included 111 patients with coronary artery disease who underwent coronary artery bypass grafting between March 1977 and March 1983 (at the Herzchirurgische Klinik der Universität Köln; Direktor: Prof. Dr. H. Dalichau). There were 10 women and 101 men, ranging in age from 36 to 75 years, mean 54 years. Group B included 112 patients in whom coronary artery disease was proved angiographically at our institution during the same period, but who were not operated on for different reasons. There were 11 women and 101 men, ranging in age from 33 to 68 years, mean 54 years.

All surgical patients were reexamined at a mean of 34 months postoperatively, range 6–74 months, while the nonsurgical patients were reexamined at a mean of 27 months after angiography.

Baseline data collected included age, sex, history of angina, history of myocardial infarction, functional class according to the criteria of the Canadian Cardiovascular Society [3], and employment status at the time of angiography as well as at the time of the follow-up study. Occupational status was coded as professional, clerical, or physical. Physical workers were those routinely involved in the performance of heavy manual labor and physical exertion, while clerical work included employment not regularly associated with heavy manual labor. Professionals were engaged in occupations that require advanced training and especially mental rather than physical work. For women who were not employed, full-time housework was equated with physical work.

A standardized progressive exercise stress test was carried out in all patients at the time of follow-up. The test was performed on an electrically braked cycle ergometer with the patients in an upright position. The initial work load on the ergometer was set at 25 W/s and increased stepwise at the end of every 2 min by 25 W/s until the patient was forced to stop through general fatigue, breathlessness, angina pectoris, or other symptoms. The test was stopped by us if frequent ventricular ectopic beats appeared on the ECG display or if there was an ST-segment depression of more than 0.2 mV.

Results

The baseline data are summarized in Tables 1–3. At the time of angiography there were no significant differences between the two groups in respect of age,

Table 1. Patient characteristics of the study groups

	Surgical group			Medical group		
	All	Group A 1	Group A 2	All	Group B 1	Group B 2
Number of patients	111	53	58	112	44	68
Mean age (years)	54±6.8	53±7.5	56±5.8	54±7.8	52±7.0	56±5.2
Men	101	87%	95%	101	84%	94%
Women	10	13%	5%	11%	16%	6%
History of myocardial infarction	51%	38%	64%	61%	45%	72%

Table 2. Job classification and employment status

	Surgical group			Medical group		
	All	Group A 1	Group A 2	All	Group B 1	Group B 2
Occupational status Professionals	25.2%	45%	10%	9.9%	25%	0%
Clerical workers	26.1%	25%	29%	42.8%	39%	46%
Physical workers	48.7%	30%	61%	47.3%	36%	54%
Time out of work preop. (months)	8.4±13.5	3.0±4.2	13.4±16.9	–	–	–

Table 3. Functional class and exercise capacity of the study groups

	Surgical group			Medical group		
	All	Group A 1	Group A 2	All	Group B 1	Group B 2
Functional class Angiography	2.7±1.2	2.8±1.1	2.7±1.3	2.7±0.9	2.5±1.1	2.9±0.7
Follow-up	1.6±1.3	0.9±0.9	2.0±1.4	2.4±1.0	1.9±1.1	2.6±0.9
Exercise capacity (W/s)	94±47	112±42	77±45	78±42	98±43	66±34

sex, functional class, or employment status. At the time of angiography 70% of the patients in group A had been employed, compared to 65% in group B. At the time of follow-up 48% of those who had undergone coronary artery bypass surgery were still working, compared to 39% of those who had not undergone surgery.

In the patients operated on there was a close inverse relation between resumption of work after surgery and the time interval the patients had not worked before surgery. While 75% of those who had still worked 2 months before operation did resume their work postoperatively, only 27% of those who had stopped working more than 2 months before surgery were working at the time of follow-up and only 1 out of 18 who had stopped working more than 1 year before surgery (Fig. 1). Of those who did not work after surgery, 88% stated that they had stopped working for cardiac reasons; 3% had quit their jobs because of age and 9% because of some other disability or reasons unrelated to health.

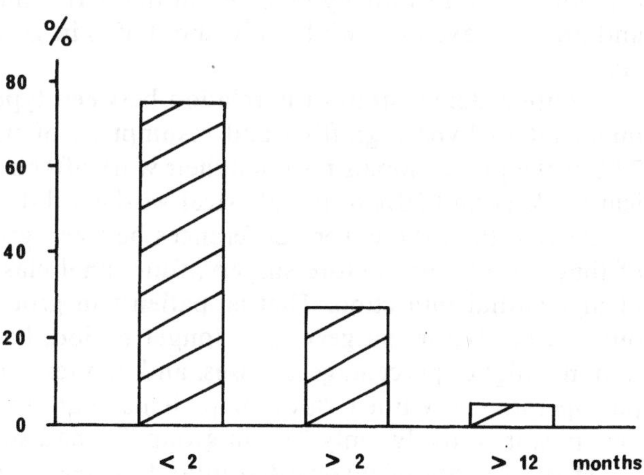

Fig. 1. Relation between length of sick leave preoperatively and resumption of work postoperatively

Comparing the patients of group A who worked postoperatively (group A 1) to those who did not (group A2), it became apparent that there were no substantial differences in respect of functional class before surgery, mean duration of angina, and time interval between angiography and surgery. There was just a slight difference in respect of age, though there was a tendency to quit working with increasing age. While only 41% of patients 55 years or older were working at the time of follow-up, 54% of patients younger than 55 years were doing so.

Substantial differences existed, however, in respect of type of work performed before surgery (Fig. 2). Patients in group A1 had on average a higher level of education and less strenuous jobs. While in this group more than 40% of the patients were professionals, only about 10% were professionals in group A2.

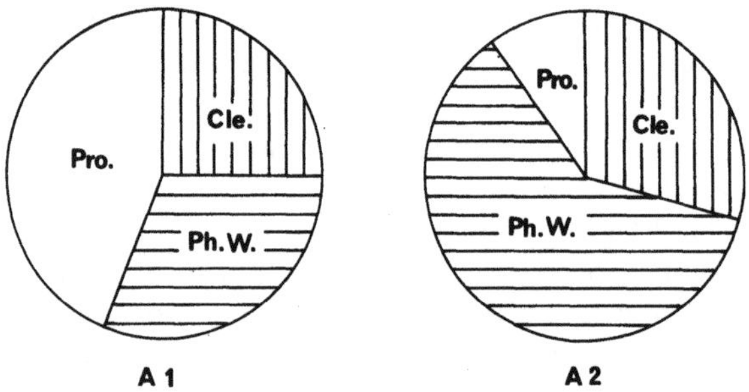

Fig. 2. Type of occupation preoperatively (*Pro.*, professionals; *Cle.*, clerical workers; *Ph. W.*, physical workers)

On the other hand, more than 60% of the patients in group A2 were physical workers and routinely involved in the performance of heavy manual labor and physical exertion, while only about 30% in group A1 were physical workers.

Figure 3 demonstrates the relation between type of work done before coronary artery bypass grafting and resumption of work postoperatively. While 79% of the professionals resumed their work after surgery, only 41% of the clerical workers and 30% of the physical workers did so.

Beyond that, there were differences between groups A1 and A2 in respect of time out of work before surgery, functional class after surgery, and history of myocardial infarction. That is, patients in group A2 on average had been out of work before surgery for a longer period, had had a myocardial infarction in a higher percentage of cases, and had less improvement in anginal pain postoperatively. While 63% of the patients in group A1 had a functional class 0 or 1 postoperatively, only 33% in group A2 had such a class.

That a history of myocardial infarction seems to be an important determinant in respect of vocational rehabilitation after coronary artery bypass grafting is illustrated by the fact that only 33% of those who had had a myocardial

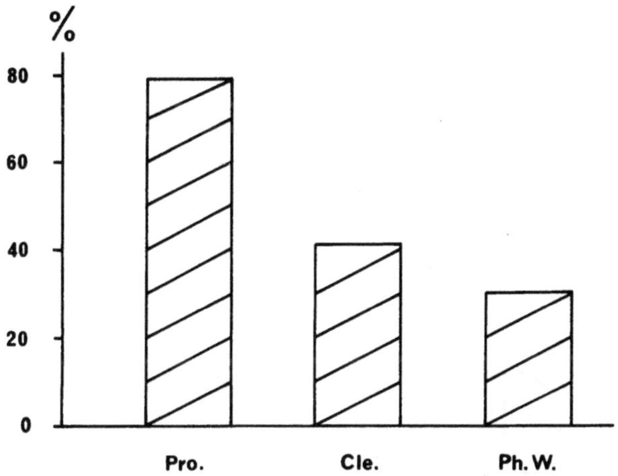

Fig. 3. Proportion of professionals *(Pro.)*, clerical workers *(Cle.)*, and physical workers *(Ph. W.)* working postoperatively

infarction worked postoperatively, while 61% of those who had not had a myocardial infarction resumed their work.

Finally, patients in group A1 on average had a better exercise tolerance than those in group A2. At the time of follow-up the exercise capacity of the patients in group A1 averaged 112 W/s, whereas that of the patients in group A2 averaged 77 W/s. In accordance herewith, 82% of the patients in group A1 stated that their physical capability after surgery was good or even very good, compared to only 55% in group A2.

Comparing groups A and B it becomes apparent that a functional improvement could also be documented in the nonsurgical group; the magnitude of improvement as well as return to an asymptomatic state was, however, considerably greater in the surgical group. The most important difference between the surgical and the nonsurgical group was that 29% of the surgical patients were asymptomatic at the time of follow-up, compared to only 5% of the nonsurgical patients. A patient was considered asymptomatic if he was able to carry out unrestricted activities without being limited by any cardiac symptoms. The exercise capacity in the nonsurgical patients was on average 78 W/s, compared to 94 W/s in the surgical patients.

Comparing the patients in group B who worked at the time of follow-up (group B1) to those who did not (group B2), it was seen that patients in group B1 – like those in group A1 – had a slightly lower age, a lower functional class at the time of follow-up, better exercise tolerance, and a less frequent history of myocardial infarction. And again patients with a higher education tended to continue working, while those with a lower training tended to quit working. 100% of the professionals were still working at the time of follow-up, in contrast to 35% of the clerical workers and 25% of the physical workers (Fig. 4).

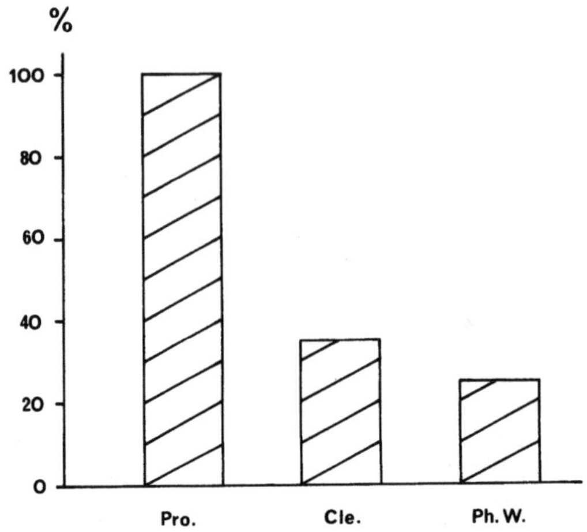

Fig. 4. Proportion of professionals *(Pro.)*, clerical workers *(Cle.)*, and physical workers *(Ph. W.)* in group B working at follow-up

Discussion

Despite functional improvement, significantly less patients worked postoperatively than before surgery. These results are similar to the experiences of other investigators [1, 6, 8, 11, 14], whereas Niles and co-workers [12] as well as Symmes et al. [17] and Wallwork et al. [18] reported a net increase in the numbers working after operation. In this respect coronary artery bypass grafting does not seem to be a very effective therapeutic intervention and possibly does not justify the enormous costs. However, it would be unfortunate to reduce medical decisions to purely economic terms. The primary goal of coronary artery bypass grafting is relief of disabling pain. Vocational rehabilitation is but one goal of surgery. Moreover vocational rehabilitation depends only partially on successful intervention, as has been shown: It is greatly influenced by several other medical and nonmedical variables that may outweigh the functional improvement accomplished by coronary artery bypass grafting.

One factor that influences vocational rehabilitation seems to be level of education, and, related to this, type of occupation and level of income. Patients with a higher vocational training seem to be more willing to return to work, probably because they are better paid and possibly because they may be more motivated and derive more fulfillment from their work than do patients with a lower vocational training and therefore probably less well paid jobs, e.g., assembly-line workers. In addition patients performing heavy manual labor may require a change in occupation or employment status postoperatively.

Though working is without doubt an important contributor to the quality of life for many patients, others may frustrated by their jobs and make use of their disease to quit working. In this respect the type and level of disability benefits as well as other socioeconomic factors are other major factors that may influence vocational rehabilitation after surgery.

Our results as well as those of other investigators show that in contrast to patients working up to the time of surgery, those who have been on disability or sick-leave before coronary artery bypass grafting usually do not return to work [8, 12, 16]. It has been postulated that these patients may have become accustomed to not working or may have difficulty reentering the job market after a prolonged absence [12].

Other problems we have not checked into, but which must be considered when studying vocational rehabilitation, are patients' self-perception of their health, the fear that work may contribute to illness, as well as the attitudes of the immediate family, close friends, and physicians toward illness and convalescence. Finally, the attitudes and policies of employers toward cardiac patients and the state of the job market, namely competition for jobs from younger, healthier persons, are certainly of importance.

While all these factors can hardly be influenced by surgery, coronary artery bypass grafting has some definite influences on vocational rehabilitation, too. The better the functional result after surgery, that is, the less the patient is disabled by anginal pain and the better the exercise capacity, the greater ist the likelihood that the patient will return to work. Because it has been shown by other investigators that there is a close relation between the completeness of revascularization and postoperative improvement in work capacity as well as reduction in exercise-induced angina pectoris [2, 7, 9, 15], one should assume that the extent of revascularization has an influence on vocational rehabilitation. Since we obtained coronary angiograms postoperatively only in a minority of patients, we were not able to assess whether completeness of revascularization had an influence on vocational rehabilitation in our patients.

Another factor that seems to influence vocational rehabilitation after coronary artery bypass grafting, and which possibly could be influenced, is the time patients are out of work before surgery or the time they have to wait for angiography and surgery. That is, the shorter is this time interval, the greater is the likelihood that patients will return to work after surgery. However, it may be that those patients who tend to return to work after surgery because of, for example, better vocational education, are more willing to work up to surgery, too, in spite of anginal pain, and that those who are less motivated to work may stop working postoperatively anyway, despite early surgical intervention.

Since in many cardiac centers patients have to wait months for coronary angiography and surgery, one may ask whether it would be justified to give preference to patients who are still working. We think the answer depends on the primary goal at which one is aiming relief of disabling anginal pain or vocational rehabilitation.

In summary, vocational rehabilitation is affected by the same medical and nonmedical factors in patients with coronary artery bypass grafting as in patients with coronary artery disease who are not operated on – in particular by work status at the time of angiography or surgery, level of education, history of myocardial infarction, and functional status. Only the latter, however, can be influenced by coronary artery bypass grafting or medical therapy.

References

1. Anderson AJ, et al. (1980) Retention or resumption of employment after aortocoronary bypass operations. JAMA 243:543-545
2. Assad-Morell JL, et al. (1975) Aorto-coronary artery saphenous vein bypass surgery. Clinical and angiographic results. Mayo Clin Proc 50:379-386
3. Campeau L (1976). Grading of angina pectoris. Circulation 54:522-523
4. Coronary artery surgery study (CASS) (1983) A randomized trial of coronary artery bypass surgery. Quality of life in patients randomly assigned to treatment groups. Circulation 68:951-960
5. Cosgrove DM, et al. (1982) Results of myocardial revascularization: A 12-year experience. Circulation [Suppl II] 65:37-43
6. Frick MH, et al. (1979) Work status after coronary bypass surgery. A prospective randomized study with ergometric and angiographic correlations. Acta Med Scand 206:61-64
7. Gohlke H, et al. (1983) Serial exercise testing up to 6 years after coronary bypass surgery: Behavior of exercise parameters in groups with different degrees of revascularization determined by postoperative angiography. Am J Cardiol 51:1301-1306
8. Hammermeister KE, et al. (1979) Effect of surgical versus medical therapy on return to work in patients with coronary artery disease. Am J Cardiol 44:105-111
9. Lawrie GM, et al. (1977) Results of coronary bypass more than 5 years after operation in 434 patients. Clinical, treadmill exercise and angiographic correlations. Am J Cardiol 40:665-672
10. Lawrie GM, Morris GC (1982) Survival after coronary artery bypass surgery in specific patient groups. Circulation [Suppl II] 65:43-48
11. Love JW (1980) Employment status after coronary bypass operations and some cost considerations. J Thorac Cardiovasc Surg 80:68-72
12. Niles NW, et al. (1980) Return to work after coronary artery bypass operation. J Thorac Cardiovasc Surg 79:916-921
13. Oberman A, et al. (1982) Employment status after coronary artery bypass surgery. Circulation [Suppl II] 65:115-119
14. Rimm AA, et al. (1976) Changes in occupation after aortocoronary vein-bypass operation. JAMA 236:361-364
15. Siegel W, et al. (1975) The spectrum of exercise test and angiographic correlations in myocardial revascularization surgery. Circulation [Suppl I] 51/52:156-162
16. Smith HC, et al. (1982) Employment status after coronary artery bypass surgery. Circulation [Suppl II] 65:120-125
17. Symmes JC, et al. (1978) Influence of aortocoronary bypass surgery on employment. CMA J 118:268-270
18. Wallwork J, et al. (1978) Return to work after coronary artery surgery for angina. Br Med J:1680-1681

Incidence of Return to Work in Relation to Invasive, Noninvasive, and Social Parameters

M. Skupin, N. Reifart, and P. Satter

Only a few patients return to work after undergoing coronary bypass grafting, despite improvement in the quality of life and prognosis [2, 4]. To analyze the reasons, a survey was conducted among patients who had undergone bypass surgery in our hospital during the last 11 years.

Patients and Methods

Between January 1973 and February 1984, 1032 patients underwent bypass grafting in our department. The questionnaire sent to the 1032 patients covered topics related to the patient's educational status, work status, and preoperative and postoperative symptoms as defined by the New York Heart Association classification (Fig. 1). Up to February 1984 (deadline), we received information concerning 451 patients, i.e., 44% of the total number. In the meantime, we have received information from 80% of the patients. The information from the additional 36% of the patients corresponds well with the results of the 451 patients presented here.

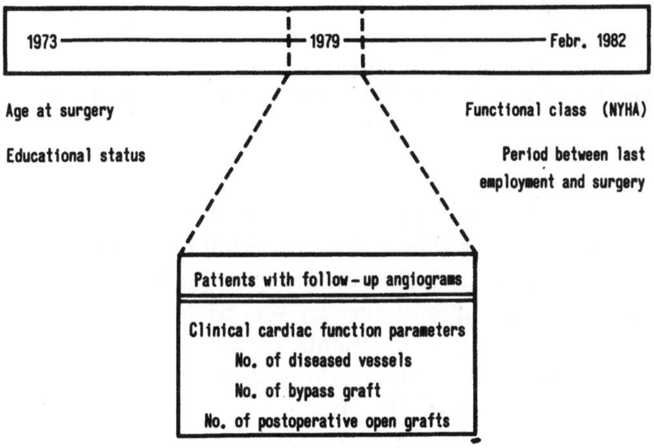

Fig. 1. Patients undergoing CABG at the J. W. Goethe Universität Frankfurt/Main, Topics covered in the questionnaire. Clinical cardiac functions were compared from patients from 1979 with follow-up angiograms

In addition to the results of this survey, a more detailed study of 112 consecutive patients who were operated upon in 1979 shall be presented. In this subgroup cardiac catherization 1–6 months following CABG was performed to assess cardiac function as well as revascularization factors such as the number of diseased vessels, the number of bypass grafts, and the number of patent grafts at the time of the postoperative angiogram.

Statistical evaluations were performed using the chi-squared test and the two tailed *t*-test for unpaired data. Differences with $P<0.05$ were considered significant.

Results

Table 1 contains a summary of the results.

Table 1. Analyzed parameters in group I (working as of February 1984) and group II (retired between surgery and February 1984), with the statistical significance levels (*P*)

Ventricular function	
Ejection fraction	NS
LVEDP	NS
EDV	NS
Degree of revascularization	
No. of diseased vessels	NS
No. of bypass grafts	NS
No. of patent grafts	NS
Age at surgery	$P<0.001$
Period between last job preoperatively and surgery	$P<0.001$
Educational status	$P<0.001$
Functional class improvement (NYHA)	$P<0.001$
Complete symptomatic relief or symptoms during high work load (NYHA class I/II)	$P<0.001$

Figure 2 shows the distribution of the 451 patients regarding working status. Of the 451 patients, 69 were excluded from further study since they were already retired at the time of surgery (group III). The average age of these 69 patients at the time of surgery was 63.7 years.

The remaining 382 patients were divided into two groups: Group I contains 153 patients who were working as of February 1984, the time of the survey. Group II contains 229 patients who worked preoperatively but retired before February 1984. Of these 229 patients in group II, 31 patients returned to work following their operation but retired before February 1984. Twenty-seven of the 31 patients retired early, but not all of them did so because of their cardiac symptoms. Four of the 31 retired at the regular retirement age. However, the

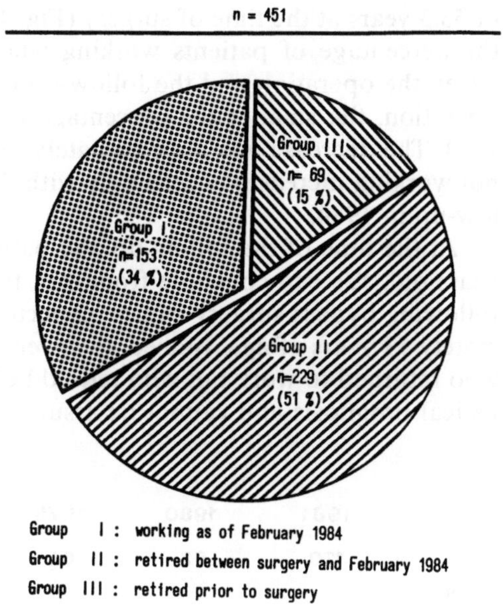

Fig. 2. Patient distribution in the follow-up survey in February 1984. One-third of the patients returned to work after surgery and were working in Feb. 1984 *(group I)*. Half of the patients were retired in Feb. 1984 *(group II)* and the rest were retired before surgery

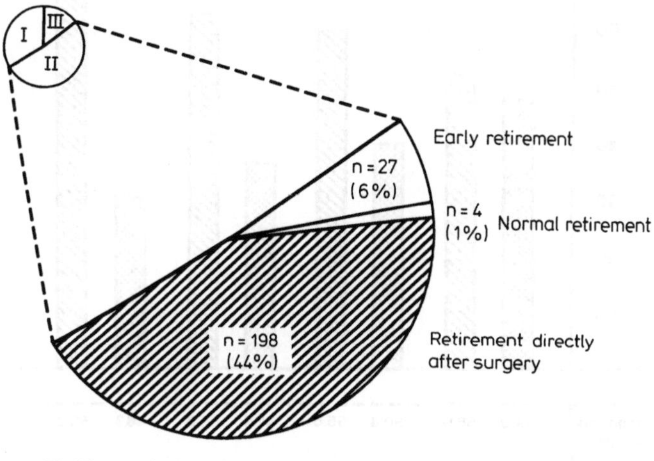

Fig. 3. Differentiation of *group II*. The majority of patients in *group II* retired directly following surgery, but 31 of the patients returned to work before retiring

vast majority of the patients in group II did not return to work at all following surgery (Fig. 3).

Age

There is a significant difference in the average age at the time of surgery between the two groups ($P<0.001$). The patients who continued working were younger, with an average age of 49.1 years. The second group was an average of 53.3 years at the time of surgery (Fig. 4). Figure 4 shows a steady decrease in the percentage of patients working when mapped against the time-span between the operation and the follow-up in February 1984. The further back the operation, the smaller the percentage of the patients working as of February 1984. The decrease was approximately 5% per year. The percentage of patients not working increases accordingly with the time span between surgery and follow-up in 1984.

At the time of the follow-up, the patients in group I were an average of 53 years old. We can conclude from this, that the patients who returned to work following bypass surgery can be expected to continue working up to approximately 53 years of age. Indeed, the average age at retirement of the 31 patients who returned to work but who retired before 1984 was 53.4 years. This is a statistical prognosis and cannot be assumed for every patient.

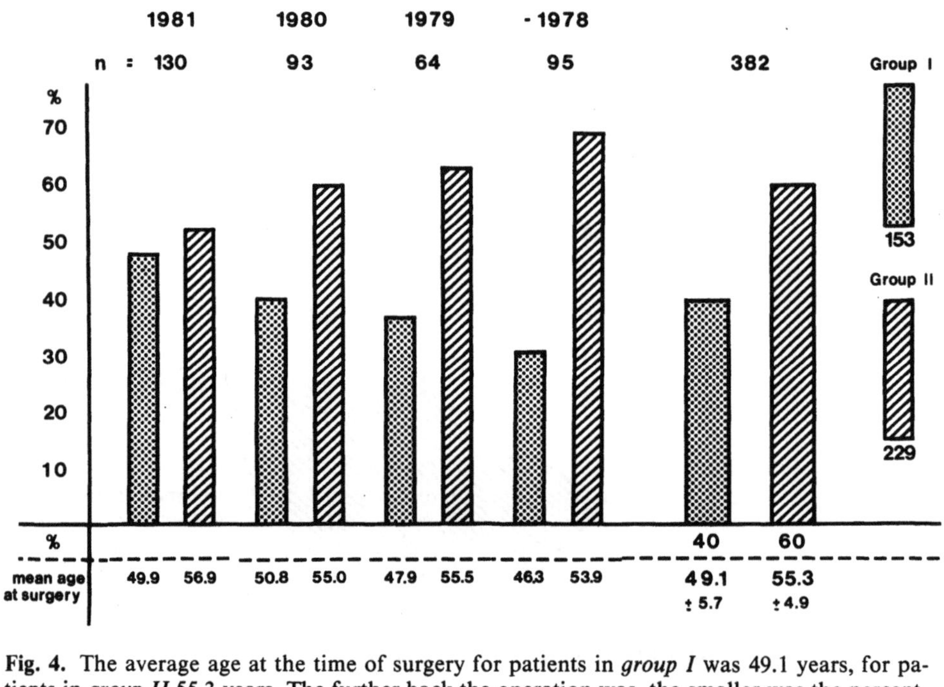

Fig. 4. The average age at the time of surgery for patients in *group I* was 49.1 years, for patients in *group II* 55.3 years. The further back the operation was, the smaller was the percentage of patients working in Feb. 1984

Education

The educational status of the patients in groups I and II is shown in Fig. 5. Of the patients in group I 25% had at least a high school (gymnasium) "degree", as against only 8% of the patients in group II ($P < 0.001$).

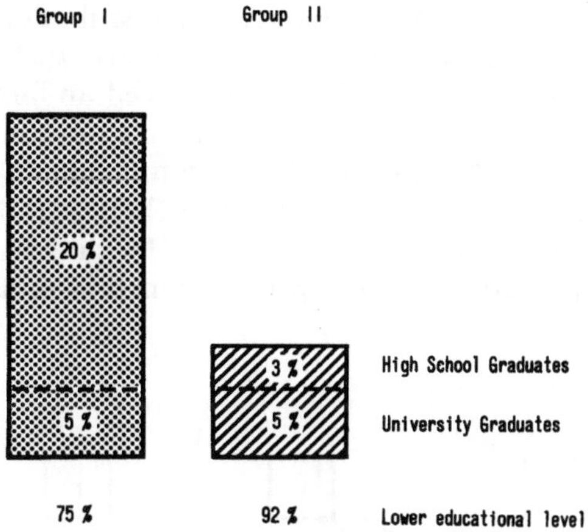

Fig. 5. Educational Status. 25% of the patients in *group I* had at least a high school degree vs. only 8% in *group II*

Gap Between Onset of Severe Symptoms and Operation

The average time between stopping work prior to the operation is 3.2 months in group I and 12.5 months in group II ($P < 0.001$) (Fig. 6). Within the relatively long period of time in group II, these patients were not retired but continued to receive payments from the health insurance companies. The patients who returned to work did so after an average of 7 months following surgery. The shorter time span between stopping work and surgery supposedly played a role in the patient's decision to return to work after the operation.

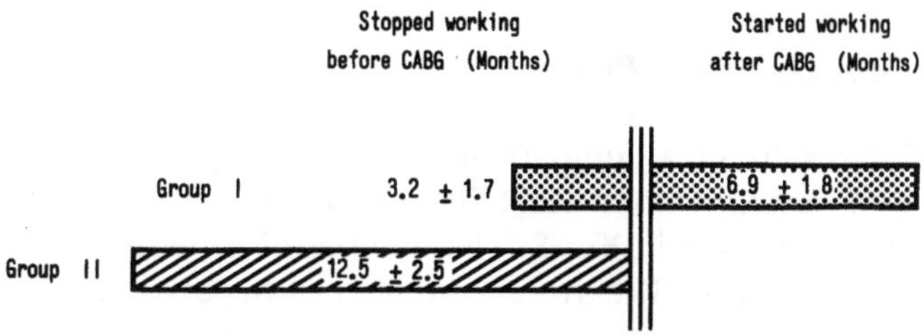

Fig. 6. Last preoperative work and first postoperative work in relation to CABG surgery. The time span between stopping work and surgery was considerably shorter for the patients who returned to work

Functional Status (NYHA)

The changes in the clinical symptoms of the patients pre- and postoperatively, classified using the NYHA system, were also compared. There is no significant difference in the preoperative distribution of the functional classes between the two groups. However, postoperative differences are evident (Fig. 7). Of the patients in group I 76% experienced an improvement in their clinical symptoms, whereas only 37% of the patients in group II improved. 89% of the patients in group I were nearly free of complaints (NYHA class 1 or class 2), in contrast to 67% of the patients in group II ($P < 0.001$). 11% of the patients in group I had considerable complaints (NYHA class 3) postoperatively, whereas one-third of the patients in group II remained in class 3 or class 4.

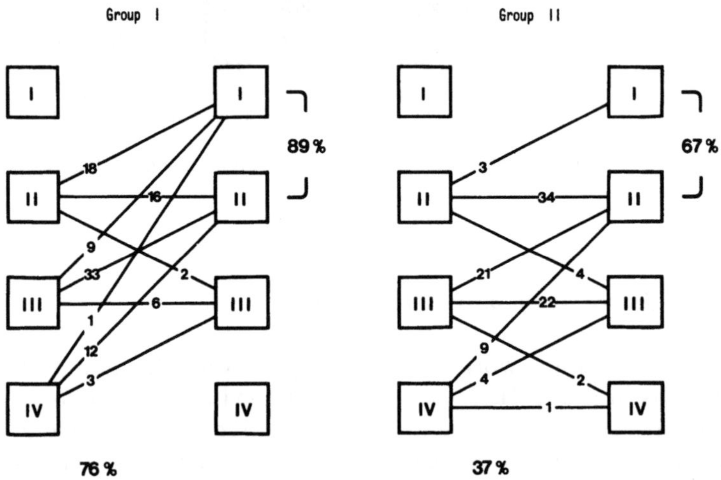

Fig. 7. Changes in the functional class (NYHA) preoperative and postoperative. The distribution of patients in the NYHA classes 1–4 preoperatively is similar in both groups. The postoperative distribution shows that 89% of the patients in *group I* were nearly free from complaints (classes 1 and 2) compared to 67% of the patients in *group II*

Coronary Artery Bypass Grafts

The results of a comparison of the average number of hemodynamically altered vessels with at least 70% obstruction and the average number of patent grafts is shown in Fig. 8. The number of diseased vessels per patient is similar in both groups. The average number of bypasses differs from 2.08 in group I to 1.86 in group II, and the average number of patent bypasses in the postoperative angiogram is slightly less in group II. None of these differences is significant at the 5% level.

Left Ventricular Function

In the subgroup of 112 patients who were operated upon in 1979, cardiac function parameters were evaluated invasively: the ejection fraction, the left ventricular end-diastolic volume, and the left ventricular end-diastolic pressure. The

	Group I n = 48	Group II n = 64
Diseased vessels / pat.	2.38 (± 0.9)	2.35 (± 0.8)
Bypasses / pat.	2.08 (± 0.7)	1.86 (± 0.6)
Open bypasses at follow-up	89 %	79 %

Fig. 8. Extent of revascularization and return to work of the 112 patients operated upon in 1979 (M ± SD). The revascularization parameters of the two groups differed only slightly from each other

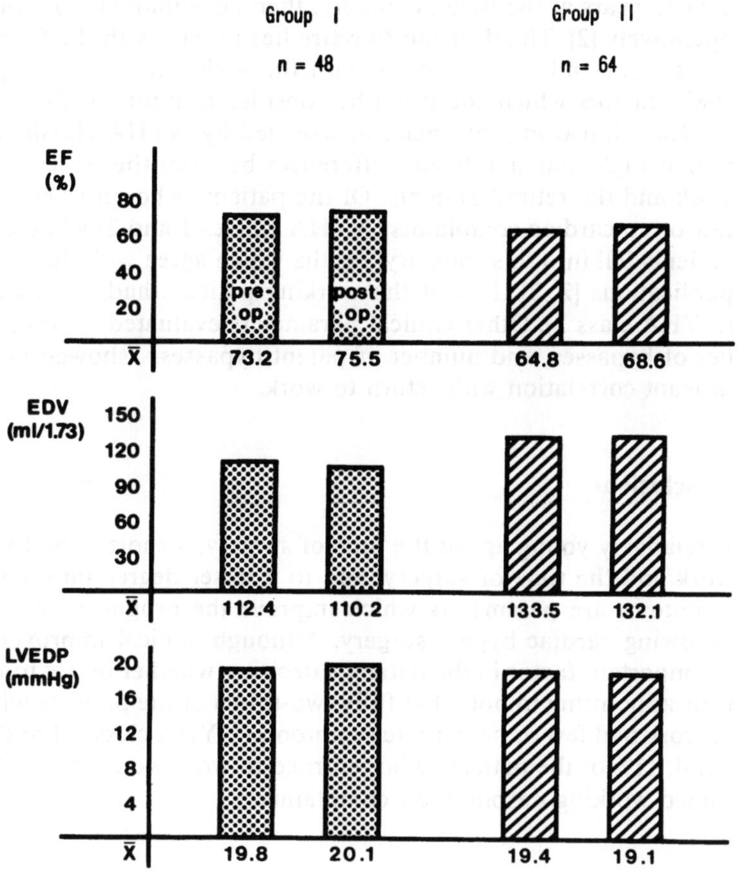

Fig. 9. The left ventricular function of the 112 patients operated upon in 1979 differed only slightly from each other

preoperative results of all three parameters differed only slightly from the postoperative results in both groups (Fig. 9). The ejection fraction and the left ventricular end-diastolic pressure were slightly lower and the left ventricular end-diastolic volume was slightly higher in group II. However, none of the differences was significant at the 5% level.

Discussion

Of the 85% of the patients who were working preoperatively, only 48% returned to work. This percentage, while not unusual in Germany, is small in comparison to the USA [4] and England [5] and can be attributed to the longer waiting lists and the different social security systems. Patients younger than 53 years seem to have a good prognosis as well as those with at least a high school (gymnasium) degree, findings which are supported in other publications [1, 3, 4]. The time span between stopping work and surgery is another important factor. If the patient has been off work longer than 6 months preoperatively and is over 53 years at the time of surgery, then he is unlikely to return to work postoperatively [2]. The decision to retire lies in part with the German social security system and more recently with the higher rate of unemployment (7% in 1983), factors which could not be considered in this study.

The clinical improvement, as assessed by NYHA classification grades, revealed slight but significant differences between the patients who returned to work and the retired patients. Of the patients who returned to work, 89% had few or no cardiac complaints (NYHA classes 1 and 2) while 67% of the retired patients fell into this category, results which agree with those reported in other publications [2, 3]. 11% of the working patients had considerable complaints (NYHA class 3). Other clinical parameters evaluated - cardiac function, number of bypasses, and number of patent bypasses - showed no statistically significant correlation with return to work.

Conclusions

A relatively young age at the time of surgery, a short period between stopping work and the time of surgery, and to a lesser degree improvement of clinical symptoms are parameters which improve the prognosis of returning to work following cardiac bypass surgery. Although clinical improvement (NYHA) is an important factor in the patient's decision whether or not to return to work, it is disappointing to note that fully two-thirds of the patients who did not return to work had few or no cardiac symptoms (NYHA classes 1 and 2). On the other hand, 11% of the patients who returned to work were class 3 (NYHA) but continued working despite their complaints.

Summary

Despite improvements in the quality of life and prognosis which coronary artery bypass surgery (CABG) offers, relatively few patients return to work following revascularization. A retrospective study of patients undergoing bypass grafting within the past 11 years at our hospital shows that the combination of relatively young age at the time of surgery, the improvement of clinical symptoms, and the short period of time between stopping work and surgery significantly increase the incidence of returning to work.

Clinical improvement alone does not determine whether the patient returns to work: two-thirds of the patients who did not return to work had few or no cardiac symptoms (NYHA class 1 or 2) and 11% of those who returned to work had considerable cardiac complaints (NYHA 3).

References

1. Barnes GK, Ray MJ, Oberman A, Kouchoukos NT (1977) Changes in working status of patients following coronary bypass surgery. JAMA 238:1259–1262
2. Hacker RW, Torka M, von der Emde J (1982) Revaskularisation des Myokards durch aortokoronaren Bypass. Dtsch Ärzteblatt 47:23–28
3. Niles NW, Vander Salm TJ, Cutler BS (1980) Return to work after coronary artery bypass operation. J Thorac Cardiovasc Surg 79:916–921
4. Oberman A, Wayne JB, Kouchoukos NT, Charles ED, Russell RO, Rogers WJ (1982) Employment status after coronary artery bypass surgery. Circulation [Suppl II] 65:115–119
5. Wallwork J, Potter B, Caves PK (1978) Return to work after coronary artery surgery for angina. Br Med J 2:1680–1681

Postoperative Exercise Performance Determines Return to Work

H. Gohlke, K. Schnellbacher, H. Steinrücken, L. Samek, and H. Roskamm

Coronary artery bypass grafting (CABG) improves symptoms of exercise-induced angina pectoris and the objective parameters of exercise performance for at least 6 years after bypass surgery [7], but the effect of CABG on the return-to-work rate has generally been disappointing [1, 3, 5, 10, 11]. The objectives of the present study we are to evaluate factors that are related to the return-to-work rate in a patient population undergoing a comprehensive program of rehabilitation before and after coronary artery bypass grafting.

Patients and Methods

Patient Selection

The retrospective analysis of factors related to the return-to-work rate was performed in consecutive male patients who had undergone coronary artery bypass grafting between 1973 and 1979 without other associated procedures. Information on the work status of these patients was obtained by written questionnaire.

Depending on the physical job demands, patients were classified as blue-collar or white-collar workers; in addition, patients were categorized according to the type of employment as laborers, employees, civil servants, or self-employed. In order to minimize the influence of older age on the return-to-work rate, patients had to be 60 years or less at the time of the questionnaire for inclusion in the study. Patients who were already on, or had applied for, disability pension before surgery were excluded from analysis. 481 patients remained in the study.

Exercise Testing

Supine exercise testing with measurement of pulmonary capillary wedge pressure at rest and during exercise was performed with an electrically braked bicycle ergometer [5]. Exercise tolerance was recorded as well as the occurrence of angina pectoris during exercise.

Angiography

Pre- and postoperative coronary angiography was performed by the Sones or Judkins technique. A greater than 50% luminal diameter reduction of a bypassable vessel was considered a significant lesion. The completeness of revascularization was assessed by postoperative angiography, as recently described [6].

Left ventricular function by angiography was assessed by a scoring system evaluating segmental wall motion in the RAO projection [5].

Statistical Analysis

Forty-one pre- and postoperative variables relating to body size, age, myocardial function, coronary angiographic findings, and exercise hemodynamics before and after CABG, as well as variables related to the educational level, type of employment, physical job demands, and duration of absence from work before surgery were analyzed. The correlation between these variables and work status after CABG was determined by use of univariate and multivariate stepwise logistic regression analysis [4]. Calculations were performed on a PDP 11/45 computer.

Results

As stated above, 481 male patients constituted the study population; mean age at surgery, pre- and postoperative exercise tolerance, the number of diseased vessels, the number of constructed distal anastomoses, and the LV scores are given in Table 1.

Of the 481 patients, 328 (68.2%) were employable after coronary artery bypass grafting (CABG). 311 of these (64.6% of the study population) were actually working, 13 were unemployed, and 4 were being trained for more skilled

Table 1. Preoperative and postoperative patient characteristics

Preoperative	
Number of patients (male)	481
Mean age at surgery (yrs)	48.2 ± 4.5
Exercise tolerance (W)	64.6 ± 32.0
Number of diseased vessels/pt.	2.4 ± 0.7
LV score	8.3 ± 3.7
% of patients with transm. MI	51%
Duration of absence from work (months)	5.8 ± 4.5
Postoperative	
Exercise tolerance (w)	96.0 ± 29.0
Number of distal anastomoses/pt.	2.6 ± 1.0
LV score	9.2 ± 4.7

and physically less demanding jobs. 153 patients (31.8%) were retired after surgery. The rate of employment remained quite stable up to 7 years after bypass surgery.

Several factors influenced the return-to-work rate after CABG. As might be expected, younger patients had a higher return-to-work rate than older patients. The return-to-work rate decreased from 85% in patients under age 40 to 59% for patients aged 52 and older ($P<0.02$). Similarly, the duration of absence from work before surgery influenced the return-to-work rate: the longer the preoperative absence from work, the lower the return-to-work rate ($P<0.0001$). The return-to-work rate was also determined by the type of employment: Employees returned to their job in 78% of cases, compared to 71% of self-employed, 65% of civil servants, and 59% of laborers. These differences were highly significant at the 5 per mille level.

The strongest determinant of postoperative gainful employment, however, was exercise tolerance after bypass surgery: only 30% of patients with an exercise tolerance of 50 W or less went back to work, compared to more than 85% of patients with an exercise tolerance of 100 W or more (Fig. 1) ($P<0.000001$).

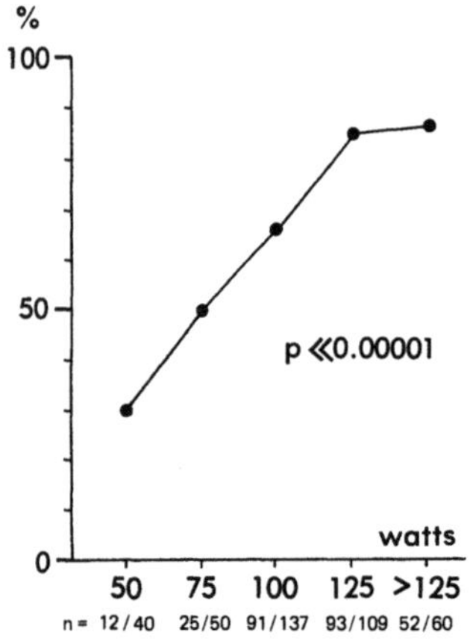

Fig. 1. Relationship between postoperative exercise tolerance and return-to-work rate in 481 patients after bypass surgery. The employment rate varies from 30% in patients with an exercise tolerance of 50 W or less to more than 85% in patients with an exercise tolerance above 100 W

The results of univariate and multivariate analysis of the most important variables for a group of 315 patients in whom all these variables were known is shown in Table 2. Exercise tolerance after surgery and the occurrence of angina during exercise are the most important variables for return to work after CABG. The third important variable is completeness of revascularization.

The next five variables which are important for return to work are not related to the success of CABG: They are, in descending order of importance, duration of absence from work before surgery, physical job demands, age at operation, type of employment, and educational level.

Table 2. Univariate and multivariate analysis of factors correlating with return to work after DABG among, blue- and white-collar workers ($n = 315$)

	Univariate analysis χ^2 value	*DF*	*P* value	Multivariate analysis *P* value
Exercise tolerance after CABG	62.98	2	0.0000	0.0000
AP during exercise after CABG	42.22	3	0.0000	0.0064
Completeness of revascularization	12.44	3	0.006	0.0445
Duration of absence from work before surgery	10.92	3	0.0121	
Physical job demands	5.98	1	0.0144	
Age at operation	8.36	2	0.0153	0.0075
Type of employment	7.94	3	0.0473	0.0272
Educational level	6.81	3	0.0782	

The results of the multivariate analysis show that exercise tolerance, occurrence of angina during exercise, age at operation, completeness of revascularization, and the type of employment provided independent information with respect to the return-to-work rate (Table 2).

In order to determine if different variables may be important for the return to postoperative gainful employment in patients with different physical job requirements, we performed a separate univariate and multivariate analysis of these variables for blue- and white-collar workers. In blue-collar workers (Table 3) exercise tolerance after CABG was by far the most important variable, followed by the completeness of revascularization and the age of the patient. In white-collar workers (Table 4) the exercise tolerance was again the most important variable; however, the second in order of importance and far more decisive than completeness of revascularization or age was the type of employment: employees having the highest return to work rate, followed by self-employed and civil servants. Thus, in blue-collar workers functional and angiographic results of the bypass operation are of greater importance than in white-collar workers.

Table 3. Univariate and multivariate analysis of factors correlating with return to work after CABG among blue-collar workers ($n = 167$)

	Univariate analysis χ^2 value	*DF*	*P* value	Multivariate analysis *P* value
Exercise tolerance after CABG	23.49	2	0.0000	0.0000
AP during exercise after CABG	12.21	3	0.0067	
Completeness of revascularization	11.90	3	0.0078	0.0078
Duration of absence from work before surgery	3.46	3	0.3265	
Age at operation	12.70	3	0.0018	0.008
Type of employment	3.37	3	0.3265	
Educational level	4.34	3	0.2268	

Table 4. Univariate and multivariate analysis of factors correlating with return to work after CABG among white-collar workers ($n = 158$)

	Univariate analysis			Multivariate analysis
	χ^2 value	*DF*	*P* value	*P* value
Exercise tolerance after CABG	31.14	2	0.0000	0.0000
AP during exercise after CABG	13.29	3	0.0041	
Completeness of revascularization	5.81	3	0.1211	0.0120
Duration of absence from work before surgery	7.57	3	0.0558	
Age at operation	5.40	2	0.0672	0.017
Type of employment	22.91	3	0.0000	0.0000
Educational level	4.92	3	0.1775	

Discussion

Our study shows that within the framework of a comprehensive rehabilitation program the return-to-work rate is highly correlated with the functional results after CABG, which were of greater importance than the angiographically determined completeness of revascularization. The employment rate remained constant for up to 7 years after surgery. This correlates with the recently shown persistent improvement of exercise performance up to at least 6 years after CABG [7]. In white-collar workers nonmedical factors are of greater importance for the return-to-work than in blue-collar workers. The variation of the return-to-work rate depending on the type of employment may reflect to some extent differences in retirement benefits. For some patients it is not financially advantageous to return to work, and it may even mean a loss of net income and a decrease of retirement benefits. Others cannot return to work because of company policies concerning patients after cardiac surgery.

Despite these limitations the postoperative exercise performance was the most important factor for the return to work. This is in contrast to previous publications on German patients, where the medical outcome did not correlate with return to work after CABG [2, 9]. Whether these differences are due to differences in patient selection, symptomatic improvement after surgery, or differences in the rehabilitative efforts remains unclear.

Although our results are far from satisfactory, they indicate that efforts to maintain and secure employment in the perioperative period will help the medical outcome of bypass surgery to play an important role in determining who returns to work.

References

1. Barnes GK, Ray MJ, Oberman A, Kouchoukos NT (1977) Changes in working status of patients following coronary bypass surgery. JAMA 238:1259–1269
2. Blümchen G, Scharf-Bornhofen E, Brandt D, VandenBergh C, Bierck G (1979) Clinical results and social implications in patients after coronary bypass surgery. In: Roskamm H,

Schmuziger M (eds) Coronary heart surgery - a rehabilitation measure. Springer, Berlin Heidelberg New York, pp 370-374
3. CASS principal investigators and their associates (1983) Coronary artery surgery study (CASS): A randomized trial of coronary artery bypass surgery; quality of life in patients randomly assigned to treatment groups. Circulation 68:951-960
4. Cox DR (1970) The analysis of binary data. Methuen, London
5. Gohlke H, Schnellbacher K, Samek L, Stürzenhofecker P, Roskamm H (1982) Long-term improvement of exercise tolerance and vocational rehabilitation after bypass surgery: a 5 year follow-up. J Cardiac Rehabil 2:531-540
6. Gohlke H, Samek L, Betz P, Roskamm H (1983) Exercise testing provides additional prognostic information in angiographically defined subgroups of patients with coronary artery disease. Circulation 68:979-985
.7. Gohlke H, Gohlke-Bärwolf C, Samek L, Stürzenhofecker P, Schmuziger M, Roskamm H (1983) Serial exercise testing up to 6 years after coronary bypass surgery: behaviour of exercise parameters in groups with different degrees of revascularization determined by postoperative angiography. Am J Cardiol 51:1301-1306
8. Hammermeister KE, DeRouen TA, English MT, Dodge HT (1979) The effect of surgical versus medical therapy on return to work. Am J Cardiol 44:105-111
9. Lichtlen P, Liese W, Leitz K, Borst HG (1978) Postoperative Klinik nach aorto-koronarem Venenbypass in Relation zum Ausmaß der Revaskularisation. Z Kardiol 67:83-91
10. Oberman A, Kouchoukos NT (1979) Working status of patients following coronary bypass surgery. Am Heart J 98:132-133
11. Rimm AA, Barboriak JJ, Anderson AJ, Simon JS (1976) Changes in occupation after aortocoronary vein-bypass operation. JAMA 236:361-364

Predictability of Postoperative Resumption of Work

P. Sergeant, E. Lesaffre, W. Flameng, and R. Suy

The physician's primary intention has always been the restoration of the patient's health, defined for the coronary patient as a longer survival and a better quality of life. The current economic crisis which is devastating Western Europe has modified the different aspects of medicosurgical treatment of coronary patients. The restoration of the patient's social dignity and a near normal personal income has become very important, as has the cost-containment and cost-efficiency of surgical and rehabilitation programs.

Since international studies could not be projected to the Belgian situation due to differences in social laws and circumstances, a study has been made of the preoperative and late postoperative employment status in patients submitted to coronary surgery. Clinical and socioeconomic parameters were analyzed, and we attempted to define those subgroups with a poor postoperative work resumption expectancy.

Patients and Methods

Five hundred and two patients underwent pure coronary artery bypass grafting at the University Hospital Leuven (Belgium) in 1981. Excluding women, males above 60 years old, males already retired, males disabled for a noncardiac reason, and five operative deaths, 250 patients remained for study in this report and formed the original data group. A second sample was made of the first 100 patients in 1982. Forty patients fulfilled the inclusion criteria of the original data group and formed the independent test sample.

The mean age of the original data group was 50.1 ± 5.9 years. Only 44% of the patients had a normal ventricular function, which correlates well with 46% of the patients not having had a preoperative infarction. 42% had one preoperative infarction and 12% had had two preoperative infarctions. A complete revascularization was performed in 75.6% of the patients. The perioperative infarction rate was 3.2%. Atherosclerotic pathology was found distally to more than 50% of the distal anastomoses in 25% of the patients.

Chi-square contingency analysis was performed on the preoperative and postoperative univariate data. The procedure Logist, a stepwise logistic regression procedure, of S.A.S. [3] was selected for the prediction of postoperative resumption of work. The results of this logistic regression were projected on to an independent sample.

Preoperative Status

In opposition to many studies [1–2], a very low preoperative employment status was noted, with only 30.4% of the patients at work during the last 3 weeks before surgery. 29.6% had been on sick leave for less than 6 months and 40% for more than 6 months. The high compensation paid for sick leave in Belgium might explain some of these results. No differences in preoperative employment status were found in the different groups of angiographic ventricular function ($P=0.338$) or age at the time of surgery ($P=0.561$). The influence of the number of preoperative infarctions was not quite significant ($P=0.053$). The type of employment showed a significant difference ($P=0.043$); 43% of the self-employed stayed at work till the operative data as against 28% of the employees.

Postoperative Status

In the 24 months after surgery 63.2% of the patients resumed their occupation full- or part-time and worked for longer than 3 months. This work resumption was not influenced by type of employment ($P=0.149$), by age at the time of surgery ($P=0.278$), or by ventricular function ($P=0.165$). The self-employed worked again after 3.25 ± 1.8 months, the employees after 5.47 ± 3.0 months. Two parameters did influence work resumption, one clinical, the number of preoperative infarctions ($P=0.003$), and one socioeconomic, the duration of preoperative unemployment ($P=0.001$). The preoperative sick leave is, of course, a reflection of certain other socioeconomic aspects as well as of the clinical condition. Sick leave will readily be granted to a manual worker with a strenuous job involving much physical activity, whereas a highly educated person will probably prefer to continue a desk job with responsibility, even when disabled by angina pectoris.

Prediction of the Work Status

The predictability of postoperative reemployment was analyzed in three stages. In stage one, only the preoperative parameters were taken into account for stepwise logistic regression; in stage two the operative parameters were added to the first data set; and in stage three the late postoperative data completed the two first data sets.

The ten clinical and socioeconomic preoperative parameters are: age, preoperative work status, type of employment, months sick leave immediately preceding surgery, number of preoperative infarctions, preoperative anginal classification, preoperative NYHA functional classification, angiographic ventricular function, angiographic coronary score, and end-diastolic pressure. The best results were obtained using two parameters only in the formula - adding another did not increase the accuracy. The two parameters were the preoperative work status and the number of months of preoperative sick leave.

$$\text{Probability of resumption} = \frac{e^{3.04-0.12\times\text{months}-0.40\times\text{status}}}{1+e^{3.04-0.12\times\text{months}-0.40\times\text{status}}}$$

Fixing the posterior probability threshold at 0.50, there was a sensitivity of 89.2%, a specificity of 62.2%, and 79.4% correct predictions. The number of preoperative infarctions just failed to reach the level of significance necessary for inclusion in the formula.

In a second stage, three operative and perioperative parameters were studied: the completeness of surgery, diffuse pathology distally to more than 50% of the anastomoses, and perioperative infarction. The two same parameters as in stage one were selected for the formula and therefore no changes in sensitivity, specificity, or correct predictions have been found.

The postoperative anginal class and the NYHA functional class at the time of follow-up formed the postoperative parameters. Combining the 15 preoperative, operative, and postoperative parameters in stage three, a new formula was obtained, using one preoperative and one postoperative parameter: the number of months unemployed before surgery and the NYHA functional class after surgery. The sensitivity increased to 90.5%, the specificity to 63.3%, and 80.6% of the predictions were correct (posterior probability threshold at 0.50). Modifying this threshold to 0.60 and 0.70 did not increase the number of correct predictions but caused a shift from sensitivity to specificity. At 0.60 the sensitivity was 85.4% and the specificity 70%, while at 0.70 the sensitivity dropped to 66.5% but the specificity increased to 77.8%.

The obtained formulas of stage one and stage three were projected on the independent test sample. The posterior probability threshold selected from the original data study was 0.70. Stage one (only preoperative data) produced a sensitivity of 74.0%, a specificity of 76.9% , and 75% correct predictions. Stage three (all parameters) gave 77.5% correct predictions, with a sensitivity of 88.8% and a specificity of 53.8%.

Discussion

The very low preoperative employment status encountered in this study is very typical for Belgium, where social laws guarantee an employee from 1 week to 1 month of full wages and 60% of his original income for the rest of his life till retirement, with a minimal loss in pension. Some companies have group insurance covering the full income during sick leave. The self-employed receive only a fixed allowance after 3 months without income, but most of the self-employed in the higher income brackets have private insurance. It is striking that several clinical factors like age, number of infarctions, and ventricular function had only a minimal influence on the preoperative employment status. The postoperative employment is very high at 63%, certainly considering that until recent years a myocardial infarction was considered a permanent and definitive disability, whatever the effect on the ventricular function of on the clinical condition of the patient.

The number of preoperative months of sick leave was found to be very important in the univariate and multivariate analysis; this is, of course, a reflection of many different aspects. It is influenced by the clinical condition of the patient, his personal opinion, his family, the family physician, the medical controller, work, working conditions, and the patient's level of education; it is also related to certain factors totally independent of the patient, like the waiting list for coronary angiography and surgery.

The stepwise logistic regression, based only on the preoperative parameters, enabled us to predict those patients for whom a postoperative resumption of work would be unlikely. This group would be the target group for a rehabilitation program. This would increase the cost-containment and the cost-efficiency of postsurgical rehabilitation programs. It would be interesting to see whether the economic crisis and the reduction of preoperative unemployment duration, noticed in recent years the form of a shortened waiting list for both coronary angiography and surgery, does stimulate resumption of work. This study has provided the treating physicians with a better understanding of some economic aspects involved.

References

1. Gutmann MC, Knapp D, Pollock M, Schmidt S, Simon K, Walcott G (1982) Coronary artery bypass patients and work status. Circulation [Suppl III] 66:33–42
2. Hammermeister KE, DeRouen TA, English MT, Dodge HT (1979) Effect of surgical versus medical therapy on return to work in patients with coronary artery disease. Am J Cardiol 44:105–111
3. S.A.S. User's Guide Statistics (1982) Cary, NC 27511, USA

Clinical Results and Return to Work After Coronary Heart Surgery

H. Magometschnigg, W. Klepetko, S. Hanna, and E. Domanig

For evaluation of the effect of coronary artery bypass surgery on postoperative employment status, we examined 95 patients, all of whom were admitted from one hospital and operated on at the II. Surgical Department of the University of Vienna during the years 1976–1983. Two of the patients (2.1%) had died by the time of reexamination, which was between 6 and 12 months after operation. Of the 93 survivors (81 men, 12 women; mean age 52.3 years, range 30–65) only 14 (15%) had resumed work after that period. Our main interest was focused on the connection between working status and physical capacity, which can be expressed in the results of a postoperative treadmill test; such a test was performed by 63 patients during their rehabilitation. Thirteen further patients could not be burdened for different reasons of health (hepatitis, claudication, postcardiotomy syndrome, cardial failure, aneurysm). The remaining 17 patients either did not undergo treadmill load during rehabilitation or did not join in any rehabilitation program. Out of the 30 patients (24 men, 6 women) from whom an exact measure of physical capacity was not available, only two (6.6%) resumed work after operation. Before the operation, two had already retired and the remaining 26 did so afterwards.

Of the 63 patients for whom treadmill test protocols were available, only 12 had resumed work after operation. Table 1 indicates the number of patients performing different watt levels (50–225 W) and their employment status before and after operation.

Table 1. Watt levels and employment status in the 63 patients who performed treadmill tests

Watts	Number of patients	Working before CABS	Working after CABS
50	6	5	0
75	15	15	3
100	20	14	1
125	10	9	3
150	6	5	2
175	3	3	1
200	2	2	2
225	1	1	0
	63	54	12

As can be seen, 8 of the 12 working patients (66.6%) were able to perform more than 125 W and the other four patients could do some 75–100 W. This represents a slight tendency towards resumption of work by patients with higher exercise tolerance. For a better comparison of the individual load tolerance, we have evaluated nominal values of the exercise test with the nomogram from Bühlmann [1], which includes age, sex, and height (Table 2).

Table 2. Employment status pre- and postoperatively in relation to actual exercise performance expressed as a percentage of the expected maximum

		Preoperative	Postoperative	Mean age
<50% $n=19$	Working	18 (94%)	2 (11%)	47.5
	Early retirement	1 (6%)	17 (89%)	54.0
	Normal retirement	0	0	–
50%–75% $n=21$	Working	18 (85%)	2 (10%)	50.5
	Early retirement	1 (5%)	17 (80%)	52.9
	Normal retirement	2 (10%)	2 (10%)	65.6
>75% $n=23$	Working	18 (78%)	8 (35%)	47.5
	Early retirement	5 (22%)	15 (65%)	53.6
	Normal retirement	0	0	–

Two out of 19 patients (11%) who could perform less than 50% of their nominal value, 2 out of 21 patients (10%) who performed between 50% and 75%, and 8 out of 23 patients (35%) who performed more than 75% of their expected maximum were working again ($P<0.01$). On the other hand, the majority of the patients who had retired prematurely before the operation could be found in the group with more than 75% of expected exercise performance (5=21%), compared to only one patient (=5%) in the group between 50% and 75% and one patient (=5%) in the group with less than 50% exercise performance. This indicates that the frequency of preoperative retirement was independent of physical working capacity, and postoperative retirement was lowest in the group with more than 75% of their nominal value ($P<0.01$). The mean number of bypasses was nearly identical in the three groups, with 2.1 in the lowest group, 2.2 in the middle group, and 2.0 in the highest group.

Regarding the influence of preoperative and postoperative infarction, no striking influence on employment status could be detected. Preoperative infarction occurred 6 times in the working group (50%) and 31 times in the nonworking group (61%), and all four patients suffering postoperative infarction were in the nonworking group.

The connection between employment status and NYHA (New York Heart Association) classification is indicated in Table 3. Of the working patients, 91% were in NYHA groups I and II, as against 50% of the nonworking patients.

Table 3. Employment status postoperatively in relation to NYHA class

NYHA class	Working	Nonworking
I	4 (33%)	11 (21%)
II	7 (58%)	19 (37%)
III	1 (9%)	18 (35%)
IV	0	3 (7%)

Discussion

The percentage of patients reported to work after coronary artery bypass surgery (CABS) differs widely from 80% [2] in the USA, to 60% in Canada [3] and 50% in the FRG [4]. Our result of only 15% working after operation is to be found at the far end of the scale. When considering the factors contributing to this poor result, physical working capacity seems to be of less influence than we expected. The greatest percentage of patients who returned to work after operation could be found in the group with a higher watt performance, as well as in the group with higher nominal values of treadmill load. However, this observation does not explain the strikingly high number of nonworking patients after CABS. Although pre- and postoperative myocardial infarction as well as postoperative NYHA classification had a greater influence, they cannot be responsible for the result alone. It seems that psychological and sociological factors contribute more to the result than do medical circumstandes. For instance, the difference in medical insurance systems of the above-mentioned states as well as other socioeconomic aspects, like good or bad economic circumstances, influence the frequency of resumption of work to a high degree.

References

1. Bühlmann H (1965) Klin. Funktionsprüfung d. Herzens. Schweiz Med Wochenschr 40/95:1331
2. Lawrie GM, Morris GC, Howelly JF, Spencer WH, Winters WL, Chapman DW, Ogura JW, Lie JT (1977) Clinical, angiographic and treadmill results of coronary bypass surgery, 5 to 7 years after operation. Am J Cardiol 39:270
3. David P (1979) Contributing factors preventing return to work of cardiac surgery patients. In: Roskamm H, Schmuziger M (eds) Coronary heart surgery. Springer, Berlin Heidelberg New York, pp 370–374
4. Gleichmann U, Fassbender D (1977) Probleme der Früh- und Spätrehabilitation nach Herzinfarkt. Proceedings: Int. Symposium: Der Herzinfarkt, Wien 31. 3.–2. 4. 1977

Working Capacity and Psychological Adjustment Before and After Surgery

Z. Hymowitz, D. Stein, T. Troudart, A. K. DeNour, J. Borman, A. Appelbaum, and M. S. Gotsman

Introduction

Coronary artery bypass surgery aims to improve coronary blood supply to ischemic myocardium and relieves angina pectoris. There is no evidence that it prolongs life or reduces the incidence of further myocardial infarction except in two specific subsets of patients, those with narrowing of the left main coronary artery and those with severe triple-vessel disease and reduced ventricular function [1].

Successful coronary artery surgery reduces anginal pain: it should improve physical work capacity and the quality of life and permit patients to return to work. The purpose of this paper is to study the work and the psychosocial status of patients before and after coronary bypass surgery and to determine whether they improve after the operation.

We studied the medical and socioeconomic background of 275 subjects with coronary artery disease who underwent coronary angiography and were candidates for coronary bypass surgery (CABG). Eighty of these patients underwent the operation and a subset of 30 were given a detailed psychiatric examination.

The study examined the factors which influenced return to work in the 80 patients who underwent CABG.

Patients and Methods

Eighty patients were studied. They had a personal interview before the operation. The relevant clinical, psychological, and socioeconomic data were recorded. These included: age, sex, marital status, holocaust experience, family history, social class, education, smoking history, number of previous infarctions, number of coronary arteries with greater than 50% narrowing at the time of angiography, work status, length of wait for surgery, and whether or not the patients received a disability pension.

The patients were interviewed by telephone 1 year after surgery and completed a detailed diary which included: hours worked, days absent from work, cigarettes smoked, grade of angina, grade of shortness of breath, doctor, emergency room and hospital visits, exercise regime, social activities, drug regime, and sexual intercourse.

A subset of 30 male patients underwent a psychological assessment the day before the operation. The assessment included a clinical assessment of depression by the Hamilton Rating Scale for Depression (HAM-D) [2] and three self-ratings: the Brief Symptoms Inventory (BSI) [3], the Psychosocial Adjustment and Illness Scale (PAIS) [4], and the Family Environment Scale (FES) [5]. Furthermore, they did the Shanan Sentence Completion Test (SSCT) [6], which measures coping as well as direction of investment of energy. Twenty-two of the wives were also assessed by the BSI and the FES. One year after surgery, the patients and their wives were retested with the same psychological tests.

The data were recorded on a PDP 11/34 computer and analyzed by the SPSS statistical package.

Results

Return to Work

The patients ranged in age from 36 to 75 years with a mean age of 58 years. There were 68 males and 12 females. Twenty-five had experienced the holocaust but 49 had not.

Only three patients were smoking at the time of the surgery and they smoked <1 packet/day. The patients' history of smoking is shown in Table 1.

Table 1. Smoking history

Maximum amount smoked	No. of persons
Never smoked	25
Less than 1 packet/day	16
1 packet/day	12
1½–2 packets/day	14
More than 2 packets/day	13
Total	80

Four patients had single-vessel disease, 13 had double-vessel disease, 56 had triple-vessel disease, and 7 had triple-vessel plus left main disease. Twenty-four of the patients had had no previous infarction. Twenty-nine had had one infarction, ten had had two infarctions, and seven had had three infarctions.

Sixteen patients waited 0–3 months for surgery, 29 waited 4–11 months, 19 waited 1 year, while 16 patients waited >1 year.

Social class was determined by occupation. Thirteen patients were in social class I, 27 in social class II, 31 in social class III, 2 in social class V, and 7 in social class IX (housewives and kibbutz members).

Thirty-four patients worked full-time before surgery, 18 worked part-time, 13 were retired (received a pension), 7 were housewives (only one did light housework, the others did nothing but rest at home), and 8 were unemployed (but did not receive a pension).

After surgery, there were 34 full-time workers, 22 part-time workers, 14 persons retired, 7 housewives all working at home an average of 4 h a day (which we now classify as part-time workers), and 3 persons unemployed.

After surgery, 37 patients had no anginal pain, 28 had mild pain, and 15 had severe pain.

After examining all the possible causative factors, we found that only (a) residual chest pain, (b) a wait of >1 year for surgery while receiving a disability pension, and (c) age were significant factors related to return to work. The others were not significant.

There were 15 patients with severe anginal pain after surgery. Seven returned to part-time work while eight did not return to work after surgery. If we exclude those over 65 not working, angina was a highly statistically significant ($P=0.0001$) factor in preventing return to work.

A statistical analysis was made on the patients who stopped working while awaiting surgery: We found that the longer the length of time the patient had not worked before surgery, the less likely he was to return to work ($P<0.02$).

The average age of those working was 58, while that of those not working was 61 - a difference which is probably statistically significant ($P=0.05$).

Psychological Assessment

The main results preoperatively indicated that both patients and wives had moderate psychological distress (on the BSI, T score of about 60). The profiles of both groups were similar, with patients scoring high (T score above 60) on anxiety, phobic anxiety, depression, and hostility. The wives' T score was just over 60 on anxiety and just below 60 on phobic anxiety and depression.

The total score on the PAIS was 33, which is indicative of moderate adjustment problems, and it correlated significantly ($r=0.516$, $p<0.01$) with the BSI. Active coping as measured by the SSCT was also low (16.0), with significant negative correlations with the BSI ($r=-0.648$, $P<0.01$) and the PAIS ($r=-0.686$, $P<0.05$).

Thus, the patients before operation showed all the characteristics of chronic patients (low active coping and many adjustment problems) who are in mild to moderate psychological stress as evaluated both by the self-ratings and by clinical assessment (mean score on HAM-D, 11.3).

Twenty-eight patients were followed up at 1 year after operation. Preliminary analysis of the data indicated that there was no significant change for the whole group on depression (HAM-D), psychological distress (BSI), or adjustment problems (PAIS). The group was therefore divided by the PAIS into two subgroups: good adjustment - a score of 20 or less on the PAIS (mean for this group, 11) - and poor adjustment - PAIS over 20 (mean, 45). There were 13 patients in the first group and 15 in the second. Examination of the presurgery data shows that the well-adjusted group were significantly younger (50 years compared to 57 years) ($P<0.05$) and had more education (12.2 years compared to 10.2 years). The difference in the PAIS between the two groups was highly significant before operation (19 compared to 43 respectively) ($P<0.01$). The other preoperative tests showed the same directional tendency but failed to reach statistical significance. At follow-up, however, the two groups differed significantly on psychological distress (BSI) as well as on depression (HAM-D) ($P<0.01$).

Thus, it seems that the patients' adjustment to cardiac disease is the best predictor of adjustment to bypass surgery. Patients who had adjusted well to cardiac disease gained much from the surgery. Not only did their adjustment improve but also the psychological distress decreased. On the other hand, patients who adjusted poorly to cardiac disease had further psychological and

This group of 30 patients also had a complete physical examination and a stress test (Bruce Protocol) 1 year after surgery. Patients exercised for a longer period after surgery but this was not statistically significant. However, the difference of the double product of the stress test carried out before and after surgery showed statistical significance ($P=0.007$ using a two-tailed paired t-test). There was no statistical significance in the stress test of those working and those not working after surgery. There was no correlation between ejection fraction and work status.

Discussion

Several studies have examined factors influencing return to work after coronary artery bypass surgery. David [7] found age to be an important factor, while Oberman et al. [8] found that age, severity of angina, and the presence of other adverse clinical factors were the main determinants of return to work. Hammermeister er al. [9] in the Seattle Heart Watch Registry identified five predictive variables of return to work: (1) prior working status, (2) years of education, (3) age, (4) cardiac functional class, and (5) period of time since the patient last worked. Gutmann et al. [10] reported that employment before surgery was the most significant predictor of work status after surgery. They reported that higher presurgery income and job classification, subjective improvement in tolerance for physical activity, and higher pre- and postoperative ejection fraction were positively related to return to work, while age, chronic medical problems, pressure of cardiac symptoms, and receipt of disability compensation were negative factors related to return to work. Niles et al. and others [11–14] reported that more patients continue to work after successful coronary artery bypass surgery, but others [10, 15–17] have shown a deleterious effect.

Our findings are similar to these studies. We found that preoperative anginal pain was a major factor in not returning to work, although age and the period of unemployment before surgery were also related factors. Moreover, the Israeli social systems has a very high standard of welfare for disabled patients and this tends to encourage or maintain unemployment. An early disability pension is possible and patients tend to retain these pensions after successful surgery, particularly when they have retired prematurely. Although four of the 13 retirees returned to part-time work, all continued to receive their pensions.

We found that there was an increase in the work force after coronary bypass surgery.

Conclusion

Our study has shown that after coronary artery bypass graft surgery, the number of full-time workers remained the same. There was an increase in part-time workers from 18 to 28 and a decrease in those not working from 27 to 17. We feel that the following would benefit greatly the patients' quality of life and encourage more to return to work:

1. Psychological evaluation and management
2. Early investigation
3. Early surgery
4. Vigorous rehabilitation
5. A secondary prevention program
6. Postoperative support and return to work

However, as time passes we must constantly be aware of attrition of grafts and the progress of the disease as a cause for the return of angina pectoris.

References

1. Cass Principal Investigators and their Associates (1983) Coronary artery surgery study (CASS): A randomized trial of coronary artery bypass surgery survival data. Circulation 68:939
2. Hamilton M (1960) A rating scale for depression. J Neurol Neurosurg Psychiatry 23:56
3. Derogatis LR (1975) Brief symptom inventory. Clinical Psychometric Research, Baltimore
4. Derogatis LR (1975) Psychosocial adjustment to illness scale. Clinical Psychosomatic Research, Baltimore
5. Moss R (1974) Family environment scale (form R). Consulting Psychologist Press, Palo Alto, California
6. Shanan J, Kaplan DeNour A, Garty Y (1976) Effects of prolonged stress on coping style in terminal renal failure patients. J Human Stress
7. David P (1978) Contributing factors preventing return to work of cardiac surgery patients. Cleve Clin Q 45:177
8. Oberman A, Wayne JB, Charles ED, Kouchoukos NT (1981) Which of your coronary bypass patients are likely to return to work? J Cardiovasc Med 6:1107
9. Hammermeister KE, DeRouen TA, English MT, Dodge HT (1978) Effect of surgical versus medical therapy on return to work in patients with coronary artery disease. Am J Cardiol 44:105
10. Gutmann MC, Knupp DN, Pollock ML, Schmidt DH, Simon K, Walcott G (1982) Coronary artery bypass patients and work status. Circulation [Suppl III] 66:33
11. Niles NW, Salm TJV, Cutler BS (1980) Return to work after coronary artery bypass operation. J Thorac Cardiovasc Surg 79:916
12. Symmes JC, Lenkel SCM, Berman ND (1978) Influence of aortocoronary bypass surgery on employment. Can Med Assoc J 118:268

13. Wallwork J, Potter B, Caves PK (1978) Return to work after coronary artery surgery for angina. Br Med J 2:1680
14. Crosby IK, Wellons HA Jr, Martin RP, Schuch D, Muller WH Jr (1980) Employability – a new indication for aneurysmectomy and coronary revascularization. Circulation [Suppl I] 62:79
15. Anderson AJ, Barboriak JJ, Hoffman RG, Mullen DC (1980) Retention or resumption of employment after aortocoronary bypass operations. JAMA 243:543
16. Barnes GK, Ray MR, Oberman A, Kouchoukos NT (1977) Changes in working status of patients following coronary bypass surgery. JAMA 238:1259
17. Love JW (1980) Employment status after coronary bypass operations and some cost considerations. J Thorac Cardiovasc Surg 80:68

Summary of the Discussion

K. E. Hammermeister

We heard Dr. Dudley Johnson of Milwaukee, Wisconsin, conclude that he thought that coronary bypass surgery did relatively little to either improve or prevent employment after coronary bypass surgery. However, there were some interesting subsets in his study, including a group of patients over the age of 65 who in fact had higher employment rates than the general population in the United States.

Another interesting point made by Dr. Johnson was that early in his operative experience, in 1968, those who were not working gave physical disability as the reason. However, 10 years later the most common reason was the desire to relax. This implies changes in society's attitudes and/or changes in the quality of the bypass surgery.

Mr. Magdi Yacoub from Harefield, England, also compared rates of return to work with an age-matched population in his area just outside of London and found similar results. He also noted a relationship between postoperative employment status and symptomatic status.

Dr. Nitter-Hauge was the first of several presenters to point out the relationship between postoperative work status and postoperative exercise duration. This was despite the fact that there did not seem to be any differences in left ventricular function between those working and those not working (all were studied hemodynamically postoperatively). Those not working had a significantly reduced exercise performance.

Dr. Carstens made similar observations in his group of patients in Cologne. The nonworkers following surgery were also more likely to have had a prior myocardial infarction.

Dr. Skupin from Frankfurt am Main found a rather high rate of failure to return to work, but the important factors here were age, duration of time off work, educational status, and also symptomatic status postoperatively.

Dr. Gohlke, reporting on a rather large group of patients in Bad Krozingen, again notes a rather substantial proportion who have failed to return to work. The relevant factors in failure to return to work were similar to those discussed previously: age, duration of time off work, and type of employment. In his rather elegant multivariate analysis the most important factor was exercise tolerance. Somewhat surprising to me was that exercise tolerance postoperatively was the most important factor in predicting continued unemployment in both the blue-collar workers and the white-collar workers. The latter would have seemed to me not to need the ability to exercise vigorously.

In the final paper of this session Dr. Sergeant examined a large group of patients (from Leuven, Belgium), and again notes a relatively high rate of failure to return to work. In a sophisticated and complex analysis he has shown that work status prior to surgery and the number of months unemployed were the two most important factors.

From these seven papers I draw two themes or two major factors that seem to influence continued unemployment: postoperative exercise ability and the duration of time off work.

I would comment further on the postoperative exercise duration or exercise capacity and ask the question of whether there is continued left ventricular dysfunction, particularly diastolic dysfunction, that may account for the persistent fatigue and dyspnea that so many patients complain about after surgery.

Dr. Gotsman from Jerusalem emphasized the psychological factors, but it is not clear to me from the data that we have heard today, or from what has been published previously, what the relative weights are of the psychological factors vs. subtle left ventricular dysfunction.

For example, fatigue can be a symptom both of depression and of left ventricular dysfunction.

Return to Work
After Coronary Artery Bypass Surgery
in Comparison to Heart Valve Replacement

Return to Work After Heart Valve Replacement

P. J. Walter, B. Ibe, and M. Gottwik

From a surgical point of view, the main benefits of any operation are thought to be the survival rate as well as a minimal incidence of postoperative complications [9]. However, we feel that there is a need to learn more about the value of this type of surgery in terms of return to useful employment, changes in quality of life, and occurrence of psychological as well as socioeconomic problems.

Patients and Methods

One thousand and sixty-three patients who had undergone Björk-Shiley heart valve replacement between 1970 and 1979 were contacted by letter. They were requested to come to the clinic for clinical reinvestigation, and over 700 patients complied with this request between January and August 1980. Of these, 307 unselected patients were asked to participate in an interview on their employment status and their psychosocial status. No patient who was asked refused to be interviewed. All interviews were conducted by the same person using a standardized questionnaire.

The interview focused upon the following four topics:

1. Occupational status prior to surgery, 1.5 years subsequent to surgery, and at the time of interview (mean 4.7 years). Patients were considered to have retired when they had collected retirement payment prior to or after the operation. Patients were considered to be disabled when they had been out of work for more than 1 year prior to surgery or more than 1.5 years subsequent to surgery. Persons were considered to be employed when they had been on sick leave for less than 1 year prior to surgery and less than 1.5 years postsurgery. Females who were neither employed nor disabled according to these definitions were considered housewives and regarded as belonging to the working group.
2. Level of education and preoperative work load as potential determinants of postoperative retirement.
3. Subjective evaluation of physical and emotional strain at work postoperatively.
4. Effects of the operation on the quality of social contacts and the occurrence of psychosocial problems.

Age, anatomical localization, and number of valves implanted were related to the frequency of return to work, retirement, or disability. The level of disability of all patients was expressed as class I–IV according to the classification of the New York Heart Association prior to surgery and at the time of the interview [4]. These data also were correlated with return to work. The mean interval between surgery and interview was 4.7 years, ranging from 2 to 9 years (Table 1).

For statistical evaluation of the results the chi^2-test was applied to investigate the independence of the individual parameters.

Table 1. Timing of follow-up interviews

Duration (years)	Patients	
	No.	%
2	57	18.5
3	42	13.6
4	46	14.9
5	53	17.2
6	38	12.3
7	41	13.3
8	23	7.4
9	7	2.2
Total	307	100

Results

Three hundred and seven patients, 125 women and 182 men, were interviewed (Fig. 1). Prior to the operation 83% were working, 11% were retired, and 6% were disabled. After surgery 60% were working, 35% were retired, and 5% were disabled. At the time of the interview the proportion of working persons had decreased to 55%, whereas that of those retired had increased to 40% and the proportion of disabled persons had remained stable at 5%. The fraction of women in the employed group that returned to work after surgery was 46% as compared to 67% of the male patients. At the time of the interview 39% of the women and 59% of the men were working (Fig. 2).

Concerning the relationship between age and preoperative employment status, 81% of patients less than 40 years old (group I), 62% of those between 40 and 50 years old (group II), and 57% of those beyond the age of 50 years (group III) were working preoperatively. At the time of the interview 54% of group I, 67% of group II, and 42% of group III were working. The difference in working status between patients over 50 years and younger patients was statistically significant ($P \leq 0.05$) (Fig. 3).

Fifty-four percent of patients with double valve replacement, 49% of those with mitral valve replacement, and 77% of those with aortic valve replacement were working preoperatively (Fig. 4). At the time of the interview the percentage of working patients was lowest in the group with double valve replacement

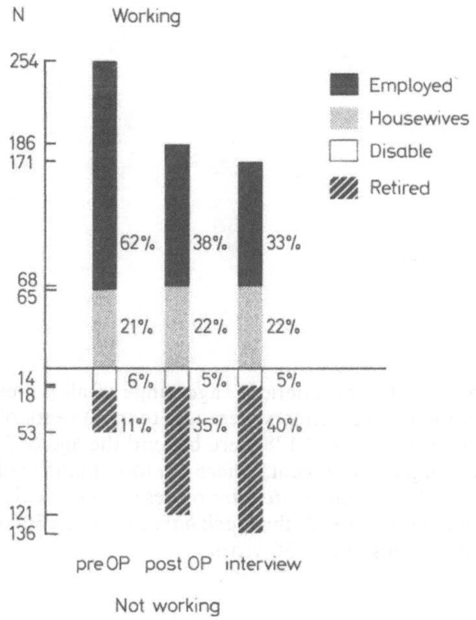

Fig. 1. The *upper part* of the figure presents the number of patients who were working, including housewives, and the *lower part* those who were retired or disabled prior to surgery, postsurgery, and at the time of the interview. The fraction of employed persons, housewives, retired, and disabled persons are given in percent prior and subsequent to the operation and at the time of the interview

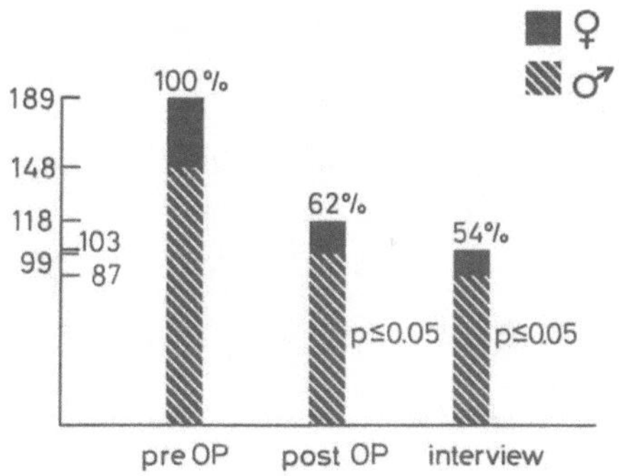

Fig. 2. Fraction of women in the employed group. Prior to surgery 41 out of 189, postsurgery 19 out of 118, and at the time of the interview 16 out of 103 were employed. When the whole group of employed persons of both sexes prior to surgery is considered to be 100%, there is a reduction to 62% postsurgery and to 54% at the time of the interview ($P \leq 0.05$)

(26%) followed by those with mitral valve replacement (55%) and those with aortic valve replacement (59%) ($P \leq 0.05$).

The clinical stage of the disease improved most in patients who worked pre- and postoperatively. At the time of the interview 93% of them were in classes I and II. Postoperatively 69% of housewives were noted to be in classes I and II. A similar figure applied to male patients who retired postoperatively (Fig. 5).

Furthermore, factors like education and working conditions played a major role with respect to employment or retirement (Table 2). The percentage of patients with a college education was significantly lower among those who retired than among those who were employed postoperatively ($P \leq 0.05$). Of the latter,

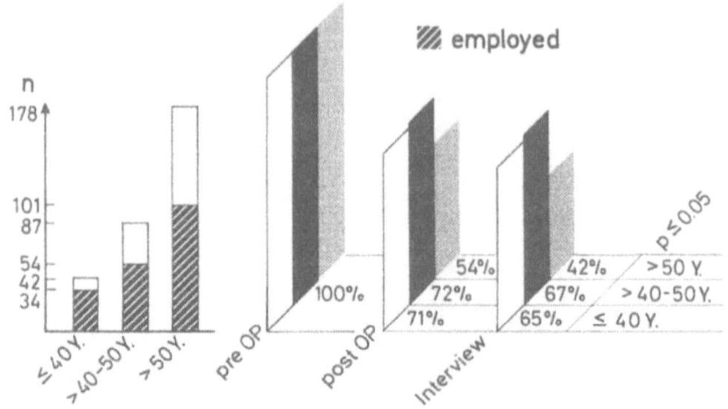

Fig. 3. The preoperative age range of all patients is related to their employment status. *Left:* A total of 42 patients were less than 40 years old. Eighty-seven patients were between 40 and 50 years old, and 178 were beyond the age of 50. *Right:* Decrease of employment subsequent to surgery in percent, where the total number of patients employed prior to surgery is considered 100%. The *white bars* represent the fraction of employed patients of the population less than 40 years old, the *black bars* the 40- to 50-year-old group, and the *dotted bars* the fraction of patients above 50 years

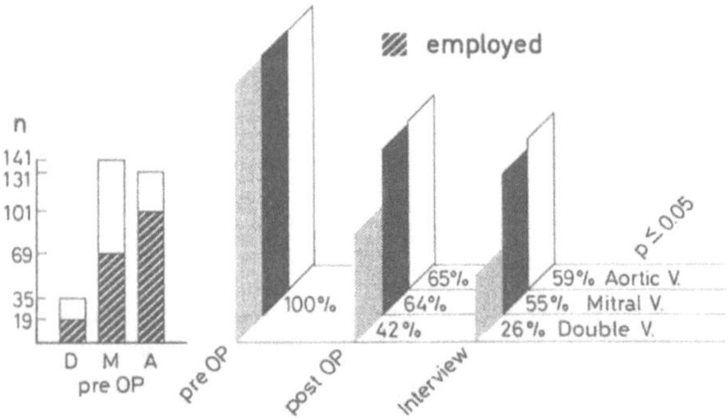

Fig. 4. Work status of patients in relation to the position of the implanted heart valve. *Left:* Total number of all patients and of the preoperative employed patients with double *(D)*, mitral *(M)*, and aortic *(A)* valve replacement. *Right:* Decrease of employment after the operation and at the time of the interview. The preoperatively employed patients were considered as 100%. *Dotted bars,* patients with double valve replacement; *black bars,* those with mitral valve replacement; and *white bars,* patients with aortic valve replacement

only 35% had to work 8 h daily preoperatively, as compared to 53% in the retired group. Patients with a college education and full-time employment prior to surgery had a higher chance of being employed at the time of the interview. The same was true if they had worked no shifts and less than 8 h per day, and, finally if they had completed an apprenticeship or vocational training course when they were young.

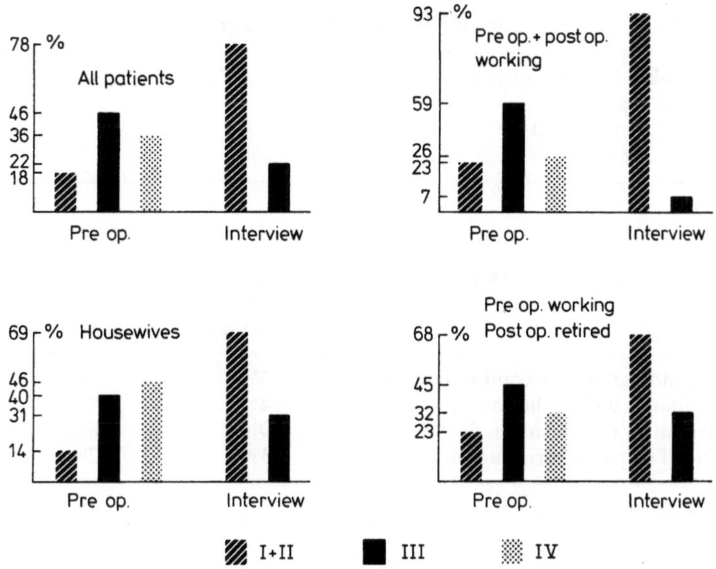

Fig. 5. Percentage of patients in the four clinical stages of disease according to the New York Heart Association classification preoperatively and at the time of the interview. *Upper left*, all patients; *lower left*, housewives; *upper right*, patients working pre- and postoperatively; *lower right*, patients working preoperatively and retired postoperatively

Table 2. Influence of education and preoperative work load on return to work

	Retired	Employed
College education	8%	24%[a]
Completed vocational training	69%	82%
>8 h work/day preop.	53%	35%[a]
Work on shifts	19%	8%
Part-time work	14%	2%

[a] $P \leq 0.05$

Subjective evaluation of the stress at work played a major role with respect to return to work after surgery (Table 3). Somewhat more than two-thirds of those employed felt no stress at work exceeding their capacity, while just over 30% did complain of strain; of these, almost one-third felt under both emotional and physical stress.

Accordingly, surgery obviously is accompanied by major emotional problems which are felt differently by retired and working persons (Table 4). Family life was considered more problematic by retired than by employed patients and housewives. Psychiatric counseling was thought to be helpful by a higher percentage of housewives and retired patients than of employed persons.

Table 3. Subjective evaluation of stress at work

Bearable for state of health	69%
Strain - physical	8%
- emotional	14%
- both	9%

Table 4. Postoperative psychosocial situation

	Retired	Employed	House wife
Would agree to second operation	63%[a]	85%[a]	70%
Isolation within the family	54%[a]	28%[a]	36%
Isolation within the environment	60%[a]	30%[a]	31%
Need of psychiatric support	25%	12%	30%

[a] $P \leq 0.01$

Discussion

In our study the fraction of patients returning to work after surgery as well as those who were employed at the time of interview is some 60%, including 22% housewives. In detail, 1.5 years after surgery just 60% were working while at the time of the interview (between 2 and 9 years after surgery, with an average interval of 4.7 years) just over half were working. On the other hand, the proportion of retired patients increased threefold from 11% to 35% from before to after the operation, and at the time of interview it had increased further to 40%. Although every seventh of the retired patients managed to find some kind of part-time job (Table 2) which gave him or her the chance to work, and the proportion of those who were doing some kind of work thus rose to some 70% at the time of interview, we feel that this group is smaller than it might have been if we take into account the high level of medical rehabilitation following heart valve replacement at our institution [9].

Different subgroups of our sample reveal social as well as clinical factors which influence reemployment.

As Fig. 3 shows, *age* plays a major role with respect to return to work. Some three to four out of every five patients under 50 years of age returned to a job, while only two out of five over 50 years did. This result is only slightly less favorable than that of David, who found 49% of his Canadian sample working beyond the age of 50 [3]. Other studies, for instance that of Niles et al., have also reported a decreasing chance of finding work in the higher age groups [6].

Sex is also important for return to work. A study from Wessex, England, revealed that after valve replacement a relatively high percentage of male patients (76) returned to work while the proportion of women was even higher since 16% of ex-housewives were now working either full-time or part-time.

However, Ross et al. count as work a wider range of activities than most other authors [7]. On the other hand, Blachly and Blachly report that 59% of their patients returned to work. However, they did not distinguish between regular employment and full-time housework [1]. In our sample just under half of the employed women returned to work postoperatively while two-thirds of the men did.

A third influential factor is the type of *heart valve replaced*. As Fig. 4 shows, only one-fourth of the patients with double valve replacement were working, while twice as many with single valve replacement worked; there was little difference in terms of the percentage working between those having undergone mitral or aortic valve surgery. Mattern et al. report that the chance of returning to work depends on the site and number of valves involved: about half of the patients with double valve replacement, 58% of those with mitral valve replacement, and 77% of those with aortic valve replacement were able to continue employment after surgery [5].

Apparently the preoperative stage of the disease does not predict return to work: 70% of the patients who underwent aortic valve replacement but 92% of those who underwent mitral valve replacement were in stage III or IV preoperatively, although a similar percentage of each group (65% and 64% respectively) returned to work. Interpretation of the figures for double valve replacement is difficult because of the small number involved.

When studying the relationship between return to work and physical condition of the patient, the nature of work for those employed must be analyzed. In general it seems that the preoperative working conditions for those retired were worse than for those who continued to work. For instance, among the retired individuals were more than 50% who had had to work more than 8 h per day, while among employed patients only 35% were in this situation ($P \leq 0.05$). Furthermore, among the retired blue-collar workers 19% had had to work shifts while this was the case for only 8% of the employed. Thirdly, one in seven of the retired patients had to do part-time work, as compared to only 1 in 50 of the group who returned to work (Table 2).

Other important factors seem to be *education and training*. While 24% of those who returned to work had a college education, only 8% of those who retired were equally well educated ($P \leq 0.05$). A completed 3-year vocational training had been achieved by 82% of the employed patients and 69% of the retired patients.

Finally, the patient's *psychosocial situation* may be an additional factor of explanatory value. We found that among the retired more than half felt isolated within their family and their wider social environment, while among the employed less than a third felt this way. Similarly, the need for psychiatric support was twice as high in the retired as in the employed group: in the former, every one patient in four felt that she or he would have liked psychiatric support while in the latter it was only every one in eight. Apparently the impact of the operation was also appreciated differently by the two groups of patients: while among the employed four out of five said that they would agree to having a second operation, among the retired only three out of five gave this answer. Thus, the psychosocial situation of patients deciding to retire seems to have deteriorated while it improved among the patients returning to work. It may also signify that the psychosocial situation may deteriorate with retirement. If so, the doctor's advice with regard to return to work might be of the utmost importance. In a Canadian valve replacement group of 31 male patients studied by David, an objective examination showed 77.5% of patients able to work but only 60.7% actually working and 39.3% not working. Of the latter group, 62.7% attributed their failure to return to work to medical advice [3]. According to Dahme, only 40% of hospital physicians, 32% of local physicians, and 22% of health insurance officials discuss return to work with their patients [2]. Therefore we surmise that the chance of returning to work may be increased if doctors talk to their patients in sufficient detail about this possibility both before and after surgery [8].

Summary

The occupational consequences of heart valve replacement using a Björk-Shiley valve and the psychological and social development of 307 nonselected patients (125 women) have been investigated. At a mean interval of 1.5 years after surgery, 60% of the patients were working, and at 4.7 years the figure was 55%.

The results are investigated with regard to six factors: education, workload, age, sex, type of valve replaced, and stage of the disease. Below 50 years of age more patients were employed while only four out of ten over 50 years retained their jobs. Double valve replacement caused a reduction in the preoperative employment status by 74%, aortic valve replacement by 41%, and mitral valve replacement by 45%. Patients who were working pre- and postoperatively showed the best clinical improvement (94% were in classes I and II, NYHA).

A significantly higher percentage of employed patients had had a college education (24% vs 18% of the nonemployed) and they usually worked less than 8 h a day. Postoperative psychosocial complications were significantly higher in retired than in employed patients.

Acknowledgements. We wish to thank Theo Becker, M. Sc. (Institute of Medical Statistics and Documentation, University of Giessen) for providing statistical analysis of these data, and Professor Hans Georg Borst, M. D. (Director, Department of Thoracic and Cardiovascular Surgery, Hannover Medical School, Hannover) and Professor Uta Gerhardt, Ph. D. (Director, Department of Medical Sociology, University of Giessen) for commenting on drafts of this manuscript in a most helpful way.

References

1. Blachly JS, Blachly AS (1968) Vocational and emotional status of 263 patients after heart surgery. Circulation 38:524–532
2. Dahme G, Dahme B, Kornemann J, Vollers A, Huse-Kleinstoll G (1980) Fulfilment of patient's expectations concerning outcome of open-heart surgery. In: Speidel H, Rodewald G

(eds) Psychic and neurological dysfunction after open-heart surgery. Thieme-Stratton, New York, pp 228–236
3. David P (1978) Contributing factors preventing return to work of cardiac surgery patients. Cleve Clin Q 45:177–178
4. Harris R (1970) Assessing the cardiac patient for rehabilitation. NY State J Med 70:511–515
5. Mattern H, Weisskirchen KJ, Fricke G, Bernhard A (1979) Exercise capacity and physical activity following prosthetic valve replacement in relation to cardio-vascular function. Z Kardiol 68:36–40
6. Niles NW, Vander Salm TJ, Cutler BS (1980) Return to work after coronary heart bypass operation. Thorac Cardiovasc Surg 79:916–921
7. Ross JK, Diwell AE, March J, Monro JL, Barker DJ (1978–1979) Wessex cardiac surgery follow-up survey: The quality of life after operation. Thorax 33:3
8. Stein B, Krasemann EO (1981) Prospective studies for the period of inability to work after myocardial infarction. Herz/Kreisl 11:526–532
9. Walter P, Schwarz F, Scheld H, Hehrlein FW (1979) Eight years of experience with the Björk-Shiley tilting disc valve prosthesis in 833 patients. Thorac Cardiovasc Surg 27:178

Return to Work After Coronary Artery Bypass Surgery in Comparison to Medical Treatment

Long Term Changes in Work Status Among Patients in the Coronary Artery Surgery Study Registry

A. Oberman, C. Fisher, L. Maynard, S. M. Mullin,
E. D. Charles Jr., and F. Tristani

Prospective randomized trials from Europe and the U.S. indicate that significant survival benefits from surgery accrue primarily to those with left main coronary artery disease and three vessel disease [2, 3, 5 A]. Most patients who have coronary artery bypass surgery have their quality of life improved, compared to medically treated patients. In the Coronary Artery Surgery Study (CASS), those patients randomly assigned to surgical therapy had significantly less chest pain, fewer activity limitations, and required less drug therapy with nitrates and betablockers [1]. But even with this improvement after surgery, employment status did not differ significantly between medical and surgical groups; the percentage of patients working decreased slightly in both treatment groups. These are not unimportant considerations, as coronary heart disease remains a predominant cause of early disability in the labor force. Of the estimated $ 25 billion spent on coronary heart disease in the United States, over 80% could be attributed to indirect health care costs associated with lost income, lower productivity, disability, insurance expenses, and workman's compensation [10].

Results from the work rehabilitation studies have generally been discouraging and have generated considerable debate on whether surgery really has an impact on indirect health costs. The CASS registry provided an opportunity to evaluate employment patterns over a 5-year period among different patient groups participating in the study. Such data permit us to evaluate prospectively this complex issue of return to work in 12863 patients meeting study criteria and less than 65 years of age with at least 1 year follow-up after baseline. Although patients are not randomized to treatment in the registry, the larger number of patients evaluated allow more detailed subgroup analyses for explanation of results. Prolonging life ist not the physician's only concern, and there is a growing recognition that proper selection of therapeutic alternatives require consideration of those factors that bear on satisfaction with one's life and productivity [6].

Methods

The study consisted of a registry of 24959 consecutive patients who underwent coronary arteriography at 15 cooperating clinical sites in the United States and Canada between 1974 and 1979. A prospective randomized study designed to compare the results of medical and surgical treatment was conducted in subsets of patients with demonstrated coronary artery disease. Not all patients or sites participated in the randomized trial portion of the study. A detailed description of the study design has been published [4].

Study Group

For these analyses, registry patients were grouped into three categories by predominant symptoms: (1) probable or definite *angina* without congestive heart failure impairment; (2) *chest pain* not considered angina and without congestive heart failure; and (3) impairment due to *congestive heart failure*. The major inclusion criteria for these analyses were the presence of at least one diseased vessel, the absence of coronary artery surgery prior to entry into the registry, and an age less than 65 years at the time of entry into CASS. Of those 24959 patients enrolled in the registry, 1781 did not meet the criteria for inclusion in these analyses because no chest pain or evidence of congestive heart failure was apparent. In addition, 8405 patients were excluded because of the lack of any significant coronary artery lesions or prior cardiovascular surgery. The 14773 remaining patients constituted the baseline population, of which 1910 patients were omitted from further analyses due to an age of 65 years or more at baseline. Furthermore, the follow-up analyses excluded those individuals attaining age 65 or more at time of evaluation due to the likelihood of voluntary retirement in such individuals.

A concerted effort was made by CASS investigators to ensure optimal surgical and medical therapy for patients participating in this trial [4]. Medical group patients became eligible for revascularization if they and their physicians desired, typically because of the development of unacceptable angina despite aggressive medical therapy. Follow-up information was collected by telephone interview or a mailed questionnaire at 1-year intervals for patients in the registry and 6-month intervals for those in the randomized portion of the study. All follow-up data presented in this report were acquired within 30 days of the scheduled follow-up date unless otherwise specified. The duration of follow-up ranged from 12 to 60 months for this report.

Definition of Terms

The patient's average level of chest discomfort during the 6 weeks before entry into the study and during follow-up was classified using the Canadian Heart Class where I = ordinary physical activity does not cause angina; II = slight limitation of ordinary activity due to angina; III = marked limitation due to angina; and IV = inability to carry on any physical activity without angina. Congestive heart failure was based on a history of congestive heart failure at baseline. Activity limitations were graded on a scale from 1 (none) to 5 (severe). Employment status at baseline was designated as "full-time" for those employed 40 h a week or more; "part-time" for those employed less than 40 h a week; "retired" for patients who had stopped working on reaching retirement age; "quit" for those patients forced to quit work prior to retirement age because of cardiac symptoms; and "other" for those currently unemployed due to economic circumstances or choice, on temporary sick leave, or disabled secondary to a noncardiac illness. Job classes were: laborer - regular working day includes routine physical exertion or heavy manual labor; clerical - employment not involved with heavy manual labor or stressful decision making; professional - occupations that require advanced training and primarily involve mental work associated with decision making, rather than physical work; homemaker - those patients who primarily work in the home with the responsibility of managing the household; other - any occupational category not encompassed by the above. The left ventricular score is a measure of left ventricular function based on the sum of scores for five segments of the ventricle defined by the RAO ventriculogram. The motion of each segment is scored as: normal - 1; moderate hypokinesis - 2; severe hypokinesis - 3; akinesia - 4; dyskinesia - 5; aneurysm - 6. A score of 5 represents a completely normal ventricle and a score of 30 is theoretically possible for those with marked left ventricular dysfunction. A vessel is considered diseased if a lesion of 70% or greater is found in the major coronary artery segments or 50% or more in the left main coronary artery. Unless otherwise noted, treatment group refers to the initial decision for medical or surgical management.

Statistical Techniques

Stepwise linear discriminant analysis was used to identify a set of potential predictors of return to work from available pertinent variables. The process was carried out in a stepwise manner so that at each step in the process, the variable which contained the most discriminating power, when added to the variables already selected for the model, would be identified. The process stopped when the remaining, unselected variables all had achieved discriminating ability that was not statistically significant ($P > 0.10$).

Then, stepwise logistic regression was used to estimate regression coefficients for those predictors. Logistic regression does not assume the predictor variables to be normally distributed and probably provides a better estimate of regression coefficients than does a discriminant analysis [9]. For each variable that entered the model, regression coefficients and constants were reported and with these numbers the probability of return to work could be computed with the logistic function.

Results

Patient Characteristics

The surgical group tended to be older, but differed little from the medical group in terms of the percentage of men, cigarette smoking habits, and occupational classes (Table 1). In addition, a higher proportion of the patients in the surgical group were categorized as Canadian Heart Class III or IV, 63.3% compared to 37.3% in the medical group. Typical angina without impairment due to congestive heart failure occurred more frequently in the surgical group; chest pain unclassifiable as probable or definite angina and without evidence of CHF impairment occurred more often in the medical group. In the medical group a higher proportion of patients had one vessel diseased and a lesser proportion three vessels diseased as compared to the surgical group. Impairment due to congestive heart failure was more frequent in the medical group, as was the percentage of patients with a left ventricular scores of 10 or more.

Table 1. Patient characteristics by treatment groups

Characteristics	Medical (%) ($n=6710$)	Surgical (%) ($n=8063$)
Age ≤54	53.0	44.9
55–64	35.9	41.3
≥65	11.2	13.8
Male sex	82.7	83.9
Cigarette smokers		
Never	18.9	21.0
Former	44.6	48.4
Present	36.6	30.6
Occupation		
Laborer	36.2	34.4
Clerical	24.0	24.0
Professional	23.8	25.8
Homemaker	9.5	8.6
Other	6.5	7.2
Canadian heart class		
No angina	11.7	2.7
I	7.6	3.9
II	34.4	21.8
III	28.0	40.3
IV	9.3	23.0
Unrelated	9.1	8.3
Symptoms		
Typical angina	79.0	90.0
Chest pain unclassifiable	7.1	1.6
Congestive heart failure	13.9	8.4
Diseased vessels		
One	40.9	18.1
Two	30.9	31.5
Three	28.2	50.4
Left ventricular score		
5	32.1	34.8
6–9	34.9	41.3
10–14	22.8	18.9
≥15	10.2	5.1

Return to Work

Because of these differing symptom-complexes, patients were grouped by predominant symptoms at entry into the registry, as well as by treatment. All groups showed a decreasing percentage of patients working as follow-up progressed through years 1, 3, and 5 (Table 2). Of those patients with typical angina, a higher percentage of the surgical group was employed at baseline but the rate of decline slightly exceeded that of the medical group, a 10.8% loss to the work force, compared to 8.7% in the medical group, over the 5 years of follow-up. The percentage of those presenting with nondiagnostic chest pain declined only half as much, approximately 5% in both medical and surgical groups. The congestive heart failure group had the lowest percentage of patients working full- or part-time at baseline, but showed only a 3.7% further decrease in the medical group and a 5.5% decrease in the surgical group at the fifth year follow-up.

Table 2. Percent of participants working at follow-up years by predominant symptoms and treatment groups at baseline

Symptom/group	Baseline	Year 1	Year 3	Year 5
Angina ($n = 12558$)				
Medical	65.6	58.9	58.2	56.9
Surgical	70.1	63.7	62.3	59.3
Chest pain ($n = 603$)				
Medical	67.8	66.1	64.4	62.5
Surgical	69.4	70.8	69.6	64.4
Congest. ht. fail. ($n = 1612$)				
Medical	49.0	38.8	42.6	45.3
Surgical	53.0	46.4	46.8	47.5

One factor possibly confounding the medical classification concerns the cross-over of patients from medical treatment to surgical treatment later in the course of their illness. This change in treatment status creates a medical-surgical group potentially altering the results attributable solely to medical treatment. Therefore, we analyzed the results separately for the medical-surgical group, termed a "cross-over" group (Table 3). The cross-over group started at a higher level of employment than the pure medical or surgical group for all three symptom classifications but unexpectedly showed a marked decline in employment over the 5 years of follow-up so that by the fifth year a lesser percentage of the cross-over group was working than the surgically or medically treated patients in the angina and chest pain groups. The results at the first year do indicate that these patients either continued to have problems when treated medically or discontinued work due to the surgical procedure because the employment status at that point in time dropped to its lowest ebb for this group. The gains over the following years, as noted above, were insufficient to compensate for this early marked decline in employment. Due to the high percentage of cross-over patients working at baseline in the congestive heart failure group, more of them were working at year 5 despite an 11.9% decrease in employment. The percentage of this group working was 54.8% versus 43.3% for the medical group and 47.5% for the surgical group.

Table 3. Percent of participants working at follow-up years by predominant symptoms and treatment groups at baseline

Symptom/group	Baseline	Year 1	Year 3	Year 5
Angina ($n=12558$)				
Medical	65.0	59.6	58.0	57.2
Surgical	70.1	63.7	62.3	59.3
Cross-over	73.6	47.7	59.6	55.8
Chest pain ($n=603$)				
Medical	67.5	66.9	66.3	64.7
Surgical	69.4	70.8	69.6	64.4
Cross-over	76.9	46.2	48.7	51.2
Congest. ht. fail. ($n=1612$)				
Medical	48.1	38.6	41.1	43.3
Surgical	53.0	46.4	46.8	47.5
Cross-over	66.7	42.9	58.3	54.8

Another way of considering these data is to examine the net change in work status; the overall numbers who went from an unemployed or part-time status to part-time or full-time status, respectively, improved; and conversely, those who went from a full-time or part-time status to a part-time or unemployed status, respectively, declined (Table 4). Using this net change as an index, 65.0% to 71.6% of the medical subgroups demonstrated no change at 1 year, 11.6% to 12.6% improved, but about twice as many declined in the angina and congestive heart failure groups with a lesser decline in those presenting with nondiagnostic chest pain. Data from the surgical group revealed similar differences. The only demonstrable benefit occurred among the surgical subgroup with chest pain. These patients exhibited a small differential gain of 2.8% (11.1 vs. 13.9) in work status at 1 year. Unfortunately, this improvement did not persist at 5-years follow-up, at which time all groups showed a net reduction in work force compared to baseline, with a percent decline of 1.4–2.5 times greater than improvement.

Figure 1 depicts the distribution of employment at 1 year by the work status at baseline. Generally, patients tended to remain in the same employment status. Most of the medical and surgical groups working full-time or part-time at baseline continued to do so. The vast majority of those retired at baseline remained in this status or became unemployed. Although some of those who had quit work or were otherwise unemployed at entry into the program resumed full- or part-time work, over 60% remained unemployed. The logistic regression analysis allowed us to adjust statistically for differences in patient characteris-

Table 4. Net change (%) in work status at follow-up by predominant symptoms and treatment groups at baseline

Treatment/work status		Angina	Chest pain	Congestive heart failure
One year				
Medical –	No change	67.3	71.6	65.0
	Improved	12.3	12.6	11.6
	Declined	20.4	15.8	23.4
Surgical –	No change	68.1	75.0	64.2
	Improved	11.6	13.9	13.5
	Declined	20.3	11.1	22.3
Five year				
Medical –	No change	61.7	58.7	60.6
	Improved	11.8	17.0	15.3
	Declined	26.6	24.3	24.2
Surgical –	No change	59.4	66.1	57.4
	Improved	11.6	10.2	15.2
	Declined	28.9	23.7	27.5

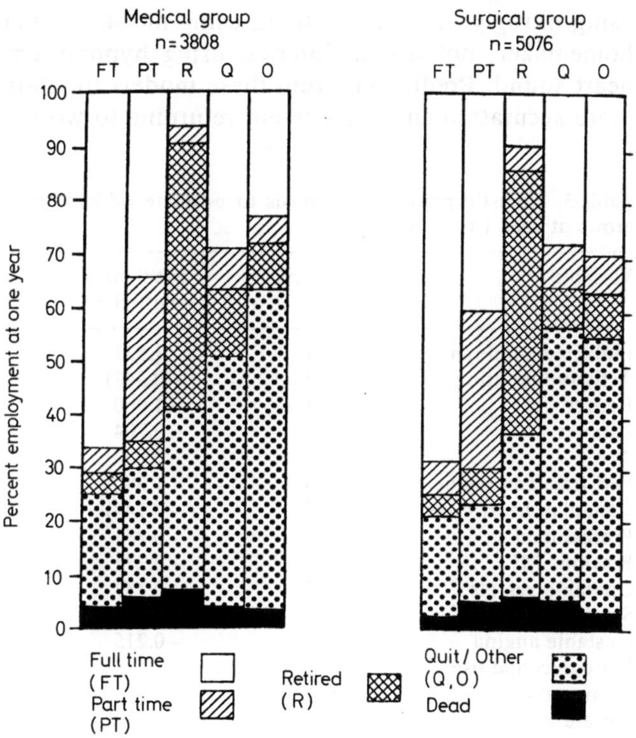

Fig. 1. Classification of work status at baseline and 1 year afterwards. This figure demonstrates that work status at baseline is clearly an important factor in predicting employment patterns after treatment. Patients from both medical and surgical groups tend to remain in their initial work status classification

tics, including disease status, and determined the best predictors of return to work and estimated the odds of returning to work for a given patient. The results were similar among all patient groups and only the data from the angina group at the first and fifth year were presented for the medical and surgical groups (Tables 5, 6). For both treatments and both follow-up years, the variables selected were remarkably similar: primarily employment status at baseline, activity limitation at follow-up, occupational class, and age. If one arbitrarily characterized hypothetical patients on the basis of these characteristics, the probability of returning to work could be estimated (Table 7). Those medical patients who had little activity limitation, were employed full-time as professionals, and were aged 40 had a 98% probability of returning to work, compared to 20% for those who had severe activity limitations, were not employed full-time, whose occupation was laborer, and were aged 60. The corresponding values for the surgical group were 79% and 2%. All other predictors in the model (Table 5) were considered the same for both "high" and "low" groups – those with likelihood of success or failure, respectively. For the medical group the patients were considered for both the "high" and "low" probability groups to be not retired, not part-time employed, Canadian Heart Class 1, without previous MI, with one operable vessel, and a non-smoker having stable angina. For the surgical group, the patients were considered not part-time employed, using nitroglycerine, not retired, using nitrates, Canadian Heart Class 1, nonhomemaker, not using diuretics, using hypoglycemics, and without a third heart sound. Predictions from these models for those returning to work were more accurate than for those not returning to work.

Table 5. Logistic regression analysis to estimate odds of returning to work for the angina group at year 1 ($n = 5657$)

Variable	Rank	Medical coefficient	Rank	Surgical coefficient
Full-time employment	1	1.531	1	1.748
Activity limitation	2	(−0.348)	2	(−0.363)
Retired	3	−1.900	7	−1.128
Laborer	4	−0.704	6	−0.677
Age	5	−0.057	5	−0.051
Part-time employment	6	1.380	3	1.271
Canadian heart class	7	(−0.144)	9	−0.173
Professional	8	0.481	14	0.266
Previous MI	9	−0.271		-
Operable vessels	10	−0.137		-
Smoking	11	−0.175		-
Unstable angina	12	−0.215		-
Nitroglycerine use		-	4	(0.967)
Homemaker		-	10	0.933
Nitrate use		-	8	(0.710)
Diuretic use		-	11	−0.281
Hypoglycemic		-	12	0.549
Third heart sound		-	13	−0.614

( ) indicates follow-up variable at year 1

Table 6. Logistic regression analysis to estimate odds of returning to work for the angina group at year 5 ($n = 5706$)

Variable	Rank	Medical coefficient	Rank	Surgical coefficient
Activity limitation	1	(−0.745)	1	(−0.657)
Full-time employment	2	1.167	2	0.893
Part-time employment	5	1.277	8	0.788
Age	4	−0.083	4	−0.083
Laborer	6	−0.572	5	−0.496
Retired	9	−1.068	7	−1.112
Smoking	13	−0.221	15	−0.179
Professional		-	9	0.481
Nitroglycerine use	7	(0.500)	6	(0.732)
Homemaker	11	0.844	3	1.349
Hypoglycemic use		-	12	0.467
Sex	3	0.665	10	0.669
LV score	8	−0.043		-
Activity limitation	10	−0.152	11	−0.080
Recreation activity	12	0.185		-
Antiarrhythmic		-	13	0.335
Proximal vessels	14	−0.151		-
Beta-Blocker		-	14	(0.178)

( ) indicates follow-up variable at year 5

Table 7. Odds of returning to work at year 1 by major predictor variables and treatment group

Predictor[a]	Probability of return to work High	Low
Class activity limit - yr. 1	1	5
Full-time employment	Yes	No
Occupation	Profes.	Laborer
Age	40	60
Treatment group		
Medical	0.98	0.20
Surgical	0.79	0.02

[a] All other predictors in the model (Table 5) were considered the same (see text) for both "high" and "low" groups

Conclusion

Patients who have coronary bypass surgery have their quality of life improved as compared to medically treated patients, but enjoy no particular advantages in returning to work. As noted in many previous studies regardless of treatment, patients show a 10% or more net loss from the work force over a 5-year period after coronary arteriography [8]. Johnson and co-workers [5] aptly point out that the trend in the general population is also in this direction, the magnitude depending greatly on age. The randomized portion of the CASS study demonstrated significant improvement in quality of life and less disability among those treated surgically, but no favorable increase in return to work [1].

These data from the CASS registry clearly indicate the similarities for the medical and surgical groups in work patterns and variables predictive of work status. Definition of surgically treated subgroups based on symptom complexes and "cross-overs" from medical to surgical treatment do not explain the downward trends in work status despite relief of chest pain, improved functional status, and diminished need for drug therapy. A further consideration is the self-perception of one's disability and medical status. Self-perceived limitations may be as important as the actual disability [6, 11]. Baseline employment status is the most powerful predictor of return to work. Activity limitations at the time of determination of employment status, occupation, and age also appear to be key variables. However, the angiographic and follow-up medical variables contribute little to these analyses for prediction of work status.

Over the next decade the age of the work force is likely to rise and expectations are for a shortage of younger workers [7]. Such anticipated developments will further exaggerate the cost of failure of patients having coronary bypass surgery to return to productive employment. Dealing with the problem now might avoid further costly demands on a society already facing difficulties in financing its health care system.

Acknowledgment. The research upon which this publication is based was supported by the National Heart, Lung and Blood Institute, Coronary Artery Surgery Study, Grant No. NHLBI-N01 HV 62922.

References

1. CASS Principal Investigators and their Associates (1983) Coronary artery surgery study (CASS): A randomized trial of coronary artery bypass surgery – quality of life in patients randomly assigned to treatment groups. Circulation 68:951–960
2. CASS Principal Investigators and their Associates (1983) Coronary artery surgery study (CASS): A randomized trial of coronary artery bypass surgery – survival data. Circulation 68:939–950
3. European Coronary Surgery Study Group (1982) Long-term results of prospective randomized study of coronary artery bypass surgery in stable angina pectoris. Lancet II:1173–1180
4. CASS Principal Investigators and their Associates (1981) National Heart Lung and Blood Institute Coronary Artery Surgery Study. Circulation [Suppl II] 63:79
5. Johnson WD, Kayser KL, Pedraza PM, Shore RT (1982) Employment patterns in males before and after myocardial revascularization surgery. Circulation 65:1086–1093

5 A. Murphy M, Hultgren H, Detre K, Thomsen J, Tokaro T, and participants of the Veterans Administration Cooperative Study 1977 Treatment of chronic stable angina. A preliminary report of survival data of the Randomized Veterans Administration Cooperative Study. N Engl J Med 297:621

6. Oberman A (1984) Role of quality of life assessment in clinical trials. In: Wenger NK, Mattson ME, Furberg CD, Elinson J (eds), Assessment of Quality of life in clinical Trials of Cardiovascular Therapies. Np: Le Jacq Publishing Inc., pp 67–86

7. Oberman A, Finklea JF (1982) Return to work after coronary artery bypass grafting. Ann Thorac Surg 34:353–355
8. Oberman A, Wayne JB, Kouchoukos NT, Charles ED, Russell RO Jr, Rogers WJ (1982) Employment status following coronary artery bypass surgery. Proceedings of the NIH Consensus Development Conference on Coronary Artery Bypass Surgery, Bethesda, Maryland, December 3–5, 1980. Circulation [Suppl II] 65:115–119
9. Press SJ, Wilson S (1978) Choosing between logistic regression and discriminant analysis. J Am Stat Assoc 73:699–704
10. Report of the Working Group on Arteriosclerosis of the National Heart, Lung and Blood Institute (1981) Arteriosclerosis 1981, vol 1. National Institute of Health, Washington D.C. (NIH Publication No. 81-2034)
11. Wayne JB, Oberman A, Reed BA, Charles ED, Cutter GR, Hale CB, Kimmerling RA (to be published) Work status, employment goals and return to work following coronary artery bypass surgery

Comparison of Employment Status Between Medically and Surgically Treated Coronary Artery Disease over 6–7 Years

K. E. Hammermeister, T. A. DeRouen, M. Zia, and H. T. Dodge

This report will describe the work status, as assessed three times over a 6- to 7-year period, of coronary artery disease patients entered into the Angiography Registry of Seattle Heart Watch. The purpose of these analyses is to determine the factors associated with continued employment and to assess the effect of form of therapy on work status. These studies have been previously reported (Hammermeister et al. 1979, 1983).

Methods

Seattle Heart Watch

Seattle Heart Watch was a multifaceted study conducted over the decade of the 1970s in the community of Seattle, Washington, with the primary goal of identifying patients at risk for sudden cardiac death. Among the several projects in Seattle Heart Watch was the Angiography Registry; the primary goal of this registry was to identify angiographic characteristics of patients dying from coronary artery disease. These analyses have been reported in detail in a monograph (Hammermeister 1983 a) as well as elsewhere (Hammermeister 1983 b).

It was the intent of the Angiography Registry to enter all consenting patients undergoing coronary arteriography for suspected coronary artery disease in Seattle during the 5-year period from 1969 to 1974. Because of special interest in the outcome of patients having coronary bypass surgery, the 1880 initially surgically treated patients represent nearly all such patients (95%) operated in Seattle during this period. However, due to limited funding the 736 initially medically treated patients represent an approximately 40% sample of such patients. Of this medical group, 248 did not have significant coronary artery disease (stenosis of one or more major vessels > 50%), leaving 488 initially medically treated patients with coronary artery disease.

Baseline characteristics from the history, physical examination, resting electrocardiogram, exercise test, coronary arteriogram, and left ventricular angiogram were recorded prospectively on data forms. Planned follow-up in regard to death and hospitalization for cardiac events was conducted by mailed questionnaire and telephone. Specially designed questionnaires to assess employment status 3 months before and 1 year after entry were sent out in 1977. Completed questionnaires were received from 238 patients in the medical cohort and 1333 in the surgical cohort, representing 81% and 85%, respectively, of living patients at that time.

Near the end of the study in 1980, a second special questionnaire to assess employment and symptomatic status was sent out. Completed questionnaires were received from 190 medically treated patients and 1261 surgically treated patients, representing 86% and 89%, respectively, of living patients.

Patient Characteristics

The entry characteristics of the group represented in the 1-year follow-up are very similar to those of the total cohort. Mean age at entry was 53 years. Patients in the surgical cohort were more symptomatic and had more extensive coronary disease than patients in the medical cohort (an average of 2.0 stenotic vessels per patient compared to 1.6). Medically treated patients generally had more evidence of left ventricular dysfunction. Job classifications at entry were similar between the two cohorts, with 39% professional or administrative, 13% clerical or laboratory, 30% skilled or factory, 14% semiskilled or unskilled, 3% homemakers, and 1% unclassified.

Data Analysis

The significance of the association between individual baseline characteristics and work status at 1 year after entry was assessed with the chi-square test. To select those baseline characteristics most predictive of continued employment 1 year after entry, a stepwise discriminant analysis was used. By entering a covariant identifying form of treatment, the stepwise discriminant analysis was also used to test for effect of form of therapy (medical or surgical) on continued employment while adjusting for any differences in baseline characteristics between the two treatment cohorts.

The significance of the difference in the proportions of patients working before and at the two intervals after entry was assessed using McNemar's test for correlated proportions.

Results

Table 1 shows the number and proportion of patients working at entry, 1 year, and 6–7 years after entry. At each follow-up period there was a reduction in the proportion of patients working. The drop in the percent working was highly significant ($P < 0.001$) between each time interval for both the medical surgical cohorts. However, there was no significant difference in the proportion working between the medical and surgical cohorts, except at the final follow-up, when slightly more medically treated patients (43%) were working than surgically treated patients (34%; $P < 0.05$).

The reasons for not working at the final assessment 6–7 years after entry are given in Table 2. Heart disease was the reason in the majority of patients, but was given more frequently in the medical cohort (61%) than the surgical cohort (51%; $P < 0.025$).

Table 1. Proportions of medically and surgically treated patients working full-time 3 months before entry and 1 year and 6–7 years after entry into Seattle Heart Watch (Hammermeister et al. 1983)

Time	Medically treated patients N/T	(%)	Surgically treated patients N/T	(%)	*P*
3 months before entry	92/124	(74)	757/991	(76)	NS
1 year	78/124	(63)	637/991	(64)	NS
6–7 years	53/124	(43)	333/991	(34)	<0.05

Abbreviations: N, number of patients working full-time at the interval; *T,* total number of patients who answered both work questionnaires; *P,* significance of difference in distribution of full-time employment between medical and surgical cohorts

Table 2. Reasons for not working full-time at the final assessment 6–7 years after entry into Seattle Heart Watch (Hammermeister et al. 1983)

Reason for not working	Medically treated patients N/T	(%)	Surgically treated patients N/T	(%)	*P*
Heart disease	67/110	(61)	387/757	(51)	
Other illness	8/110	(7)	33/757	(4)	<0.025
Nonmedical	35/110	(32)	341/757	(45)	

Abbreviations: N, Number of patients not working full-time because of indicated reason; *T,* total number of patients in treatment cohort not working full-time; *P,* significance of difference in distribution of reasons for not working full-time between medical and surgical cohorts

Baseline characteristics associated with unemployment at 1 year are shown in Table 3. Longer duration of unemployment at entry, advanced age, less formal education, and New York Heart Association Functional Class III or IV were negatively associated with continued employment in both the medical and the surgical cohorts. However, there was no difference in the proportion employed between medical and surgical cohorts even when subgrouped by the above variables. Duration of unemployment at entry was a particularly powerful predictor of continued unemployment. Only 16% of medically treated patients and 11% of surgically treated patients who had been unemployed 3 months or longer prior to entry were working full-time 1 year later.

The stepwise discriminant analysis shown in Table 4 confirms that employment status prior to entry is the most powerful predictor of continued unemployment in both the medical and surgical cohorts, explaining nearly half of the variance (R^2) in 1-year employment status. Age and duration of formal education contribute modestly, but significantly, to the predictive model in both medical and surgical cohorts.

The discriminant analysis summarized in Table 5 confirms the lack of effect of form of therapy (medical or surgical) on 1-year employment status even after adjusting for the five covariates shown.

Table 3. Factors affecting full-time employment 1 year after entry into Seattle Heart Watch (Hammermeister et al. 1983)

Factor		Medically treated patients N/T	(%)	*P*	Surgically treated patients N/T	(%)	*P*
Duration of unemployment at entry (mo)	<3	118/149	(79)		726/927	(78)	
	3–12	4/18	(22)	<0.01	23/123	(19)	<0.01
	>12	4/31	(13)		5/135	(4)	
Age (years)	≦55	96/127	(76)	<0.01	506/701	(72)	<0.01
	>55	29/74	(39)		241/497	(48)	
Education (years)	≦12	61/115	(53)	<0.01	443/752	(59)	<0.01
	>12	62/82	(76)		295/426	(69)	
Functional class at entry	I, II	81/107	(76)	<0.01	341/446	(76)	<0.01
	III, IV	29/60	(48)		346/579	(60)	
Job activity	Light	65/76	(86)		336/397	(85)	
	Moderate	36/47	(77)	NS	267/325	(82)	<0.01
	Heavy	8/12	(67)		65/95	(68)	
Number of stenotic vessels	1	83/118	(70)		219/329	(67)	
	2	31/57	(54)	<0.05	283/463	(61)	NS
	3	12/27	(44)		247/407	(61)	

Abbreviations: N, number of patients working full-time 1 year after entry with indicated characteristic; *T,* total number of patients with indicated characteristic; *P,* significance of difference in distribution of full-time employed between groups defined by characteristic

Table 4. Stepwise discriminant analysis of characteristics predictive of full-time employment 1 year after entry into Seattle Heart Watch (Hammermeister et al. 1983)

Characteristic	Medically treated patients Increment in R^2	*F*	Surgically treated patients Increment in R^2	*F*
Employed 3 months before entry	0.450	128	0.405	660
Age	0.017	4.8	0.021	35.0
Education	0.013	3.9	0.009	14.9
Functional class at entry		NS	0.007	12.3
Duration of unemployment at entry	0.013	3.7	0.006	9.8
$\sum R^2$	0.482		0.447	

Abbreviations: F, F statistic indicating significance of characteristic in predicting full-time employment 1 year after entry (*F* 3.84 equals *P* 0.05 at 1 and 100 degrees of freedom)

Other stepwise discriminant analyses (not shown) were performed deleting patients unemployed for noncardiovascular reasons or those unemployed 3 months before entry. The former analysis was done because a therapy directed at heart disease (coronary artery bypass surgery) could not be expected to improve employability in those unemployed for noncardiac reasons. In the latter

Table 5. Stepwise discriminant analysis testing for effect of surgical versus medical therapy on full-time employment 1 year after entry into Seattle Heart Watch (Hammermeister et al. 1983)

Variable	Increment in R^2	$\sum R^2$	*F*
Employed 3 months before entry	0.409	0.409	777
Age	0.020	0.429	39.8
Education	0.009	0.438	18.1
Functional class at entry	0.006	0.444	11.8
Duration of unemployment at entry	0.004	0.448	7.9
Surgery	0.000	0.448	0.9

Abbreviations: See Table 4

analysis we wished to test the hypothesis that coronary artery bypass surgery was more effective than medical therapy in maintaining employment. In neither analysis was employment at 1 year significantly associated with form of therapy.

Discussion

The results of our analyses of work status of coronary artery disease patients entered into the Coronary Arteriography Registry of Seattle Heart Watch clearly show no improvement in employment over a 6- to 7-year period for surgical therapy versus medical therapy. To the contrary, a modestly larger proportion of medically treated patients were working at 6–7 years than surgically treated patients. Our findings of no beneficial effect of surgical versus medical therapy have been confirmed by Russel et al. (1980) in an analysis of 95 patients entered into the National Cooperative Unstable Angina Study from the University of Alabama and from the much larger Coronary Artery Surgery Study (CASS Investigators and their Associates, 1983). In an assessment of 64 patients at 2 years after entry into The European Coronary Surgery Study, Frick et al. (1979) reported a higher employment rate in surgically treated patients (60% of 30) compared to medically treated patients (26% of 34). However, the statistical ($P < 0.05$) and clinical significance are limited.

The strongest predictor of subsequent work status was the employment status 3 months prior to entry. Virtually every study that has examined this issue has reported similar findings. There is, of course, considerable logic to this finding. In a competitive job market employers are more likely to hire an actively or recently employed person than one who has been unemployed for a lengthy period. Patients who have been unemployed for substantial periods adapt to the unemployed life-style with a change in daily schedule and activities. When the habits of daily living have been adapted to the unemployed status it is difficult for the patient to aggressively seek work.

A large number of reports have presented data on work status in surgically treated patients before and after surgery, but without a comparable medically treated control group. The vast majority of these studies report fewer patients working after coronary artery surgery than before. On the other hand, there is an overwhelming consensus that coronary bypass surgery improves exercise tolerance and relieves angina in patients limited by angina preoperatively. If patients are unemployed because of their coronary heart disease and if coronary bypass surgery relieves functional disability due to coronary heart disease, why has return to work been so disappointing? Can it be that the operation is not as successful as we imagine? Is it the fault of the patient, the physician, or society? We believe that a portion of the explanation can be found in a consideration of all four.

The operation is not a cure; it is palliative. Preoperative resting left ventricular systolic dysfunction is usually not improved (Hammermeister et al., 1974). Left ventricular diastolic dysfunction during exercise also is not improved with coronary bypass grafting (Hirzel et al., 1983). Thus many patients exchange exercise limitation by angina preoperatively for exercise limitation by dyspnea and fatigue postoperatively. Furthermore, there may be residual ischemic myocardium resulting in persistent angina early postoperatively in 10%–20%, increasing to 40% or more 5–7 years postoperatively.

On the other hand, dramatic symptomatic relief occurs in the majority of patients. Yet personal interviews with many patients postoperatively indicate attitudes that impede return to work. Many will blame the "stress on the job" for their disease and fear that return to even sedentary work will accelerate their disease. Others have had unstimulating or boring employment and find their surgery an opportunity to break out of an unpleasant situation. Finally, physicians need to recognize that their belief in the "goodness" of work is not always shared.

The medical profession still bears some of the responsibility for excessive unemployment following coronary bypass surgery. While physician attitudes are changing, there are still many who advise medical retirement for trivial disability if it is due to heart disease. Many physicians fail to recognize that there is little or no evidence linking employment to cardiac events, with the possible exception of work involving strenuous isometric exercise.

Finally society has to bear a substantial portion of the blame. The society that makes it possible for a successfully operated patient to have greater personal income from combined disability insurance, retirement, and social security than he would earn if fully employed cannot expect a substantial number of patients to return to work. Similarly, the fear of higher workman's compensation premiums for patients having a cardiac event on the job is a significant deterrent to the employer hiring a person with heart disease, regardless of functional status.

To conclude, we regard the failure of a substantial number of patients to return to work after coronary bypass surgery not as a failure of the operation, but as a failure to educate and change the attitudes of the patient, his physician, and society.

References

CASS Investigators and their Associates (1983) Coronary Artery Surgery Study (CASS): A randomized trial of coronary artery bypass surgery. Circulation 68:951-960

Frick MH, Harjola PT, Valle M (1979) Work status after coronary bypass surgery. A prospective randomized study with ergometric and angiographic correlations. Acta Med Scand 206:61-64

Hammermeister KE, Kennedy JW, Steward DK, et al (1974) The failure to successful aorta-coronary saphenous vein bypass grafting to improve resting ventricular function in patients with chronic angina. N Engl J Med 290:1-6

Hammermeister KE, DeRouen TA, English MT, Dodge HT (1979) Effect of surgical versus medical therapy on return to work in patients with coronary artery disease. Am J Cardiol 44:105-111

Hammermeister KE (ed) (1983a) Coronary bypass surgery. The late results. Praeger, New York

Hammermeister KE (1983b) The effect of coronary bypass surgery on survival. Prog Cardiovasc Dis 25:297-334

Hammermeister KE, DeRouen TA, Zia M, Dodge HT (1983) Effect of coronary bypass surgery on continued employment. In: Hammermeister KE (ed) Coronary bypass surgery. The late results. Praeger, New York, pp 413-423

Hirzel HO, Wegmueller R, Grimm J, Krayenbuehl HP, Senning Å (1983) Left ventricular function during exercise before and after coronary bypass surgery. In: Hammermeister KE (ed) Coronary bypass surgery. The late results. Praeger, New York, pp 311-333

Russell RO, Wayne JB, Kronenfeld, et al (1980) Surgical versus medical therapy for the treatment of unstable angina. Changes in work status and family income. Am J Cardiol 45:134-140

Return to Work After Surgical and Medical Treatment of Patients with Coronary Artery Disease

J. Jehle, P. Grossmann, L. Kampa, M. Kloke, A. Krian, and F. Loogen

It is universally accepted that bypass surgery reduces angina pectoris and improves exercise capacity. The rate of employment differs in various countries and is not a generally accepted indication for surgery. Studies have shown that in the USA about 60%–90% of all employees return to work, whereas in West Germany the rate is less than 50% [1, 2, 3]. There are only a few studies on the return to work among patients without surgery [4].

In this study we investigated retrospectively the rate of employment in two groups of patients with coronary artery disease: one group underwent bypass surgery, the other medical treatment. The aim of the study was to find out whether the rate of employment is influenced by the different forms of therapy.

Methods

The surgically treated group consisted of 204 patients, 21 of whom were women. Their mean age was 52 years, ranging from 25 to 71 years. In this group 26 patients died, 15 late postoperatively. In all patients a coronary bypass procedure was performed. Patients with sole aneurysmectomy were excluded. The medically treated group consisted of 149 patients, including 12 women. Their mean age was 50 years, ranging from 29 to 67 years. In this group 33 patients died during the observation period. In 49 patients a complete analysis of all data was not possible, mainly because no further information was available. In most of the patients treated medically there was no indication for surgery because of minor symptoms; however, indication for surgery was present in 31 patients; 26 patients refused operation, while in 5 cases the surgeons rejected the operation.

The observation period lasted from 1976 to 1983, i.e., all patients in the surgically treated group were operated in 1976. The first postoperative examination took place after 9 months and the second after 6–7 years. In all patients treated medically the exact diagnosis was established by angiography performed in 1976, too.

Results and Discussion

The status of the patients in both groups before surgery and before the diagnostic procedure is depicted in Fig. 1. There were no significant differences between patients who underwent surgery and those who did not: (a) 37% and 45%, respectively, were laborers, i.e., skilled or unskilled blue-collar workers, (b) 50% and 43% were office workers (white-collar workers), and (c) 13% and 12% were professionals.

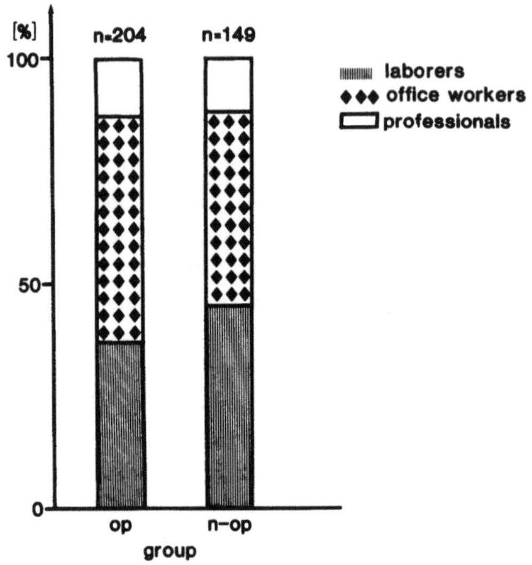

Fig. 1. "Preoperative" status of patients in the surgically treated *(op)* and medically treated *(n-op)* groups. No significant difference is seen in terms of the professions represented in the two groups

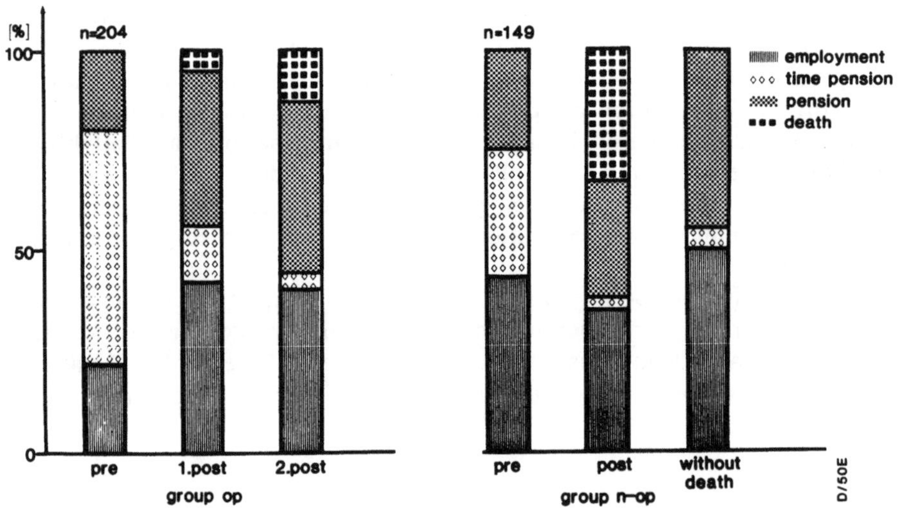

Fig. 2. Employment status in the surgically *(op)* and medically *(n-op)* treated groups before and after surgery and diagnostic angiography, respectively. Preoperatively most patients were receiving time pension; postoperatively 44% were still working. After angiography *(group n-op)* about 50% of those who did not die returned to work

Figure 2 shows the employment status of the surgically and medically treated groups. The patients were divided into four groups: employment, time pension (no final decision concerning employment status made before operation), pension, and death. In the surgical group most patients (58%) were receiving time pension, 22% were working, and 20% were receiving a pension. The rate of reemployment increased at the first examination in comparison to the preoperative rate. It remained nearly unchanged at the time of the second examination, at about 40%. The number of patients receiving time pension decreased; most of them received a pension, so that the pensioners increased from 20% to 40% postoperatively.

In the medically treated group more patients (43%) were working at the time when the diagnosis was established. This rate had not changed significantly after 7 years, even when the deceased patients were excluded. Similar results were found in patients receiving a pension. In both groups no patient receiving a pension prior to the treatment returned to work later.

The postoperative employment status of the three occupational groups – laborers, office workers, and professionals – is shown in Fig. 3. The deceased patients were excluded.

More than 50% of the laborers received a pension in both groups. Only 32% of the laborers treated surgically and 42% of those treated medically were working. Among office workers the rate of employment was higher postoperatively, at 52% and 44% respectively. No significant differences were found in the two groups. Fifty percent of the surgically treated professionals were work-

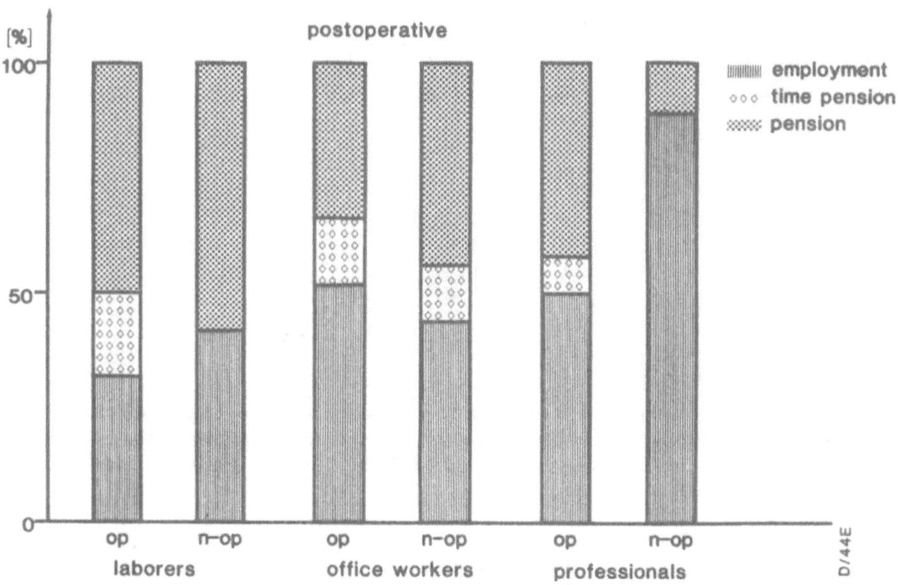

Fig. 3. "Postoperative" employment status of laborers, office workers, and professionals in the surgically *(op)* and medically *(n-op)* treated groups. In both groups most of the laborers received a pension, whereas most of the professionals were working

ing postoperatively, whereas 89% of those treated medically were still working; because of the small number of patients (26 patients in the medically treated group), the difference was not significant. These results show that about 50% of all patients – 44% in the surgically treated group and 50% in the medically treated group – returned to work, without any significant differences between the treatment groups. Laborers showed the lowest and professionals the highest rate of reemployment irrespective of the kind of treatment.

Which factors do influence the rate of employment in these two groups? One factor may be the extent of coronary artery disease. In Fig. 4 the employment status in the medically treated group is depicted in correlation with one-, two-, and three-vessel disease. The results can be briefly summarized: The rate of employment was highest in patients with one-vessel disease. About 50% of the patients with two- or three-vessel disease died during the observation period. In the surviving patients there was no difference in the rate of employment between the two examinations, i.e. before and 7 years after heart catheterization.

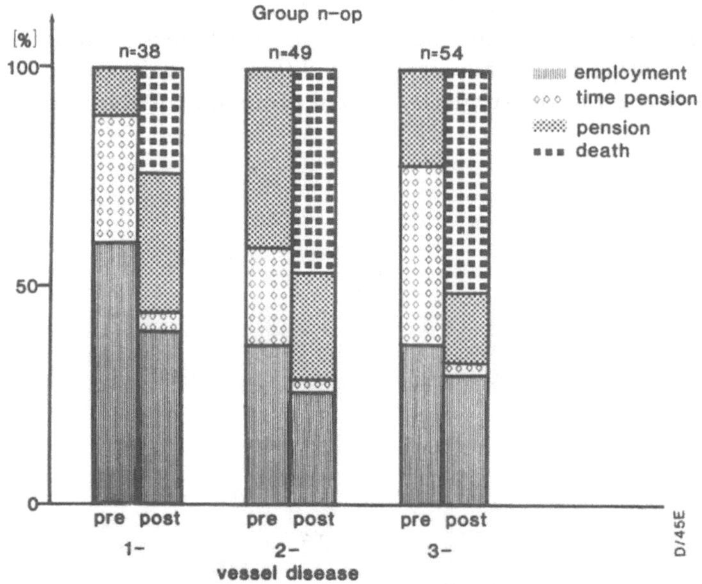

Fig. 4. Influence of the extent of coronary artery disease on employment status in the medically treated *(n-op)* group. Most patients with one-vessel disease were working. About 50% of the patients with two- or three-vessel disease died during the observation period

In the surgically treated group (Fig. 5) we found no difference in employment status in the groups with one-, two-, and three-vessel disease. Postoperatively 150 patients were reexamined by angiography. We divided these patients into two groups: complete (100%) and incomplete (< 100%) revascularization.

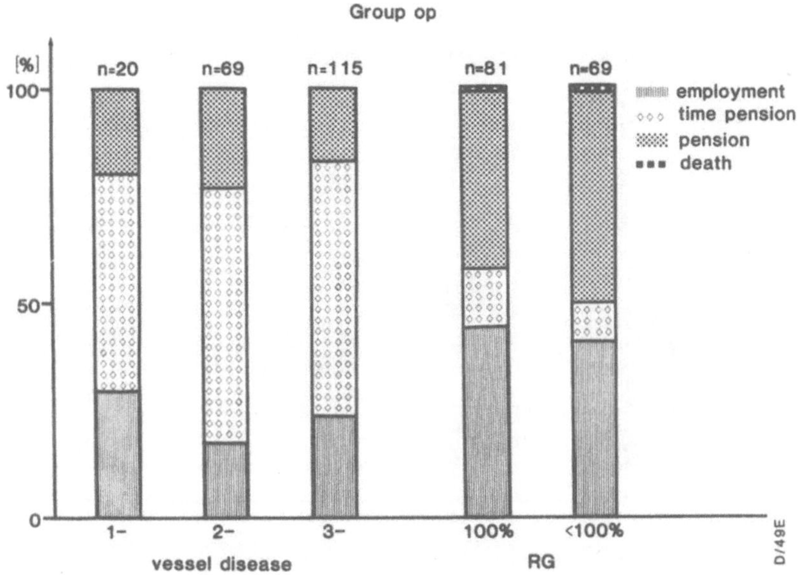

Fig. 5. Influence of the extent of coronary artery disease and the degree of revascularization on employment status in the surgically treated *(op)* group. The extent of coronary artery disease and the degree of revascularization did not influence the rate of reemployment

There was no significant difference concerning the employment status in these groups.

From these results we conclude that the extent of coronary artery disease influences the prognosis of medically treated patients and therefore the employment status of the surviving patients. The degree of revascularization did not influence the reemployment status in the surgically treated group.

The influence of left ventricular function on employment status is depicted in Fig. 6. The left ventricular function is described as good, slightly, or severely impaired. In the medically treated group there was a correlation between left ventricular function and return to work: More patients with a good or slightly impaired function returned to work than patients with severely impaired function. In the latter group most patients died during the observation period. Regarding only the surviving patients, there were no differences between the two examinations in the single groups.

In the surgically treated group less patients were working before operation than in the medically treated group irrespective of left ventricular function. After surgery about the same percentage of patients returned to work as in the medically treated group. Mortality was not significantly different in the three groups with varying left ventricular function and was much less than in the medically treated group.

These results show that left ventricular function did not significantly influence the rate of employment in the operated patients. The same result was seen in the medically treated group when only the surviving patients were considered.

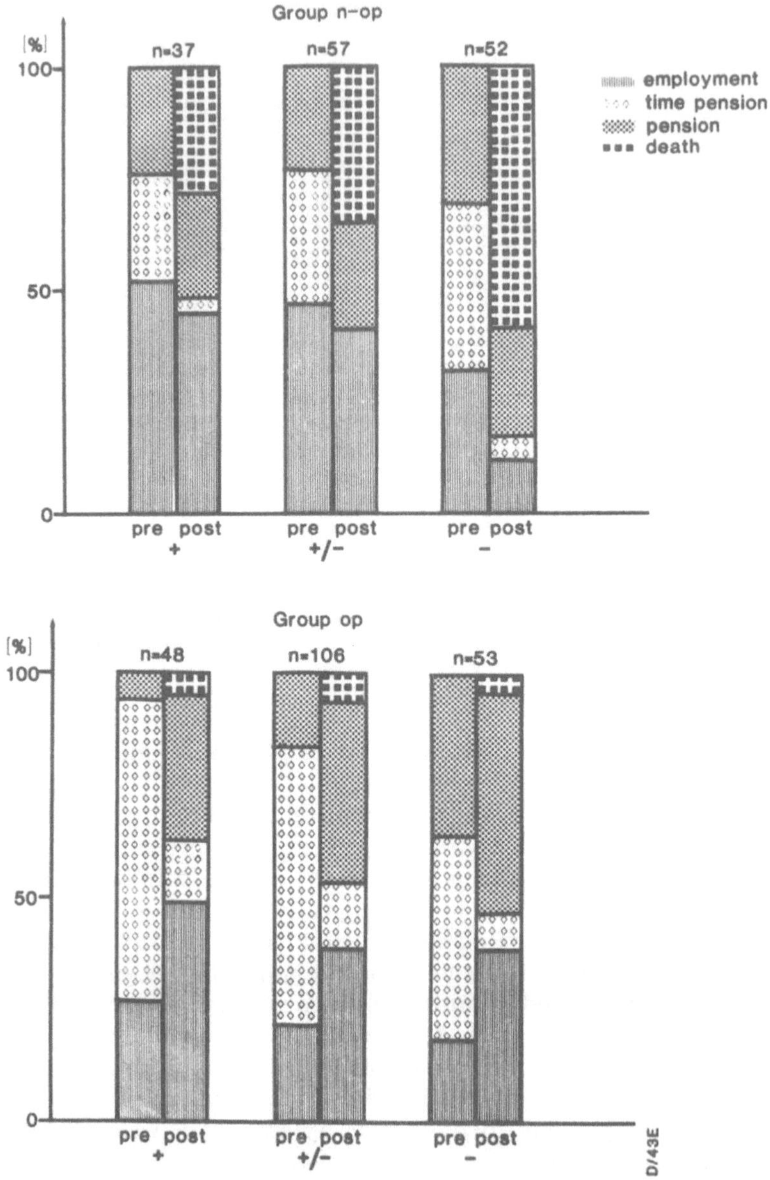

Fig. 6. Influence of left ventricular function on employment status in the surgically *(op)* and medically *(n-op)* treated groups. +, good; +/−, slightly impaired; −, severely impaired. In the medically treated group there was a correlation between left ventricular function and return to work. In the surgically treated group no differences were found

One important factor for reemployment may be the age of the patient at the time of surgery or heart catheterization or at the time of the last examination. Figure 7 shows the patients of both groups subdivided into different age groups. The age considered was that in the year of the last examination in 1983.

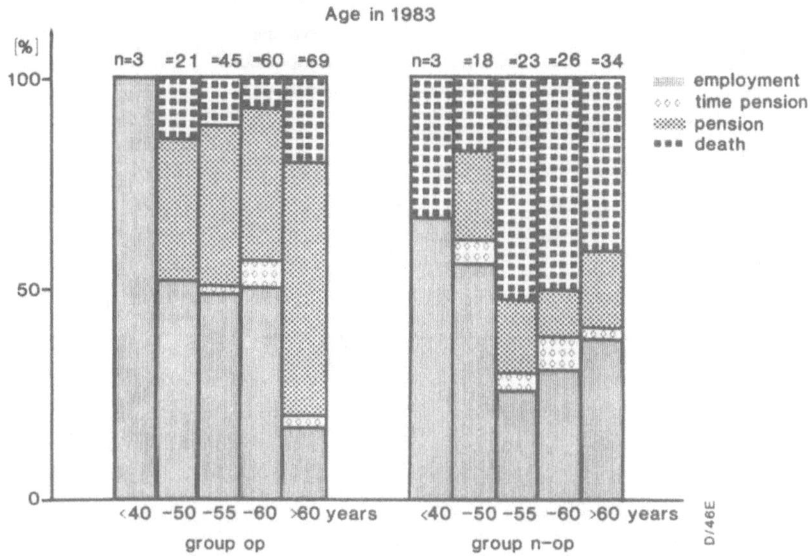

Fig. 7. Influence of age on employment status in the surgically *(op)* and medically *(n-op)* treated groups. In the former about 50% of all patients younger than 60 years were working. In the medically treated group less patients were working because of the high mortality in patients older than 50 years

In the surgically treated group about 50% of the patients younger than 60 years were working. Most patients older than 60 years were receiving a pension. In the medically treated group, results seem similar, but the lower rate of employment in patients older than 50 years was due to the high mortality in this age group. Neglecting the deceased patients, more than 50% of the older patients returned to work until 1983. The relatively high rate of employment among the older patients is caused by the large number of professionals, whereas among the laborers only younger patients returned to work.

Patients' complaints are another factor which may influence return to work. In Fig. 8 the degree of angina pectoris was correlated to the employment status. In the surgically treated group a significant improvement was seen in all patients. Patients working had less angina than did others. This difference was evident pre- and postoperatively. In the medically treated group angina did not change on average. The marked decrease in angina in the group of patients receiving a pension was due to the fact that in this group more patients with severe angina died and only patients with less angina survived. Besides these changes, it is evident that patients in the medically treated group, especially the working patients, generally had less angina before heart catheterization than the operated patients preoperatively.

The results can be summarized as follows:

1. About 50% of the patients returned to work. Coronary artery surgery did not influence this rate significantly.

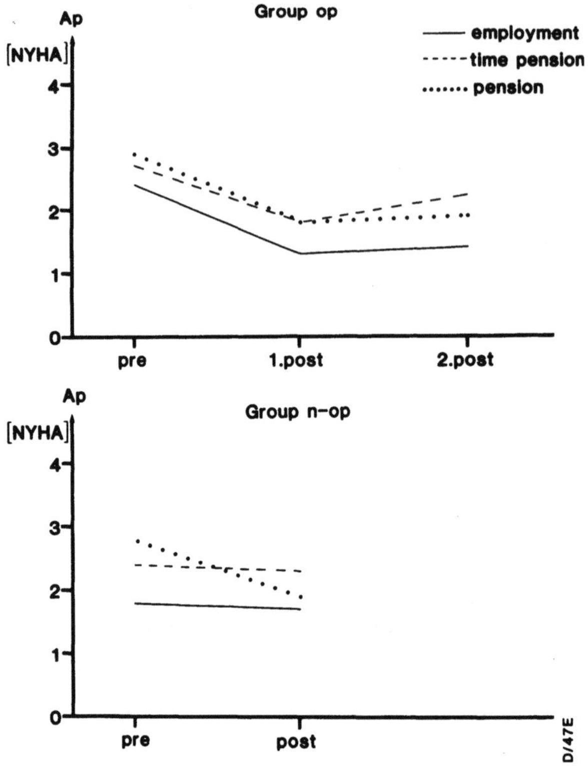

Fig. 8. Influence of the degree of angina pectoris on employment status in the surgically *(op)* and medically *(n-op)* treated groups. Patients with less angina were working in both groups with no differences "pre-" and "postoperatively"

2. The rate of reemployment in this study was not influenced by therapeutic measures – either surgical or medical – but was affected by the status and profession of the patients as well as by the degree of angina pectoris "post-operatively".

References

1. Benesch L, Neuhaus KL, Rivas-Martin J, Loogen F (1979) Clinical results and return to work after coronary heart surgery. In: Roskamm H, Schmuziger M (eds) Coronary heart surgery. Springer, Berlin Heidelberg New York
2. Blümchen G, Scharf-Bornhofen E, Brandt D, van den Bergh C, Bierck G (1979) Clinical results and social implications in patients after coronary bypass surgery. In: Roskamm H, Schmuziger M (eds) Coronary heart surgery. Springer, Berlin Heidelberg New York
3. Gehring W, Koenig W, Wrana N, Mathes P (1984) Aortokoronare Bypass-Operation. Welche Faktoren beeinflussen die Arbeitswiederaufnahme. Herz Gefäße 4:205
4. Hammermeister KE, DeRouen TA, English MT, Dodge HT (1979) Effect of surgical versus medical therapy on return to work in patients with coronary artery disease. Am J Cardiol 44:105

Return to Work After Coronary Artery Bypass Surgery in Comparison with Medical Treatment

H. Mannebach, U. Gleichmann, and H. Seggewiss

Introduction

In 1977 we conducted a first study involving all patients with coronary heart disease treated in our hospital in 1975 and 1976. A second study was done in 1983 with another cohort of patients, admitted for treatment in 1981 and 1982. We were looking for differences in working status between medically and surgically treated patients, as well as for differences over the years.

Study Population

The first study included a total of 516 patients; 134 of them had undergone bypass surgery, while 382 had been treated medically. Patients with an age above 59 or patients who had already retired before coronary arteriography or surgery were excluded. The second cohort of patients numbered 445; 117 of them had been elected for bypass surgery, and 268 had been treated medically (Table 1).

Table 1. Medical and surgical treatment in the two study populations

		Treatment	
		Medical *n*	Surgical *n*
1st study	1975	236	78
	1976	146	56
2nd study	1981	153	64
	1982	115	113
		650	311

A detailed questionnaire was sent to all patients and included questions on current state of health, present working status, and educational level. The answers were checked by the contents of their clinical records. The interval between surgery or coronary arteriography and the time of the study ranged from

6 to 18 months; the response rate was 84% in the first and 80.5% in the second study.

Results

All patients of the second cohort had undergone coronary arteriography; therefore we are able to compare the two treatment groups with respect to their coronary status.

Since the patients were not allocated at random to medical or surgical treatment, there was a considerable difference in the severity and extent of coronary artery disease between the two groups, as would be expected. The percentage of patients with two- or three-vessel disease was considerably higher in the surgical group (77.9%) than in the medical group (30.9%, $P<0.5$). Of the patients treated medically, 13% had minor coronary artery disease with a narrowing of the arteries to less than 75%. There was no left main disease in the medical group (Table 2).

Table 2. Coronary status in the surgical and medical groups (2nd study only)[a]

Disease	Surgical group $n=177$	Medical group $n=268$
One-vessel	15.8	55.9
Two-vessel	41.2	24.2
Three-vessel	36.7	6.7
Left main	6.2	–
Minor	–	13.0

[a] Results expressed as percentages

After bypass surgery the patients were readmitted to our hospital for rehabilitation. During a period of 3–4 weeks they attended a physical training program with individualized exercise prescription. Prior to discharge an exercise ECG in the upright position and pulmonary artery pressure measurements at rest and during exercise in the supine position were performed. When making a judgment about the time of return to work we relied on the results of these different exercise tests.

Within 3–4 weeks after surgery two-thirds of patients were able to exercise at a level of 75 W for 20 min, without experiencing angina pectoris or major rhythm disorders. This exercise level is usually taken to justify the discharge of the patient. During diagnostic exercise testing more than 70% of patients sustained a maximum load of 100 W or more in the upright position and more than 50% did so in the supine position. From these data it could be expected that the majority of the surgical patients would be able to return to work involving light to moderate strain (Table 3).

Table 3. Early postoperative working capacity (2nd study only; $n=177$)[a]

Maximum load	Type of exercise		
	Upright	Supine	Training
25 W	–	2.0	2.5
50 W	3.8	16.3	22.5
75 W	24.0	28.6	66.2
100 W	20.0	26.5	8.7
>100 W	51.9	26.4	–

[a] Results expressed as percentages

Table 4. Rating of subjective improvement

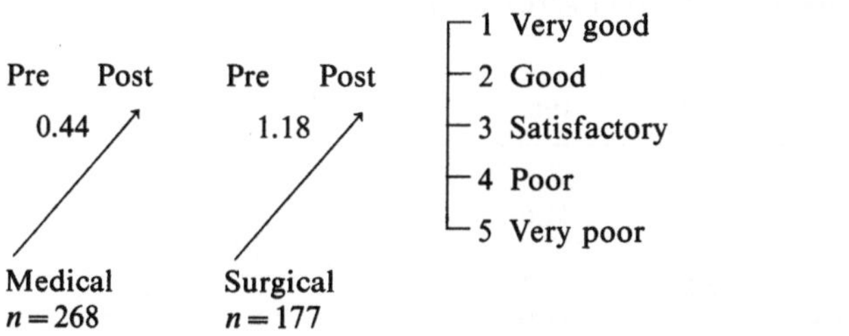

An important aspect of rehabilitation is the subjective well-being of the patient. We asked our patients to rate their state of health on a scale of 1–5 at the time of the first admission and to compare it with their present feeling. Both the medical and the surgical group reported an improvement, but the amelioration in health status was rated greater in the surgical group (+1.18 points), starting from a poorer level, than in the medical group (+0.44 points); the difference was statistically significant ($P<0.5$, Table 4).

From the first to the second study there was a significant increase in the percentage of surgical patients reporting an improvement of their health status from 49% to 78% ($P<0.1$). Concomitantly, the percentage of patients reporting a worsening of their health after surgery decreased from 24% to 5%. We believe that these data reflect on a subjective level the technical improvement of coronary artery bypass surgery in recent years. With medical treatment the number of patients reporting no changes in their health status increased from 24% to 49%, while the number of patients reporting an improvement decreased slightly from 53% to 41% (Table 5).

There were significant differences in the working status of the two groups and also significant trends from the first to the second study. The percentage of patients actually working was always lower in the surgical group than in the medical group. There was also a decrease in the percentage of surgical patients returning to work from 47% to 41% ($P<0.1$) from the first to the second study.

Table 5. Subjective improvement in health status in the medically (M) and surgically (S) treated groups (the first study contained an imcomplete report)

Year		1975	1976	1981	1982
Improved	M	53.3	48.4	45.1	41.7
	S	49.3	55.3	78.1	78.8
Unchanged	M	24.3	28.1	43.1	49.6
	S	16.4	16.0	15.6	15.9
Worsened	M	16.8	17.1	11.8	8.7
	S	24.6	21.5	6.2	5.3

Table 6. Working status following medical (m) or surgical (s) treatment

Year		1975	1976	1981	1982
Working	M	58.7	62.1	57.5	56.5
	S	47.4	48.2	40.6	41.6
Retired	M	34.9	31.4	32.7	24.3
	S	48.7	42.8	53.1	31.0
Other	M	6.4	6.5	9.8	19.2
	S	3.9	9.0	6.3	27.4

Concomitantly, the number of patients who retired after surgery increased to 53%, whereas the number of patients who retired with medical treatment did not change over the years. The lower percentage of retired patients in the cohort of 1982 results from the higher number of patients who were convalescent or ill at the time of the study. The lower percentage of surgical patients who returned to work in 1981 and 1982 despite a significant improvement in the patients' well-being clearly indicates that the changes in the economic situation between 1977 and 1983 may have influenced the decision of the patients and/ or the advise of their physicians to retire (Table 6).

This view is supported by the differences in working status when we examine the various types of occupation. In all four subgroups the number of patients working was significantly lower with surgical than with medical treatment (–4% in self employed to –23.5% in workmen). From the first to the second study there was a further decrease in working patients both in the medical and in the surgical group, but the decrease in the surgical group was significantly more marked. Especially the sharp decrease from 75% to 53% in the subgroup of self-employed patients is indicative of a socioeconomic impact on the decision to retire (Table 7).

Table 7. Return to work after CABS in different occupational groups

	% working			
	1st study		2nd study	
	M	S	M	S
Self-employed	79.6	75.0	72.5	53.6
Employees	76.7	70.7	73.7	58.7
Officials	68.9	53.8	64.6	41.7
Workmen	49.3	25.8	45.8	22.6

Table 8. Length of preoperative absence from work among those surgically treated patients who returned to work

	% working	
Months	1st study	2nd study
-1	26.9%	11.6%
-6	42.3%	51.9%
-12	25.0%	22.2%
>12	5.8%	14.3%
	$n=64$	$n=73$

Another nonmedical factor related to the return to work is the length of the preoperative absence from work. Like others, we found a significant decrease in the percentage of working patients when they had been absent from work for more than 6 months. This held for both the first and the second study. Out of the total of 311 patients who had undergone surgery, 137 patients returned to work, and two-thirds of the working patients had been absent from work for less than 6 months (Table 8). In surgical patients who returned to full-time work, the average length of preoperative absence from work was 109 days; patients who retired after surgery had a mean length of preoperative absence from work of 246 days.

In summary, our data show a marked improvement in working capacity and state of health after coronary artery bypass surgery as compared to the preoperative disability. Despite this, the percentage of patients returning to work after surgery is significantly lower than among patients treated medically. Comparing the two cohorts investigated in 1977 and 1983, we found some evidence that socioeconomic factors may have a greater impact on the working status than medical factors.

Return to Work
After Coronary Artery Bypass Surgery
in Comparison to Coronary Angioplasty

Vocational Rehabilitation After Coronary Angioplasty and Coronary Bypass Surgery

B. Meier, V. Chaves, L. v. Segesser, B. Faidutti, and W. Rutishauser

Introduction

Several studies on employment patterns after coronary artery bypass surgery (CABS) or percutaneous transluminal coronary angioplasty (PTCA) have recently appeared. Johnson et al. (1982) reported on 2229 consecutive male CABS patients. They found that in younger patients employment before and after CABS was equal. In older patients accelerated retirement with CABS became evident. The fraction of patients working without limitation, however, was increased by 20% after CABS. Almeida et al. (1983) gathered data on 2284 consecutive patients. They found that 66% of patients either working at the time of CABS or having discontinued work because of cardiac symptoms returned to work. Danchin et al. (1983) found no improvement in employment after CABS compared to medical treatment in 76 male patients randomly assigned to either therapy.

In contrast to these rather sobering results after CABS, Holmes et al. (1983) reported on 279 patients with successful or failed PTCA in a multicenter survey. Patients with successful PTCA returned to work in 99% of cases, while those with failed PTCA and subsequent surgical treatment did so in 97%.

The present study was undertaken to examine the long-term work status of patients undergoing PTCA at our center and to compare it to that of a group of CABS patients and to the literature.

Methods

The study was carried out retrospectively on 150 consecutive patients treated with PTCA before November 1983 and on 150 consecutive patients treated with CABS by one surgeon before January 1983. All patients were treated at the University Hospital of Geneva. Questionnaires were mailed to all patients thought to be alive and a telephone interview was attempted if they responded incompletely or failed to reply. Objective data were retrieved from the patients' charts.

Results

Comparison Between PTCA and CABS

Of the PTCA and CABS patients addressed, 123 (82%) and 124 (83%), respectively, responded. Of the responders, 99 PTCA patients (80%) and 113 CABS patients (91%) had worked until the intervention or had stopped working for cardiac reasons less than 2 years prior to the intervention. These patients were theoretically supposed to resume work after their intervention, providing the outcome was favorable.

Table 1 compares the baseline characteristics, while Table 2 compares the outcome of these patients after elimination of the 16 patients with failed PTCA.

Table 1. Baseline characteristics of patients supposed to resume work

	PTCA ($n=83$)	CABS ($n=113$)	*P*
Age (years)	51±7	55±8	0.001
Male (%)	92	90	NS
Follow-up (months)	14±12	26±9	0.0001
Vessels involved	1.4±0.6	2.4±0.7	0.0001
Infarction (%)	54	66	NS
Ejection fraction (%)	63±10	58±15	0.01
LVEDP (mmHg)	12±5	17±7	0.05
Angina class	3.0±0.8	2.7±1.0	NS
Cardiac drugs	2.3±0.9	3.0±1.0	0.0001

Table 2. Outcome of patients supposed to resume work

	PTCA ($n=83$)	CABS ($n=113$)	*P*
Work resumed (%)	81	87	NS
- same or more (%)	43	49	NS
- less (%)	38	38	NS
Delay (days)	79±113	148±103	0.001
Hospital stay postintervention (days)	3±2	17±29	0.0001
Angina class postintervention	1.2±1.5	0.7±1.3	0.01
Cardiac drugs postintervention	2.6±1.4	2.1±1.3	0.05
Satisfied (%)	84	94	0.05

Table 3 stratifies the patients into those who had stopped working for cardiac reasons and those who worked up to intervention. The 10 PTCA patients and the 20 CABS patients disabled for cardiac reasons less than 2 years prior to their intervention provide two interesting cohorts. Only 40% of either cohort had a physically demanding profession. They had stopped working a mean of 101 ± 104 (mean ± SD) days (PTCA) and 130 ± 143 days (CABS) before their intervention (NS). Three (30%) of the PTCA patients but 14 (70%) of the CABS patients resumed work after their intervention ($P = 0.04$). However, 9 of these 14 CABS patients resumed work only at a reduced level. Looking at patients returning to at least the same level of work they maintained prior to their cardiac problem, the return to work ratio was 2/10 (20%) in the PTCA group and 5/20 (25%) in the CABS group (NS).

The actual loss of working power due to the interventions themselves can be expressed by the patients working up to the intervention but failing to resume work afterwards. This constellation was found in 9/73 (12%) PTCA patients and 8/93 (9%) CABS patients (NS).

Table 3. Preintervention work status of patients supposed to resume work

	PTCA	CABS
Stopped work for cardiac reasons <2 years prior to intervention	10	20
Worked until intervention	73	93
Total	83	113

Factors Affecting Return to Work Rate

In the search for factors influencing the capacity to work after a revascularizing cardiac intervention, both PTCA and CABS patients were separated into patients resuming an equally or more demanding work (group A) and patients not resuming work or resuming work at a lower level only (group B).

PTCA. Of the PTCA patients 36/83 (43%) qualified for group A and 47/83 (57%) for group B. There was no difference between A and B in terms of age, sex, follow-up time, preintervention ejection fraction or left ventricular end-diastolic pressure, angina class pre- or postintervention, cardiac drug intake preintervention, or continuation of smoking. The parameters probably associated with return to normal work are listed in Table 4.

CABS. Of the CABS patients 55/113 (49%) qualified for group A and 58/113 (51%) for group B. There was no difference between A and B in terms of age, sex, type of work, follow-up time, vessel involvement, history of myocardial infarction, preintervention ejection fraction or left ventricular end-diastolic pressure, angina class pre- or postintervention, hospital stay postintervention, or continuation of smoking. Parameters probably associated with return to normal work are listed in Table 5.

Table 4. Factors associated with return to normal work in PTCA patients

	Back to same or more work ($n=36$)	Back to less or no work ($n=47$)	*P*
Cardiac drugs postintervention	1.8 ± 1.2	3.1 ± 1.2	0.0001
Previous infarction (%)	39	67	0.02
Satisfied (%)	94	77	0.03
Physical work (%)	33	53	0.07[a]
Hospital stay postintervention (days)	2.5 ± 1.6	3.4 ± 2.8	0.08[a]
Vessels involved	1.2 ± 0.4	1.5 ± 0.8	0.08[a]

[a] *P* values between 0.10 and 0.05 are considered to show tendencies only

Table 5. Factors associated with return to normal work in CABS patients

	Back to same or more Work ($n=55$)	Back to less or no work ($n=58$)	*P*
Cardiac drugs postintervention	1.8 ± 1.0	2.5 ± 1.4	0.01
Cardiac drugs preintervention	2.8 ± 1.0	3.3 ± 1.0	0.02
Satisfied (%)	98	89	0.06[a]

[a] Considered to show tendency only

Discussion

The return to work rate was not different after PTCA or CABS. Of the PTCA patients 81% and of the CABS patients 87% resumed work. Discounting patients resuming work only at a level inferior to that before the intervention, the figures are 43% for PTCA and 49% for CABS. The overall loss in the potential work force of about 15% with both PTCA and CABS comprises about 10% not resuming work although they had worked up to the procedure (disability directly linked to the procedure) and 5% not resuming work who had previously been disabled (failure of procedure to remedy disability). It is of interest that successful PTCA produces as much disability as CABS. Only psychosocial factors can account for that.

In the small subgroup of CABS patients previously disabled, return to work was found more often than in the respective subgroup of PTCA patients. Yet, most CABS patients resumed work at a reduced level. This signifies a superior potential of CABS to restore some degree of work capacity but an equally poor potential of both procedures (20% PTCA, 25% CABS) to restore normal work capacity.

Almeira et al. (1983) have found in a cumulative literature review of about 7500 patients that the percentage of patients working before and after CABS was 60% and 63%, respectively. The range of patients working before CABS (22%–91%) was much wider than after CABS (51%–74%). This reflects the differences in definitions of pre-CABS work status. Johnson et al. (1982) found a decline of the percentage of working patients after CABS, which they at least partially explained by a normal decline with time and coronary heart disease. While the results in our CABS patients are in keeping with most studies in the literature, the results in our PTCA patients are inferior to those reported by Holmes et al. (1983), who described a decline of only 2% in patients working after PTCA. This must be explained by differences in patient selection, post-procedural guidance of patients, and local socioeconomic factors but not by PTCA technique, since the cited study showed no difference in terms of the success or failure of PTCA.

Our PTCA data correspond fairly well to those reported in an abstract on 163 PTCA patients and 151 CABS patients by Jang et al. (1982). However, the superiority in the return to work rate of PTCA over CABS described there was not found here. This speaks even more in favor of our CABS results considering that the groups of PTCA patients and CABS patients compared in this paper have significant differences in their baseline characteristics (Table 1) which are unfavorable to CABS patients: CABS patients were older, had a longer follow-up time, had involvement of more vessels, had a worse ejection fraction and higher end-diastolic left ventricular pressure before the intervention, and took a larger number of different cardiac medications before the intervention.

Our CABS patients fared better than our PTCA patients in terms of having less angina, taking fewer cardiac medications, and being more often satisfied after their intervention (Table 2). However, they paid for their improvement more dearly, which is expressed by a five times longer hospital stay and a twice as long delay before resuming work.

The factor associated most closely with failure to resume normal work was the number of different cardiac medications taken at the time of the postinterventional survey. This was not paralleled by anginal pain, which may indicate overprotection by physicians tending to treat the patients more vigorously than needed and to keep them away from work longer than necessary. A similar phenomenon has to be suspected of being behind the long delays before resuming work of 79 days after PTCA and 148 days after CABS, which especially in the case of PTCA are totally unjustified by the intervention per se and reflect a certain lack of confidence in this relatively new mode of therapy.

We conclude that neither PTCA nor CABS improved the overall ability to work of an unselected group of patients in Geneva. PTCA brought patients back to work sooner, but CABS showed a more impressive improvement in a number of subjective and objective follow-up findings.

References

Almeida D, Bradford JM, Wenger NK, King SB, Hurst JW (1983) Return to work after coronary bypass surgery. Circulation 68-II:205–213

Danchin N, David P, Bourassa MG (1983) Coronary artery surgery as a measure of vocational rehabilitation: an analysis of the working status of patients with mild angina randomly assigned to medical or surgical treatment. Eur Heart J 4:687–690

Holmes DR, Vlietstra RE, Mock MB, Smith HC, Dorros G, Cowley MJ, Kent KM, Hammes LN, Janke L, Elveback LR, Vetrovec GW (1983) Employment and recreation patterns in patients treated by percutaneous transluminal coronary angioplasty: a multicenter study. Am J Cardiol 52:710–713

Jang GC, Gruentzig AR, Block PC, Cowley MJ, Dorros C, Holmes DR, Kent KM, Leatherman LL, Myler RK, Stertzer SH, Sjolander M, Williams DO (1982) Work profile of patients following coronary angioplasty or coronary bypass surgery: results from a national cooperative study [Abstr]. Circulation 66-II:123

Johnson WD, Kayser KL, Pedraza PM, Shore RT (1982) Employment patterns in males before and after myocardial revascularization surgery. Circulation 65:1086–1093

Return to Work After Coronary Angioplasty

C. Vallbracht, G. Kober, D. Scherer, and M. Kaltenbach

Introduction

Considerable advances have been made in transluminal coronary angioplasty (Mock et al. 1982) since Grüntzig introduced the technique in 1977 (Grüntzig et al. 1977). Once steerable dilatation catheters became available to treat difficult-to-reach stenoses, cases of multiple-vessel disease were gradually added to the patient population.

As experience was acquired, the indication for single coronary bypass was less frequently established than was that for TCA, and single bypass surgery has already become the exception. The extent to which a similar trend is to be expected for multiple-vessel disease cannot be adequately assessed at present.

More than 800 transluminal coronary angioplasties (TCA) were performed between October 1977 and May 1984 at our hospital in Frankfurt. The experience of the first few years is reflected in the rapid rise of both the absolute values and the acute success rate (defined as at least a 20% reduction in the degree of stenosis), which rose from an overall rate of 36% initially to 73.9% at present and is approximately 80% for stenoses in the LAD (Fig. 1).

The complication rate with dissection and subsequent emergency bypass operation, however, remained between 4.5% and 5.8%: results that agree with

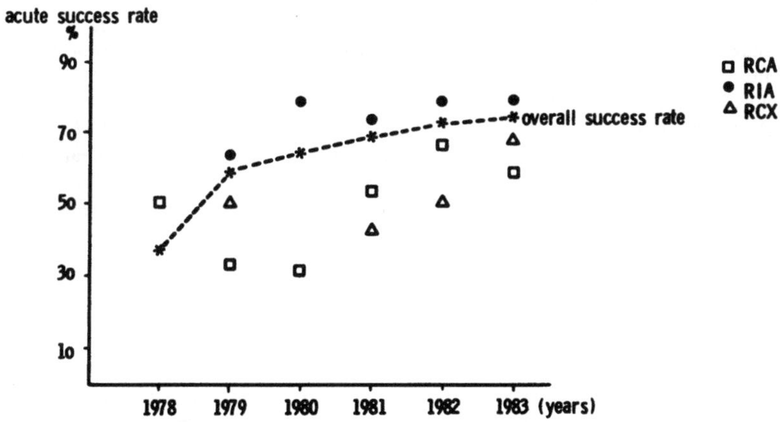

Fig. 1. Acute success rate of transluminal coronary angioplasty in Frankfurt, 1978–1983 (definition: 20% reduction in % diameter stenosis)

those reported by other study groups (Stertzer et al. 1982; Mock et al. 1982; Margolis 1982). Recurrence rate statistics, by contrast, still vary considerably; 33.6% of the 557 patients followed by coronary angiography and included in the NHLBI registry for TCA (November, 1983) suffered a recurrence.

Using the same definition of recurrence (maintenance of less than 50% of acute success *or* restenosis of more than 30%), we found only a 17% recurrence rate in 439 follow-up angiographies. Most of these recurrences were already recognizable on angiograms made 3 months after TCA.

The purpose of our study, which is still going on, was to analyze the length of occupational disability, symptoms, and occupational rehabilitation 4-6 years after TCA in comparison with bypass surgery.

Patients and Methods

The first long-term results were obtained by surveying 104 patients who underwent coronary dilatation in Frankfurt between 1978 and 1980 (54 with initial success and 50 without initial success), and who had either been working before therapy or had stopped work for cardiac reasons.

The 54 patients who were dilatated with initial success were questioned about current angina symptoms and subsequent bypass surgery or redilatation, and the answers compared with those of 52 patients who underwent bypass surgery during the same period and had also been working before therapy or had stopped for cardiac reasons (Table 1). Other important factors investigated were occupational rehabilitation with return to previous employment or disability retirement (Table 1).

Table 1. Characteristics and outcome of patients 4-6 years after TCA or bypass surgery

	TCA	Bypass surgery
Number	54	52
Mean age	55.6 years	58.4 years
Male	84%	86%
Questionnaires answered	88%	84%
Return to work	33 (61.1%) mean age 52.7 years	13 (25%) mean age 55.2 years
No return to work	21 (38.9%) mean age 58.5 years	38 (75%) mean age 61.5 years

Results

Of the 54 patients with coronary angioplasty between 1978 and 1980, 33 (66.1%) returned to full-time employment - 29 (53.7%) to their previous job and 4 (7.4%) to another occupation. The mean age of those who returned to work was 52.7 years and that of those who did not return to work, 58.5 years.

Of the 52 patients who underwent bypass surgery during the same period, 13 (25%) returned to full-time employment: 11 (21.1%) to their old job and 2 (3.8%) to a different occupation. The mean age of those returning to work was 55.2 years and that of those who did not return to work, 61.5 years.

The overall mean length of occupational disability in the TCA group was 24.2 weeks: 16.8 weeks before and 7.4 weeks after dilatation. The overall mean length of occupational disability in the bypass surgery group was 63.5 weeks: 25.4 weeks before and 38.1 weeks after bypass surgery (Table 2, Fig. 2).

Table 2. Return to work after TCA or bypass surgery

	TCA	Bypass surgery
Number	33 (66.1%)	13 (25%)
Mean age	52.7 years	55.2 years
Occupational disability before intervention	16.8 weeks	25.4 weeks
Occupational disability after intervention	7.4 weeks (2/3 0–3 weeks)	38.1 weeks (70% 13–24 weeks)
Mean length	24.2 weeks	63.5 weeks

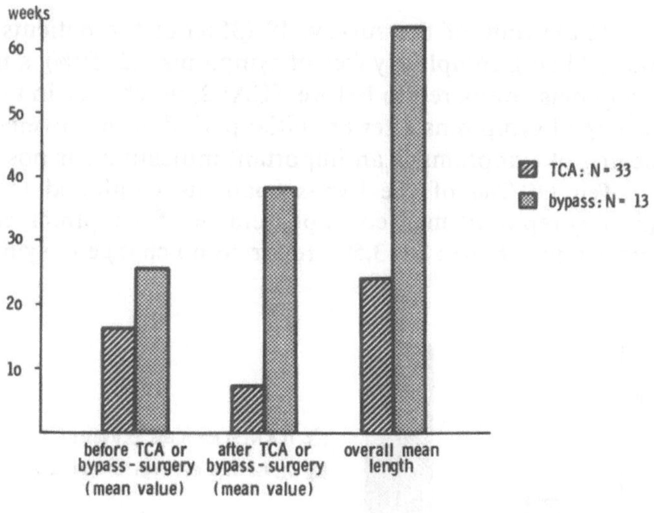

Fig. 2. Occupational disability before and after TCA and bypass surgery

A closer analysis of the length of occupational disability after TCA indicated that two-thirds of the patients had already returned to work within 0–3 weeks after TCA; this corresponds more or less to the 2-week convalescent period we recommend at discharge (Fig. 3).

Analysis of the length of occupational disability after bypass surgery revealed that approximately 70% of the patients who returned to work reported a sick leave of 13–24 weeks and 30%, considerably longer leaves (Fig. 4).

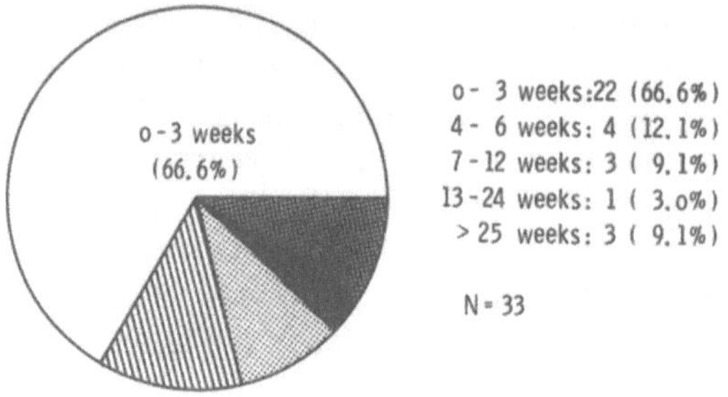

Fig. 3. Occupational disability after TCA

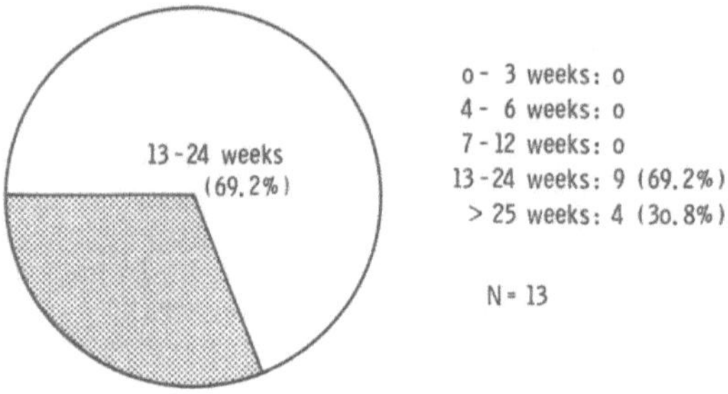

Fig. 4. Occupational disability after bypass surgery

At the time of the survey, 19 (35%) of the patients in the TCA group reported being completely free of symptoms; 32 (59%), a marked improvement in symptoms compared to before TCA; 2, no change in symptoms; and 1, a worsening of symptoms after an initial period of improvement. This return or worsening of symptoms is an important indication for possible recurrence.

Ten (19.2%) of the bypass patients continued to be symptom free; 30 (57.7%) reported marked improvement of symptoms compared to the period preceding surgery; 7 (13.5%) reported no change in symptoms; and 5 (9.6%) re-

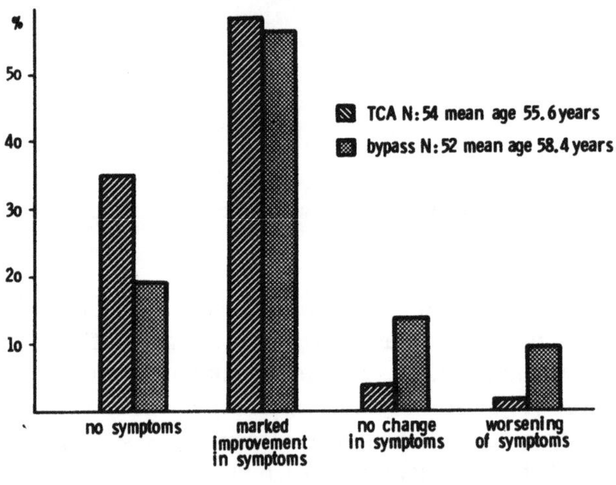

Fig. 5. Symptoms 4–6 years after TCA or bypass surgery

ported a return or worsening of symptoms after an initial period of improvement (Fig. 5).

Discussion

The role played by psychosocial and economic aspects, in addition to many other factors, in the comparison of two different methods of treating the same disease should not be underestimated. One important question in this regard is the different lengths of occupational disability, a factor which, in some cases, could be crucial for reintegration in the workplace.

Even though statistics on the percentage of patients from both groups who returned to work are considerably influenced by the age differences (some patients in the bypass group had reached retirement age), there was a greater tendency for retirement in the bypass surgery group, even in the younger patients; this was possibly due to external influences, such as advice from a family physician or colleagues, or to the impressive experience of thoracic surgery. For obvious reasons, it is virtually impossible to confirm this thesis. Thus we cannot say whether there is a significant difference in return to work after TCA and bypass surgery at present.

With regard to the patients with a continued marked improvement of symptoms, the frequency of which was roughly the same in both groups, the significance of the impressively high number of patients with continued absence of symptoms in the TCA group is qualified somewhat by the age difference and the higher incidence of two- and three-vessel disease in the bypass group. Continued improvement or absence of symptoms, however, seems to be an important indication for a good 5-year, long-term result of TCA.

The most important finding, in our opinion, was the considerably shorter sick leaves after TCA: two-thirds of patients had already returned to work within 0–3 weeks after coronary dilatation. This observation, which was recently also reported by the study group in Krotzingen (Stürzenhofecker et al. 1983), could encourage the trend to extend the indications for TCA.

References

Grüntzig A, Myler R, Hanna E, Turina M (1977) Transluminal angioplasty of coronary artery stenosis. Circulation [Suppl] 84:55–56

Margolis JR (1982) The role of the percutaneous intraaortic balloon in emergency situations following percutaneous transluminal coronary angioplasty. In: Kaltenbach M, et al (eds) Transluminal coronary angioplasty intracoronary thrombolysis. Springer, Berlin Heidelberg New York

Mock MB, Kent KK, Bentivoglio LG, Block PC, Bourassa M, Cowley MJ, Detre K, Dorros G, Gosselin J, Grüntzig A, Myler R, Simpson J, Stertzer SH, Williams DO, Mullin SM, Costa B, Mitchell H, and participating Medical Centres (1982) The National Heart, Lung, and Blood Institute percutaneous transluminal coronary angioplasty registry: The first 1116 cases. In: Kaltenbach M, et al (eds) Transluminal coronary angioplasty and intracoronary thrombolysis. Springer, Berlin Heidelberg New York

Stertzer SH, Myler RK, Wallsh E, Bruno MS (1982) Transluminal coronary angioplasty: results, complications, follow-up and consideration of indications. An analysis of 409 procedures. In: Kaltenbach M, et al (eds) Transluminal coronary angioplasty and intracoronary thrombolysis. Springer, Berlin Heidelberg New York

Stürzenhofecker P, Petersen J, Betz P, Schnellbacher K, Roskamm H (1983) Coronarangioplastie versus Bypass-Operation bei coronarer 1-Gefäßerkrankung. Vergleich von funktionellem Resultat, beruflicher Wiedereingliederung und Risiko. Herbsttagung der Deutschen Gesellschaft für Herz- und Kreislaufforschung, Ulm/Neu-Ulm

Work Status and Percutaneous Transluminal Coronary Angioplasty

F. Boulay, P. David, P. R. David, and M. G. Bourassa

Since the first successful percutaneous transluminal coronary angioplasty (PTCA) was performed in man in September 1977 (Grüntzig 1978), the results of this nonoperative approach to the treatment of patients with coronary artery disease have been increasingly positive. Although coronary artery bypass graft surgery (CABG) appears to improve the quality of life and to prolong survival in selected subsets of patients, it has apparently failed to affect employment and recreational status (National Institutes of Health Consensus - Development Conference Statement 1981; Oberman et al. 1983; CASS Principal Investigators and Their Associates 1983, p 939–950). This new alternative to CABG may provide greater beneficial effects on cardiac rehabilitation in selected patients. To assess the potential socioeconomic impact of this new technique, we evaluated prospectively the work status of our first 158 patients before and after PTCA.

Material and Methods

Between February 1980 and March 1982, PTCA was attempted at our Institution on 177 coronary segments in 158 consecutive patients with severe angina pectoris, objective evidence of transient myocardial ischemia, a recent coronary angiogram showing at least one coronary artery stenosis of 70% or more, suitable for CABG, and several of the commonly accepted angiographic criteria for PTCA (Grüntzig et al. 1979).

Our patient population included 114 men and 44 women with a mean age of 50 ± 10 (range 30–76) years. The baseline clinical and angiographic profile of the patients is shown in Table 1.

Coronary angiograms in multiple views were performed before and after the procedure and PTCA was carried out through a percutaneous femoral approach using Grüntzig's technique (Grüntzig et al. 1979). Successful PTCA was defined as a persistent increase in luminal diameter of 20% or more, with a residual mean transstenotic pressure gradient less than 20 mmHg.

Baseline and follow-up data forms similar to those used in the National Heart, Lung, and Blood Institute PTCA Registry were completed before and 6 months and 1 year after PTCA. Work status was coded as full-time (40 h per week or more), part-time (less than 40 h per week), retired (age related), or unemployed. Time to return to work was the interval from the date of PTCA to the date of return to work. Information on recreational status and disability

Table 1. Clinical and angiographic profile of 158 patients in whom PTCA was attempted

Age: $\overline{X} \pm SD$, years	50.3 ± 10.2	(30–76)
Sex: men/women	114/44	
Duration of angina: $\overline{X} \pm SD$, months	18.1 ± 26.1	(1–120)
Duration of present level of symptoms: $\overline{X} \pm SD$, months	4.3 ± 5.7	(25–52)
Anginal symptoms:		
Stable effort angina, functional class[a] I–II	64	41%
III–IV	37	23%
Variant angina	15	9%
Unstable angina (variant angina excluded)	42	27%
Medical history		
Prior myocardial infarction	18	11%
Prior unstable angina	45	28%
Prior bypass surgery	11	7%
Extent of coronary artery disease		
1-vessel disease	130	82%
2-vessel disease	22	14%
3-vessel disease	5	3%
Left main disease	1	0.6%
Ventricular function at rest		
Normal	120	76%
Abnormal	31	20%

[a] Canadian Cardiovascular Society Classification (Campeau 1976)

was also recorded. Life-style was coded as active (physically demanding activities or sports) or sedentary. Limitation by disease was defined as a restriction of activity by the patient's medical condition.

Of these 158 patients, 15 retired before PTCA and 1 suffered a myocardial infarction after PTCA and died suddenly 2 weeks later. Thus, work status data were available at 6 months and at 1 year in 142 and 103 consecutive patients respectively.

Statistical differences were determined by chi-square tests for discrete variables and *t*-tests for continuous variables. A P value of less than 0.05 was considered statistically significant.

Results

Work Status Before and After Successful or Unsuccessful PTCA

Employment patterns for all patients are shown in Table 2. In these consecutive patients, 84% were working before PTCA, 79% at 6 months, and 89% at 1 year. The percentage of patients working full-time did not differ before and after PTCA. Of 119 patients who were working before PTCA, 5 stopped working upon reaching retirement age, while 19 (16%) and 95 (80%) respectively were not working and working 6 months later. Among 23 patients unemployed at baseline, 1 retired, 5 remained unemployed and 17 (74%) returned to work (4 only part-time).

Table 2. Work status of patients before and after PTCA with or without CABG

	Baseline		Month following PTCA 6		12	
	$n=142$		$n=142$		$n=103$	
Working full-time	113	80%	106	75%	84	81%
Working part-time	6	4%	6	4%	8	8%
Retired	0		6	4%	2	2%
Unemployed	23	16%	24	17%	9	9%

Work Status and the Initial Results of PTCA

Among our first 158 patients, PTCA was unsuccessful in 55 (35%); 71% of them underwent CABG, which was performed within 24 h of attempted PTCA in 88% (urgent CABG in 49%). Among the clinical and angiographic variables, two significant pretreatment determinants of successful PTCA were observed in this group: stable versus unstable angina (68% versus 50%, $P<0.05$) and normal versus abnormal left ventricular function (71% versus 42%, $P<0.005$).

Work status was assessed in the following three subsets according to the initial results of PTCA: (1) 94 patients with successful PTCA, (2) 12 patients with unsuccessful PTCA who received subsequent medical therapy, and (3) 36 patients with unsuccessful PTCA who underwent CABG, performed within 24 h of attempted PTCA in 86%.

The employment patterns for patients in these three subsets are shown in Table 3. There were no differences in occupational status before PTCA. In patients with successful PTCA, 87% were working before treatment, 81% at 6 months, and 91% at 1 year, as compared with 81%, 83%, and 89%, respectively, of PTCA plus CABG patients. In the smaller group of medically treated patients, lower percentages of patients at work were observed before and after PTCA (67% and 50% respectively).

Of 82 successfully treated patients who were working before PTCA, 4 stopped working upon reaching retirement age, while 11 (13%) and 67 (82%) re-

Table 3. Employment patterns before and after PTCA according to initial results and subsequent treatment

	% of patients working according to initial PTCA result		
	Successful PTCA	PTCA plus CABG	PTCA plus medical therapy
Baseline	87% $n=94$	81% $n=36$	67% $n=12$
At 6 months	81% $n=94$	83% $n=36$	50% $n=12$
At 1 year	91% $n=69$	89% $n=27$	71% $n=7$

spectively were not working and working 6 months later. Among 12 successful PTCA patients unemployed at baseline, 1 retired, 2 remained unemployed, and 9 (75%) returned to work.

Variables Influencing Return to Work After Successful PTCA

Although the numbers are small, there was no major pretreatment difference in age, sex, previous infarction, limitation by disease, life-style, or work status between successfully dilated patients working and not working at 6 months (Table 4). In all 103 successfully treated patients coronary angiograms were repeated 6 months after PTCA or whenever there was clinical suspicion of recurrence. Recurrence of stenosis was defined as a restenosis of 30% or more with regard to the immediate post-PTCA angiogram. Restenosis was documented in 31 of 103 successfully dilated patients (30%). A second PTCA was successful in 21 of 23 patients (91%). During follow-up, recurrence of angina, limitation by disease, and/or restenosis with or without a second PTCA did not alter the return to work at 6 months (Table 5).

Table 4. Pretreatment variables and return to work 6 months after successful PTCA

Variables	Return to work	
	Number/ total patients	%
Age (yrs) <50	41/53	77
≧50	35/41	85
Sex Male	56/70	80
Female	20/24	83
Prior myocardial infarction		
Absent	67/84	80
Present	9/10	90
Limitation by disease		
Present	61/78	78
Absent	15/16	94
Life-style		
Active	57/71	80
Sedentary	19/23	83
Work status before PTCA		
Working	67/82	82
Not working	9/12	75

Time to Return to Work

The time delay between attempted PTCA and return to work was significantly shorter in the successfully treated group than in the PTCA plus CABG group

Table 5. Follow-up variables and return to work 6 months after successful PTCA

Variables	Return to work	
	Number/ total patients	%
Angina during follow-up		
Absent	42/54	78
Present	34/40	85
Limitation by disease		
Absent	58/72	81
Present	18/22	82
Restenosis		
Absent	48/63	76
Present	28/31	90
Repeat PTCA		
Absent	56/72	78
Present	20/22	91

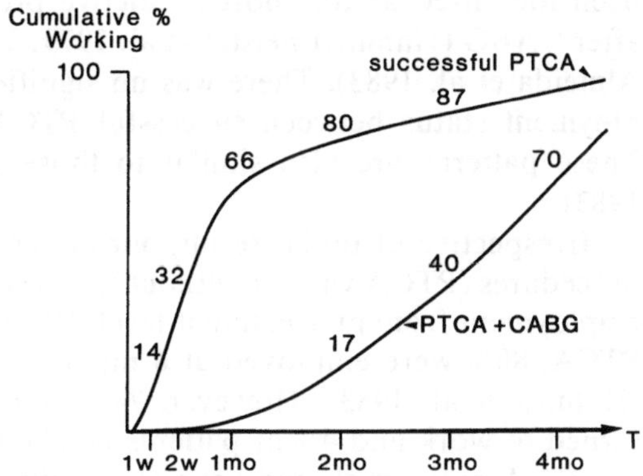

Fig. 1. Time to return to work after successful PTCA and PTCA plus CABG. Cumulative percentage of patients working against time

(41.2 ± 42.2 days versus 119.7 ± 37.6 days, $P < 0.001$). The time to return to work of medically treated patients was also short (36.8 ± 46.1 days). In successfully dilated patients, 14% returned to work within 1 week and 66% within 1 month, whereas in PTCA plus CABG patients, 60% returned to work after the third month (Fig. 1).

Discussion

Work status and factors influencing return to work after CABG have been well studied (Boulay et al. 1982; Johnson et al. 1982; Smith et al. 1982; Almeida et al. 1983). Despite relief of angina and advances in the medical management of postoperative patients, CABG has apparently not succeeded in returning more patients to gainful employment (Oberman et al. 1983). In the CASS randomized collaborative study, similar employment and recreational patterns were observed after medical and surgical therapy of patients with stable ischemic heart disease despite improvement in quality of life in the surgical group (CASS Principal Investigators and Their Associates 1983, p 951–960).

PTCA is an alternative treatment for highly selected patients. According to the initial selection criteria, it was estimated that 5%–10% of patients undergoing CABG are potential candidates for PTCA (Gosselin et al. 1980; Hamby and Katz 1980). A randomized assignment to either PTCA or CABG would provide the most reliable information for comparisons of the impact of these procedures on work status. In June 1979, the NIH PTCA workshop group concluded that because of the rapidly changing technology, the need for further refinement of indications, and the limited number of suitable patients, a randomized clinical trial would be premature. Pending such a trial, this preliminary analysis, based on our first 158 cases, provides useful information for comparisons of percentages of employed patients and time to return to work after successful PTCA and unsuccessful PTCA plus CABG.

The selection criteria of patients and the 65% success rate of PTCA are similar to those reported in previous studies during the same period (Grüntzig et al. 1979; Vlietstra et al. 1981; Kent et al. 1982). Preoperative work status has been identified as the most predictive pretreatment factor of return to work after CABG (Hammermeister et al. 1979; Boulay et al. 1982; Smith et al. 1982; Almeida et al. 1983). There was no significant difference in pretreatment employment status between successful PTCA and PTCA plus CABG patients. These patterns are also similar to those previously reported (Holmes et al. 1983).

Irrespective of initial result, our patients who underwent revascularization procedures (PTCA with or without CABG) did not have an overall reduction in employment from pretreatment level. Of the patients who were working before PTCA, 80% were employed at 6 months, a lower rate than in another report (Holmes et al. 1983). However, 74% of patients unemployed at baseline returned to work and 4% of patients reached retirement age during follow-up.

PTCA patients should have an excellent rate of return to work because of the selection criteria and a low prevalence of protracted disability or unemployment before treatment (Holmes et al. 1983). High percentages of employment were observed in successful PTCA and PTCA plus CABG patients (81% and 83% at 6 months, and 91% and 89% at 1 year, respectively). In the somewhat smaller group of PTCA plus CABG patients, the postoperative employment rate is similar to that reported in our previous studies (Boulay et al. 1982). Slightly lower percentages were reported in a previous larger study (Holmes et al. 1982). In another report, the PTCA patient group ($n = 163$) had a significantly higher employment rate than a comparable group of CABG patients ($n = 151$) after a mean follow-up of 19 ± 7 months (Jang et al. 1982).

The effect of pretreatment variables on work status following successful PTCA could not be demonstrated, probably because of the small number of patients. At 6 months, 85% of patients with angina during follow-up were working. Similarly, restenosis with or without repeated PTCA did not alter return to work (90% of these patients were employed at 6 months).

Patients who had successful PTCA returned to work significantly sooner than did PTCA plus CABG patients. A shorter time to return to work for patients with successful PTCA has previously been reported (Jang et al. 1982, Holmes et al. 1983).

The impact of selection biases on the results is uncertain, although the patient groups (successful PTCA and PTCA plus CABG) appeared to have similar baseline clinical profiles. Larger studies are needed to identify the variables influencing work status following PTCA, and a randomized trial would provide the most reliable information.

Conclusion

The present analysis of our initial PTCA experience did not indicate an improvement in work status after successful PTCA alone or after unsuccessful PTCA followed by elective CABG. However, a marked difference in the time to return to work between the two groups suggests a socioeconomic benefit in the short and mid-term management of successful PTCA patients.

References

Almeida D, Bradford JM, Wenger NK, King SB, Hurst JW (1983) Return to work after coronary bypass surgery. Circulation [Suppl II] 68:205–213

Boulay FM, David P, Bourassa MG (1982) Strategies for improving the work status of patients after coronary artery bypass surgery. Circulation [Suppl III] 66:43–49

Campeau L (1976) Grading of angina pectoris. Circulation 54:522–523

CASS Principal Investigators and Their Associates (1983) Coronary artery surgery study (CASS): A randomized trial of coronary artery bypass surgery. Survival data. Circulation 68:939–960

Gosselin AJ, Fisher L, Judkins MP, Ryan TJ, Vliestra RE, Kemp HC, Gillespie MJ, Mock MB (1980) Percutaneous transluminal angioplasty: an estimate of the number of possible candidates for the CASS registry. In: Proceedings of the workshop on percutaneous transluminal coronary angioplasty. (NIH Publication No. 80–2030) National Institute of Health, Washington DC, p 89

Grüntzig AR (1978) Transluminal dilatation of coronary artery stenosis. Lancet I:263

Grüntzig AR, Senning Å, Slegenthalter WE (1979) Non-operative dilatation of coronary-artery stenosis: percutaneous transluminal coronary angioplasty. N Engl J Med 301:61–68

Hamby RI, Katz S (1980) Percutaneous transluminal coronary angioplasty: its potential impact on surgery for coronary artery disease. Am J Cardiol 45:1161–1166

Hammermeister KE, DeRouen TA, English MT, Dodge MT (1979) Effect of surgical versus medical therapy on return to work in patients with coronary artery disease. Am J Cardiol 44:105–111

Holmes DR, Vlietstra RE, Mock MB, Smith HC, Cowley MJ, Kent KM, Detre KM (1982) Follow-up of patients undergoing percutaneous transluminal coronary angioplasty (PTCA): a report from the NHLBI PTCA Registry. Am J Cardiol 49:916

Holmes DR, Vlietstra RE, Mock MB, Smith HC, Dorros G, Cowley MJ, Kent KM, Hammes LN, Janke L, Elveback LR, Vetrovec GW (1983) Employment and recreation patterns in patients treated by percutaneous transluminal coronary angioplasty: a multicenter study. Am J Cardiol 52:710–713

Jang GC, Grüntzig AR, Block PC, Cowley MJ, Dorros G, Holmes DR, Kent KM, Leathermann LL, Myler RK, Stertzer SH, Sjolander M, Williams DO (1982) Work profile of patients following coronary angioplasty or coronary bypass surgery: results from a national cooperative study. Circulation [Suppl II] 66:123

Johnson WD, Kayser KL, Pedraza PM, Shore RT (1982) Employment patterns in males before and after myocardial revascularization surgery. A study of 2229 consecutive male patients followed for as long as 10 years. Circulation 65:1086–1093

Kent KM, Bentivoglio LG, Block PC, Cowley MJ, Dorros G, Gosselin AJ, Grüntzig A, Myler RK, Sympson J, Stertzer SH, Williams DO, Fisher L, Gillespie MJ, Detre K, Kelsey S, Mullin SM, Mock MB (1982) Percutaneous transluminal coronary angioplasty. Report from the registry of the National Heart, Lung, and Blood Institute. Am J Cardiol 49:2011–2020

National Institutes of Health Consensus - Development Conference Statement (1981) Coronary artery bypass surgery. Scientific and clinical aspects. N Engl J Med 304:680–684

Oberman A, Wayne JB, Kouchoukos NT, Charles ED, Russel RO, Rogers WJ (1983) Employment status after coronary artery bypass surgery. Circulation [Suppl II] 65:115–119

Smith HC, Hammes LN, Gupta S, Vlietstra RE, Elveback L (1982) Employment status after coronary artery bypass surgery. Circulation [Suppl II] 65:120–125

Vlietstra RE, Holmes DR, Smith HC, Hartzler GO, Orszulak TA (1981) Percutaneous transluminal coronary angioplasty: initial Mayo Clinic experience. Mayo Clin Proc 56:287–293

Return to Work After Thrombolysis According to the Subsequent Treatment

C. Coustry-Degré, E. Stoupel, P. Vandermoten, J. L. Leclerc, J. Struyven, and S. Degré

Introduction

The rate of return to work after thrombolysis followed by medical or surgical treatment was retrospectively analyzed in comparison with the rate in patients who had suffered an infarction and been treated according to the usual management but without a physical rehabilitation program.

Material

Of 270 patients suffering an acute myocardial infarction who were admitted to the C.C.U. in 1982–1983, 54 underwent thrombolysis by the intracoronary route:

- Three patients died during the first few hours after thrombolysis.
- Twenty patients were not operated after thrombolysis because they suffered from a one-vessel disease other than that of the left descending artery.
- Three patients were submitted to percutaneous transluminal coronary angioplasty during the 48 h, after thrombolysis.
- Twenty-eight patients were operated within 72 h.

Results

In the patients at work before their acute myocardial infarction (50%), we analyzed their professional situation 4–6 months after thrombolysis and various forms of accompanying treatment:

- 93% were at work after thrombolysis and surgery.
- 100% were at work after thrombolysis and PTCA.
- 66% were at work after thrombolysis and medical treatment.

These percentages were very similar to those observed retrospectively in the patients with an acute myocardial infarction who had been treated in the usual way:

- 90% of patients returned to work 4–6 months after myocardial infarction and coronary bypass surgery performed between the second and third month after the infarction.

- 70% of patients returned to work in the same conditions after myocardial infarction but without surgery.

No statistical differences were observed between the different groups of patients according to age, job, or psychological and economic status. The criteria for surgical treatment were the same in the different groups. The physical working capacity was statistically greater in the surgical groups with or without thrombolysis.

Conclusions

At mid-term follow-up, surgical treatment seems to be an important factor in the return to work; this fact can be related to better physical working capacity, psychological well-being, and quality of life. The short time lapse between the acute event and surgery or PTCA also plays a significant role.

Summary of the Discussion

P. G. Hugenholtz

Chairman: There is one technical question to you, Dr. Meier. You used the word able to work. Do you mean one *should* be able to work in your point of view? What exactly was the definition by which you considered them fit to work?

Meier: Those patients who worked up to the time of the treatment. Of course, they should be able to work again after the intervention, unless one treated them badly. And as for those patients who stopped working because of their cardiac problem, if you are able to fix their cardiac problem, they should go back to work. We only looked at those patients, not at retired people, or individuals who had been out of work for years.

Chairman: So basically your definition is: people whom **you** considered fit before and able to work after you had fixed whatever was wrong with them.

Satter: I am really surprised to hear that PTCA does not have a much better success rate than surgery, because there is no question that the morbidity of this procedure is much less. Maybe it is due to the fact that the success rate is defined as a decrease of the stenosis by 20%. If you would increase this, maybe to 50% reduction in stenosis, then the superiority of this procedure should be quite clear.

Chairman: Well, I wonder whether we all agree with you that the definition is just the reduction in gradient or the improvement in angiographic appearance. I thought we were talking about the relief of symptoms. Isn't PTCA measured by that mainly?

Satter: Right, because if you consider a reduction of a stenosis of 20% successful and the patient still has angina, I doubt whether this can be called a successful procedure.

Chairman: As far as symptoms are concerned on the average, bypass surgery yields greater relief of symptoms that PTCA can at present, but we are not talking about the same anatomy. I would give the figures worldwide for relief after successful PTCA defined by symptom relief in the neighborhood of 80%, depending on the vessel affected, and a little on the clinic, since results still depend on the experience of the operator. For bypass surgery the figure is closer to 90%.

Q: I wanted to say if one could consider an anatomical reduction of 50% a success, then one should have 100% success rate with complete disappearance of clinical symptoms in PTCA. This would be, I think, a goal which all of as would want to achieve.

Meier: I agree with the point that when we say here successful PTCA we do not always mean that it really has solved the patients problem. But I do not agree that if we change the definition, which by the way was taken up by the NIH and has worked nicely so far, from 20% to 50%, it would change a lot of things. This is because you would still call a PTCA successful according to this definition in a patient where there may be another stenosis around which you did not attempt. Or in the condition where you have increased that other lumen considerably but some flow impairment remains, with a pressure gradient. Then you would still wind up with 10%–20% of the patients continuing to have some chest pains.

Chairman: In comparing the results of PTCA to surgical treatment of coronary artery bypass grafting have you compared the pre-operative characteristics, particularly in relation to the severity of disease between the two groups? And are you justified to compare those sorts of things?

Boulay: No, on one of my slides I indicate that the determinants of initial success were mainly anatomic. Two clinical characteristics were different between these two groups: left ventricular function and unstable angina. So it is wise to say that in terms of these two clinical variables, the two groups I compared were different.

Furthermore, I think what Dr. Yacoub wants to hear is that we should do a study where surgeons and cardiologists sit together and decide what the anatomy is. Together we decide whether it is a patient who can be managed by PTCA. Next we should randomize to surgery or PTCA. Only then could you really have a comparative group and I think that we should keep that design in mind. All of us who are enthusiastic about PTCA are not claiming that we can do the same that the surgeon can do. What we are claiming, however, is clearly demonstrated in the previous talk: much reduced morbidity and cost, and I hope, also a much better and earlier return to work. But never do we want to leave the impression that one can compare PTCA in anatomical correction terms with bypass grafting; the situation is mostly quite different.

Chairman: The patients who were treated primarily with a bypass graft are different patients from the patients in whom we currently do PTCA. You can do operations in nearly all patients who need revascularization, but from these patients you can only treat a certain, although increasing, number with PTCA. And this is the difference between the patient groups compared in these three papers. Dr. Meier and Dr. Vallbracht compared two different groups treated with either primarily bypass surgery or PTCA. Dr. Boulay looked at the results of patients who could be treated with PTCA. Some of these patients were unsuccessful PTCA patients.

Q: I have a question for Dr. Meier. Is it correct that more than 80% of your patients returned to work after bypass surgery? You would have the best results we have heard today. Can you explain or can you give some information about the profession of your patients?

Meier: We only looked at those patients who either worked up to bypass surgery or had recently stopped working.

Q: This is why I asked for the definition; it is a very strict one. Were they working up to the very last moment? And did you get 80% relief? Only in the Geneva group are equally good results reported. And in Geneva they may have a very Calvinistic work ethic. Perhaps they have a greater motivation to return to work.

Chairman: There is a low rate of unemployment in Switzerland around 1%.

Q: But this still means that of those patients on whom you performed bypass surgery to solve their cardiac problems, 12%–14% are not returning to work. So even though you did bypass surgery to improve their lot, and they had worked up to or shortly before that intervention, 12% did not return to work.

Chairman: Yes, but we all agree that these figures are the lowest of any presented today.

Vermeulen: I heard a high figure in one of the presentations, of immediate operation after PTCA. I think then when we are in that area, this procedure becomes pretty dangerous. When we have to operate acutely on these patients after PTCA, most of them are in danger. They have a dissection or an acute occlusion or something equally unpleasant. And there is at least the danger of impending infarction. So, I think that these patients may have a shorter hospitalization time, but on the other hand some are in greater danger than they would be on normal heart-lung machines for bypass.

Chairman: Do you want to answer this question, Dr. Meier?

Meier: Well, the only answer we can give is the statistics. In all of the large centers performing PTCA these days, the percentage of the patients you were alluding to lies between 2% and 6%. In larger centers it is closer to 2% and in the smaller centers closer to 6% of all PTCA patients.

Vermeulen: One of the papers, definitely had a higher number of acute operations.

Chairman: But I think all would agree that this is an exception. For the audience, it ought to be clearly stated that the complication rate requiring urgent bypass grafting lies in the 2%–4% range. And you are right that it is a procedure-related complication and one always must weigh whether it is an acceptable situation. But I do think, personally, that the 95% who go scot-free and do not require a thoracotomy or 6 weeks hospitalization are the factors in the balance, which makes the whole thing tip positively towards PTCA.

Wenger: Dr. Meier, I think, raises a very important point and that is the need for continuing medication. Both the surgeons and the cardiologists have learned that with the low rate of occlusion of graft vessels, it is rather reasonable to stop most medication early: We still have some concern with early re-stenosis. And therefore, I think, at least in the early weeks, it is probably appropriate that some of our patients stay on medication. Dr. Meier, I think your two challenges therefore will be: can you or any of us do anything prospectively to evaluate or assess that subset of patients which is most likely to re-stenose? Is there going to be a clue to that group so that perhaps we may be able to differentiate with our medication regime?

The other thing that I would be most interested in as your series gets longer in time, is, will the primary care physician caring for the patients on whom you did PTCA after the first 3 or 6 months decrease the amount of medication? Will you possibly see an increase in return to work in that regard like the Canadian group did? Because if my memory serves me correctly, the Canadian group saw more return to work at 1 year than they did earlier on. And the main question is, is any of this possibly related to reassurance or to the persistence of effect of the PTCA?

Meier: The first suggestion you made will keep me busy for another few years, and to answer the second question, whether I think that more of the PTCA patients return to work (I am talking about the Geneva patients now), I am afraid not. If somebody at 14 months after a benign intervention such as a PTCA, which involves, 3 days hospitalization and intubation in the groin, has not returned to work and remains on a lot of medication, I don't think that this situation will change spontaneously for the good. But I do agree that some of those medications are imposed upon the patient by the physician, because he is not sure about what to do with the patient. And the patient himself taking three or four different medications thinks he cannot possibly go back to work.

Chairman: I think that this matter of education should also be looked at in the light that Dr. Meier has thrown on it. We are still in the experimental stages with PTCA. Let us not let this audience think that this is as far as we are with bypass grafting, where we have a reasonable standard way of operating. And here there is still argument about the timing, about the number of vessels to attack, about the extent to which you should inflate, whether or not you should do additional procedures, and so on. I find it difficult to place a definite value on that procedure so soon. What one can say, however, is that the morbidity is less. The peripheral physician does not quite know what to do with this type of patient yet. We have to teach him this and what could happen in terms of restenosis. So it comes right back to the question that you and I do not know how to answer now. What is atherosclerosis anyway? Do we actually, with the PTCA and with the ballooning, enhance that process in some? Or do we rather reduce it in others? There are more questions there than I care to answer in the few minutes we have left.

Marcus: I would like to ask Dr. Meier something about medication. What are, your main explanations for the fact that PTCA patients are on a higher cardiac medication regime? Is it due to the uneasiness of the general practitioner rather than to a lesser efficacy of the treatment?

Meier: There was no correlation between angina at follow-up and medication in the PTCA group or in the CABG group. That is why I implied that there are several factors accounting for the amount of medication. I am sure that angina is one of the main factors, but there are others.

Chairman: The other participants in the panel discussion are Drs. Crosby, Bentall, Mathes, Rothlin, and Coustry-Degré.

Q: I would like to take exception to one of Dr. Wallwork's statements, that in Germany it would be impossible for the patient to return to work after transplantation. Actually in our small series of patients that underwent transplantation we have a 50% return to work rate. One patient who was actually operated on by you 4 years ago in Stanford, is actively enjoying life and is back to work.

Wallwork: I think my point was misunderstood. I thought that in Germany, once you were registered disabled it was very difficult to become de-registered and go back to work. And in general, I would have thought that most transplantation patients would have been registered disabled by that stage. But I accept your point and I am very glad that he is doing well.

Q: We have a series of four transplanted patients who went through our rehabilitation program and they show very nicely the typical pitfalls of the German social system. The first one was forced into retirement by the social system. The second, previously a hospital orderly, is now working in the telephone exchange. The third, the most interesting, was also forced into retirement as a truckdriver; but as you can well imagine, he has suffered a drastic loss of income. And so from time to time he takes his truck from Hamburg to Sicily to put himself back into financial shape. As for the last patient, return to work is not yet decided.

Wallwork: I am becoming increasingly sorry that I made that comment, but I think the point is that for many of the patients, return to work, even in our setup, is not possible, partly because some of the patients say, "Well, look, I can read Reader's Digest. I know my 5-year survival chances and so I am not going to waste this new lease on life. I am going to go learn how to water ski or something." Now the other thing, of course, is that there are many people who would like to work after cardiac transplantation but cannot get work. One of the nice things about cardiac transplantation is that if they do well, they do very well. Very few chronic invalids, survive transplantation. Many of those patients cannot go back to work because companies don't want to employ people who have had transplants. So they have great difficulty, and the reason that I said all of that was just to highlight the fact that I don't think return to work is a very good measure of their quality of life.

Floor: I should like to add some other results in our hospitals. Six patients survive of the eight who have had transplants. And of these six – with a follow-up of 6 months to 2 years – four are living a normal life and are working. The first two patients are not working now, but they were overprotected and did not benefit from rehabilitation.

Chairman: You take over now, Dr. Crosby, and lead the panel discussion in specifics. Why don't you stay here, Dr. Wallwork? We may need you for other purposes, like distinguishing between sex and gardening!

Crosby: I think that it has been very interesting to accept that return to work is a very poor yardstick of the success of any type of medical treatment. Similarly, recreational activities are not good indicators, even though there are regional differences. And although my colleague here says that people in the south of London have more interest in gardening than in sex, that would not necessarily apply to the rest of the world.

We have had 35 speakers and that excludes some of the key discussion from the floor, but it has been quite apparent to me that return to work is not influenced by the relief of angina. If you get an early relief of angina of 90%, and all the graft patencies you talk about show that, how come only 70% of the people go back to work early after surgery? There are obviously a lot of societal factors involved.

I think that the philosophical questions are perhaps the most difficult ones. Is any person required to support himself throughout life? If he does not want to work, is he entitled to food, housing, medical care, etc.? I think that Dr. Varnauskas's approach was that if someone has coronary disease and does not want to work, then we should let him not work. That philosophical point is very difficult for us to make a decision on. It is not our decision to make. It increases your taxes if you want someone to live from the age of 35 until 75; that person is going to need a continuum of care. He may need PTCA. He may need lots of medicine. He may need streptokinase therapy. He may need coronary surgery. He may need repeat surgery, repeat PTCA. Your goal of therapy is to get that person to live from 35 for another 40 years. And I think of the attitude that some people have about breast cancer, that you never cure it, but you prolong the survival, and if they survive 30 years that is wonderful.

So I think there are a lot of social and governmental policy decisions that need to be made, and this is not the platform to make those decisions. I think those are the most important ones, not just whether we should make that person go back to work or not.

Chairman: Should we take you up on that point and say that we would like this audience to leave here tonight no longer thinking that the return to work is the only thing to go for, but rather to go for what we have heard Dr. Smith define as the sum of all the satisfactions which determine the quality of life? Could we agree on that new definition? I think it is terribly important to shift. Each time I meet someone in the Netherlands in the social services, the question is: "Did he go back to work?" It is the parameter of my success or the patient's success. I would like to have the back of that wrong concept broken once and for all and I think that this may well be the panel and the time to do so.

Crosby: I agree with that wholeheartedly. I think that as physicians our goal is to treat people and to treat them to the best of our ability, to improve the quality of their lives and to improve the length of their lives. And you cannot measure that by asking them if they work or not.

Chairman: Are there people in the room who strongly disagree with this shift in emphasis from return to work to the new parameter of enhancement of the quality of life and trying to be a good doctor to your patients? Well, maybe it was not even an issue. We all seem to agree.

Crosby: I am sorry I wasted your time with a non-issue.

Chairman: Well, I do not think it is a non-issue. Think of the discussion about rehabilitation a number of years back. What is the goal of rehabilitation in general, not only after surgery? Is it improvement in the quality of life or is it what the social insurance people would like to hear? Or increased return to work? Evidently the increased return to work was the initial incentive for all of the money that was put into rehabilitation, but now we come out to say that as physicians we are primarily concerned about the quality of life. And if working is one of those aspects, I think, then we will all agree that this is the desirable definition.

Q: I think it is very important that you bring up the point that the incentive for the whole rehabilitation effort came in part from the social services throughout the world. And let us not forget that there is an increased relief of symptoms, increased work capacity, and yet the return to work is just not there. So, maybe the premise was there, maybe that was the reason to begin, but that does not mean that we have to go on.

Are you afraid of the departments of health and social services and so forth, Dr. Mathes? Are you afraid that the clinic may have to close because you cannot prove that the people go back to work?

Mathes: I think that the historical proof is that the conservative approach in rehabilitation has increased the return to work of patients after their first coronary event. And this is the basis for the development of rehabilitation, at least in our country, and I think in others too. And now we have tried to add surgery as another means of rehabilitation. What we see is that it has achieved great success in improving the quality of life, but that it has failed to meet our expectations in terms of return to work. So I think we have to accept this as physicians, and regard this, as Dr. Varnauskas told us, as possible self-protection on the part of the patient who, after going through the coronary invasive diagnosis and the surgery, may well put the reason for all of his troubles into his specific work situation. And it makes a great deal of difference whether you go back to work as a physician or a professional, or whether you make your money digging ditches. And this, I think, is the point we all more or less agree upon.

Crosby (?): I would like to return to the recommendation of changing the criteria of return to work, the influence of that, and take it one step further. If you have such enormous waiting lists for surgery and if you have 60 days to go back to work after PTCA, and if everyone is living longer, ultimately someone has to be generating the money to feed people and give them medical care. And I believe that men and women's luck in life is to work. Now, if they have a genuine reason for not working, whether it is asthma or orthopedic problems, etc., then I think it is important to remove them from the work force. But I think the attitude of physicians has to change with regard to coronary artery disease patients. If they are well, they are free to go back to work and should be encouraged to do so. If they are not well, then they should be classified as disabled, but just having the stamp of coronary artery disease should not prevent him from ever working again.

Chairman: I totally subscribe to that particular notion. Dr. Varnauskas has a comment.

Varnauskas: To add to what Dr. Mathes said, I would like to just recall the definition of the goals of rehabilitation which were put forward by WHO. Actually this definition did not include return to work, but rather return to a meaningful life, which is quite a different thing. I think this is what very nicely has been brought up by you in the panel.

Bentall: I don't wish to suggest for a moment that British people are better either morally or in any other aspect to Americans, Germans, or French citizens, but one should not lose sight of the fact that the reports from the United Kingdom in general have shown a very much higher return to work than in Germany. It is not only higher early on but also over a 5 year period. Mr. Yacoub, for example, referred to an 87% return to work at 2 years, admittedly deteriorating later, but even then it is still close on 75% at 5 years.

In other words, a high return to work rate is possible. It may relate to the fact that to get the most satisfaction from life the British patient requires to work. I am not saying it is good or bad, I am stating it as a fact. I don't think we should lose sight of the fact that for some people work is a good thing.

Chairman: The point, I think, has already been made, that we should no longer make it the single goal.

Bentall: I agree with that completely, of course.

Yacoub: Mr. Chairman, in response to your statement that there are limitations to return to work as a parameter, I think we should not go too far, because it still is a parameter, inaccurate as it might be. It certainly does not equate with quality of life, but it is at least something that we can measure, and most parameters we measure have their inaccuracies. We should not throw it out, but perhaps we should use it more intelligently than we have done.

Chairman: Well, I would like to take issue on that with you. I think you are right that we shouldn't throw it out altogether, because it belongs to the whole story of the patient. What I am afraid of, and the reason why I would like to have it removed from its top heading to something of a minor position, is that the social services, at least in the Netherlands, judge the efficacy of the doctor by the measure to which he returns patients to work.

To be confronted with a man who comes and inspects the patient's course and says "He did not go back to work after you spent so much money on him?", reflects a bad attitude on the part of government agencies.

Psychosocial and Behavioral Aspects of Coronary Artery Bypass Surgery

The Discrepancy Between Social and Medical Rehabilitation of Patients with Coronary Heart Disease

U. Gerhardt

Although the rate of retirement after coronary bypass surgery seems to vary in different countries between some 60% and 25% (Niles et al. 1980; Walter et al. 1983; Yacoub and Guvendik 1984; Sergeant et al. 1984, this vol p. 108), its tendency to depend upon the state of the economy poses a problem for the definition of rehabilitation. While medical rehabilitation, i.e., the decrease of angina pectoris and the improvement of cardiac function, is reported for the overwhelming majority of CABS patients, return to work, which indicates social rehabilitation, is much less universally achieved; nevertheless, the former is less likely to be accepted as a sufficient criterion for the successful outcome of the operation. The discrepancy between medical and social rehabilitation invites a critical discussion since the long-term cost-effectiveness of the operation as a mode of treating coronary disease is calculated by contrasting the savings in state benefits effected through the patients' return to work with the cost of unemployment incurred in the case of their retirement (Love 1980). A tacit assumption seems to be made that the high cost of surgery might be somewhat wasted if the operation leads to loss of occupational status which, in turn, necessitates further cost in terms of social security benefits.

However, the question may be asked whether the definition of rehabilitation ought to remain the same. I wish to argue that to define the success of CABS through social rehabilitation in terms of return to work may underestimate the importance of medical rehabilitation for the patient's well-being and may even jeopardize the latter by supporting the notorious type A pattern of behavior, which is said to be instrumental in the development of myocardial infarction. Three findings are basic to my argument:

1. Blue-collar workers find it more difficult than white-collar workers to return to work after revascularization or coronary bypass surgery. This is especially true for age groups beyond the age of 50 (Bennesch et al. 1979; Borst 1981; Loose et al. 1983; Love 1980).

2. It is not only in West Germany that there is a linear relationship between the length of the preoperative waiting period and the likelihood of retirement from work after surgery (Hammermeister et al. 1979; Niles et al. 1980; Borst 1981). In this vein, Blachly and Blachly (1968) stipulate a "law of 1 year"; that is, they showed 15 years ago that the likelihood of return to work decreases drastically after a 1-year period of pre- and postoperative absence from work.

3. The clinical status of coronary or arterial functioning is worse for retired patients than for patients who return to work.

Expanding upon point 3, the most recent study of German bypass patients found a higher proportion of patients with serious handicap among the retired, and this was more obvious among those who retired from blue-collar jobs (Loose et al. 1983). It is not clear, however, whether this is due to the fact that those who are more ill are more likely to retire. It may also be that retirement has an adverse effect on health. In fact, both effects may combine. Those who are more ill may, particularly in blue-collar jobs, decide to retire; they may then face the prospect of a worsening of their condition due to the effect of job loss on their physical and psychological health. A negative effect of retirement upon psychological health was shown by the Giessen data, which reveal a higher rate of dissatisfaction and complaints among the retired (Walter et al. 1983). On the other hand, Stocksmeier et al. (see this vol p. 386) argue that early retirement may prolong life in CABS patients; in a 6-year follow-up of patients with myocardial infarction who underwent coronary angiography, these authors found that the 16% of their sample who died were exclusively from the group who returned to work after myocardial infarction. Thus, while extended absence from work pre- and postoperatively plus a blue-collar type of job are factors which favor retirement, and retired patients are in a worse state of health, it may not be concluded for cardiac functioning but only for psychological well-being that its deterioration could be due to retirement. An adverse effect of retirement on clinical status, if it exists, seems not to influence the patient's life expectancy after surgery.

Many doctors seem to be aware of this situation. Several studies have reported that the majority of patients who retired were advised to do so by their doctors (Lamendola and Pellegrin 1979, Loose et al. 1983), and if no advice was given regarding work the patients often felt uneasy and insecure (Dahme et al. 1980). However, recent programs have attempted to prove that systematic guidance of the patient by the doctor towards resuming work results in a nearly 100% rate of return to work (Stein and Krasemann 1981). This presupposes, in my opinion, that reliable knowledge exists on the medical outlook rather than merely the social advantages for the patient who returns to his job. Unfortunately, there seems to be no research which keeps the clinical state of the disease constant and investigates the effect of postoperative work status on life expectancy as compared with that of early retirement. Until such research becomes known, we may conclude from the data of Stocksmeier et al. (this vol p. 386) that retirement may have a negative effect only on the social rehabilitation of the patient, while it has a positive effect on his medical rehabilitation and, consequently, longevity.

If we look for a plausible hypothesis to explain the relationship between return to work and life expectancy, we must focus upon the so-called type A behavior personality. It is now well known that type A behavior is rightly called coronary-prone, and the questionnaire eliciting it focuses not primarily on the person's work load but rather on his style of relentlessly rushing himself and others (Rosenman 1978). The composite pattern of type A reactions comprising "intense striving for achievement, competitiveness, easily-provoked impatience, time-urgency, abruptness of gesture and speech, hyperalert posture, tense facial musculature, overcommitment to vocation or profession, and excesses of drive and hostility" (Jenkins 1978; p 25) has been further analyzed in terms of separate dimensions, central features, and physiological correlates (Dembrowsky et al. 1978, 1983). The relationship between behavioral pattern and work environment has recently been stressed by Matthews (1982), who showed that type A behavior is elicited through a certain type of circumstance, namely, work situations which "(a) are moderately competitive, (b) are uncontrollable, (c) require endurance, (d) require slow, careful work, and (e) use a broad focus of attention" (Matthews 1982; p 317). From this perspective, type A may be recognized as a habitualized style of unadapted behavior meeting a work environment which requires intelligence, diligence, and a certain capacity for postponement of gratification as well as a certain tolerance of lack of control. The suspected sex difference in type A behavior has proved an artifact due to the use of a questionnaire originally tested for males only, and the close relationship between types of demand in the work environment and type A behavior as an inadequate response to them seems to hold for males and females alike (Chesney 1983). If the reactive nature of type A behavior depending upon certain aspects of the work environment becomes clear, a hypothesis may be ventured regarding the difficulties encountered by patients returning to work after myocardial infarction. Meeting the same work environment as before, they might find themselves in a situation where they continuously have to defend their more moderate postinfarction work behavior against others' expectations that they will resume their coronary-prone behavior of the past. Kornfeld et al. (see this vol p. 224) report that 80% of the employed nonsurvivors in their sample were type A and had failed to change their behavior after the infarction and return to work.

Moreover, recent research has focused upon depressive tendencies in patients with coronary disease in general, and during the year prior to infarction in particular (Henry and Stephens 1977; Appels 1982). The joint display of time-urgency and competitiveness, on the one hand, and depressive tendencies towards withdrawal, on the other, seems to point in the direction of a reactive pattern of which type A behavior is only one side. The hypothesis may be raised that type A persons drive themselves hard *because* they are denying their depressive tendency; that is, they push themselves to the limit in a work situation which demands more than they feel able to offer and which requires more control than they can muster while, at the same time, they realize their basic inadequacy and respond with depression on a more or less subconscious level. If this hypothesis holds, the depressive tendency with its physiological correlates in coronary heart disease is as equally rooted in the work experience as type A behavior, with its totally different and somewhat antagonistic physiological patterns (Henry and Stephens 1977; Schmidt 1982). In fact, the joint activation of both physiological mechanisms seems to be particularly dangerous (Selye 1970). If they are both stimulated by the same work environment, the "coronary-prone" nature of the latter needs no further explanation. The relationship between return to work and probable reduction of life expectancy, on the one hand, and retirement and increased longevity, on the other, may have its roots in this double mechanism.

My argument so far has contrasted two aspects of the discrepancy between medical and social rehabilitation of patients with coronary artery bypass surgery. While the psychosocial functioning of the patient was maintained to be worse under conditions of unemployment, his medical condition was said to allow for increased longevity in spite of the fact that the general state of health is worse among the retired, who primarily come from the group of older blue-collar workers. On the other hand, social rehabilitation, which includes return to work, was suspected to have an adverse effect on life expectancy since the state of the patient's medical rehabilitation may be unduly eroded through work circumstances which provoke the same type A behavior in the patient as existed before the myocardial infarction. However, it ought to be mentioned that both effects may be mitigated or strengthened by the patient's family. In fact, it has been argued that the family should be the basic reference unit for the analyis of social rehabilitation (Gerhardt und Friedrich 1982). Friedrich, Kleinspehn and Ziegeler (1980, Verläufe von chronischen Krankheiten in Abhängigkeit von Folgeerscheinungen in der psychosozialen Umwelt – am Beispiel von Herzinfarkt und Diabetes, 2 vols, unpublished work) discuss the psychological impact of the family. They show how the perceptions of a husband's heart disease by the wife and by the husband may be conducive to any one of (a) a denial of symptoms and relentless resumption of preinfarction activities, (b) anxious avoidance of expenditure of energy due to a fear of exhaustion and death, (c) a wise compromise between too much and too little, or (d) a conflict-prone discrepancy between the spouses, where the husband and wife follow different perceptive patterns. Each of the four types of illness perception may be related to the twin pattern of type A behavior and depressive withdrawal. The resultant picture of family processes explains some of the lack of psychological functioning after retirement, and it elucidates some of the "coronary-prone" circumstances after resumption of work.

Finally, another mechanism of social rehabilitation involving the family may be mentioned. Gerhardt (to be published) shows for a sample of patients with chronic renal failure, particularly those from a lower-class origin, that their longevity is increased when the wife participates in the family's social rehabilitation by taking up full-time employment additional to or instead of her husband–patient. A similar process may occur with CABS patients. Crosby et al. (this vol p. 19) were able to demonstrate that the income of blue-collar patients does not suffer in spite of the patient's retirement, since the spouse or other family members take up employment as part of the family's rehabilitation efforts.

If the family is taken as the unit of social functioning, it is no longer useful to define social rehabilitation by the patient's return to work; compensating changes of family life may offset the deprivation caused by a patient's abandonment of gainful employment. Nor is it fair to overlook the patient's efforts to adapt his life-style to his illness even if they do not include his return to work; as Safilios-Rothschild (1970) points out, the conditions of economic life are so different in the upper and the lower classes that patients face circumstances which are far from equal. Therefore, the only realistic measure fo success of coronary artery bypass surgery seems to be the degree of relief of symptoms, and the improvement of the patient's clinical condition. That is, medical rehabilitation ought to be perceived as sufficient justification of the cost of the operation. Why should the nearly universal achievement of medical rehabilitation be given second place as the criterion of success of the surgery? The prevailing criterion of social rehabilitation, if defined by return to work, is far from independent of such medically uncontrollable factors as the state of the national economy and the mechanisms of a family's coping with illness. Why should cardiac surgery make itself answerable to such nonmedical issues?

Acknowledgment. I am indebted to Dr. B. Klapp for some most helpful comments.

References

Appels A (1982) Das Jahr vor dem Herzinfarkt. In: Köhle K (ed) Zur Psychosomatik der Koronaren Herzerkrankungen, Boehringer, Mannheim, pp 1–14

Bennesch L, Neuhaus KH, Rivas-Martin J, Loogen F (1979) Clinical results and return to work after coronary heart surgery. In: Roskamm B, Schmuziger M (eds) Coronary heart surgery. Springer, Berlin Heidelberg New York, pp 379–384

Blachly PH, Blachly RN (1968) Vocational and emotional status of 263 patients after heart surgery. Circulation 38:524–532

Borst HG (1981) The problem of coronary surgery – German experience. Thorac Cardiovasc Surg 29:65–70

Chesney MA (1983) Occupational setting and coronary-prone behavior in men and women. In: Dembrowski TM, Schmidt TH, Blümchen G (eds) Biobehavioral bases of coronary heart disease. Karger, Basel, pp 79–90

Dahme G, Dahme P, Kornemann J, Vollers A and Huse-Kleinstoll G. (1980) Fulfillment of patient's expectations concerning outcome of open-heart surgery. In: Speidel H, Rodewald G (eds) Psychic and neurological disfunctions after open-heart surgery. First International symposium. Thieme, Stuttgart, pp 228–236

Dembrowski TM, Weiss SM, Shields JL, Haynes SG, Feinleib M (eds) (1978) Coronary-prone behavior. Springer, New York Heidelberg Berlin

Dembrowski TM, Schmidt TH, Blümchen G (eds) (1983) Biobehavioral bases of coronary heart disease. Karger, Basel

Gerhardt U (to be published) Patientenkarrieren. Suhrkamp, Frankfurt

Gerhardt U, Friedrich H (1982) Familie und chronische Krankheit. In: Angermeyer M, Freyberger H (eds) Chronisch kranke Erwachsene in der Familie. Enke, Stuttgart, pp 3–25

Hammermeister KE, DeRouen TA, English WT, Dodge HT (1979) Effect of surgical versus medical therapy on return to work in patients with coronary artery disease. Am J Cardiol 44:105–11

Henry JP, Stephens PM (1977) Stress, health, and the social environment. Springer, New York Heidelberg Berlin

Jenkins CD, Zyzanski SJ, Rosenman RH (1978) Coronary-prone behaviour: One pattern or several? Psychosom Med 40:25–43

Lamendola WF, Pellegrin RV (1979) Quality of life and coronary artery bypass surgery patients. Soc Sci Med 13 (A):457–461

Loose DA, v Ferber C, v Ferber L, Klocke A, Schmoe J (1983) Rehabilitationserfolg nach gefäßchirurgischen Eingriffen. Einhorn, Reinbek

Love JW (1980) Employment status after coronayry bypass operations and some cost considerations. J Thorac Cardiovasc Surg 80:68–72

Matthews KA (1982) Psychological perspectives on the type A behavior pattern. Psychol Bull 91:292–323

Niles NW, Vander Salm TJ, Cutler BG (1980) Return to work after coronary artery bypass operations. J Thorac Cardiovasc Surg 79:916–21

Rosenman RH (1978) The interview method of assessment of the coronary-prone behavior pattern. In: Dembrowski TM et al (eds) Coronary Prone Behavior. Springer, New York Heidelberg Berlin, p 55–70

Safilios-Rothschild C (1970) The sociology and social psychology of rehabilitation. Random House, New York

Schmidt T (1982) Koronares Risiko und Typ-A-Verhalten. In: Köhle K (ed) Zur Psychosomatik von Herz-Kreislauf-Erkrankungen. Springer, Berlin Heidelberg New York, pp 15–43

Selye H (1970) The evolution of the stress concept. Am J Cardiol 26:289–299

Stein G, Krasemann EO (1981) Prospektive Untersuchungen zur Dauer der Arbeitsunfähigkeit nach Herzinfarkt. Herz/Kreisl 11:526–32

Walter P, Thies B, Gerhardt U (1983) Wie viele Patienten nehmen nach einer Koronaroperation ihre Arbeit wieder auf? Med Klin Prax 78 8:46–57

Psychosocial Predictors of Work Status

M. C. Gutmann, D. N. Knapp, and M. L. Pollock

Introduction

The potential impact of coronary artery bypass surgery (CABS) on work status is of major social, psychological, and economic concern. In the United States alone, approximately 170 000 CABS were performed in 1983, at an average cost of $ 15 000 per procedure. Studies indicate that employment rate declines after CABS, despite improvement in symptoms and physical activity (Oberman et al. 1982; Smith et al. 1982). A variety of medical, occupational, and psychosocial factors have been found to be related to employment status after CABS (Gutmann et al. 1982; Stanton et al. 1983; Davidson 1983). However, the combined variables were able to explain only 50% of the total variance in postoperative employment status. In order to design appropriate interventions, additional research is needed to improve the ability to predict employment change after CABS.

Method

In March of 1980, a survey questionnaire was sent to all patients who underwent CABS in two Milwaukee area hospitals during 1979. A total of 570 questionnaires were sent, and 358 (63%) were returned. The mean interval between surgery and completion of the questionnaire was 12.5 months (range, 4–22 months). The survey questionnaire consisted of multiple-choice and open-ended items covering demographic information, occupational history and job characteristics, general medical and cardiac history, risk factors, knowledge of heart disease, and perceptions of surgery and rehabilitation. After preliminary univariate analysis, discriminant function analysis was performed on a subsample of 171 subjects, selected for completeness of data.

The subsample consisted of 153 males and 18 females. Mean age was 55.4 years. Within this subsample, 135 (79%) of the subjects were working prior to surgery. Of these, 115 (85%) returned to work after surgery, while 20 (15%) were unemployed or retired at follow-up. Of the 36 subjects who were not working before surgery, 31 (86%) remained unemployed at follow-up, while only 5 (14%) resumed work after surgery. Discriminant function analysis was performed to identify variables that best predicted membership in the various work status groups. The last group was not included in the statistical analysis because of the small sample size.

Results

Preliminary univariate analyses showed that preoperative employment status was the single most significant predictor of work status after surgery (Gutmann et al. 1982). Results from the discriminant function analysis indicated that younger patients who were employed in professional or skilled jobs with light physical demands were more likely to be working before surgery. However, patients who were off work 6 months or more before surgery were more likely to perceive themselves as unemployed or retired ($P<0.005$). Since few of the previously unemployed patients return to work after CABS, the major objective was to identify factors that predict failure to resume work among patients who were working before surgery. Results of the discriminant function analysis are summarized in Table 1.

Table 1. Factors related to failure to resume work among those working before CABS

Work factors:	Time off work >1 mo. Receipt of disability compensation More physically demanding jobs
Medical factors:	Lower postoperative LVEF Longer time between Dx and CABS No cardiac rehabilitation
Perceptions and behavior:	Less perceived benefits from surgery on physical tolerance Better medication compliance Dietary failure due to family eating patterns

Work Variables

In this subsample, three work variables were significantly related to work resumption after CABS.

1. Length of time off work prior to surgery not only defined presurgery employment status, but was highly predictive of changes in employment status after surgery. Among patients working before surgery, an absence of 1 month or more significantly increased the rate of failure to resume work ($P<0.05$). This suggests a shorter critical interval than the 6 months previously reported in the literature (David 1978).
2. Failure to resume work was also significantly associated with the receipt of disability insurance compensation ($P<0.005$). Among patients who were working before surgery, 58% of those who failed to resume work were receiving disability compensation, compared to 17% of those who did return to work by follow-up. Sixty-nine percent of the patients who were not work-

ing before or after surgery were receiving disability compensation. Thus, nonemployment at follow-up was associated with high rates of disability compensation, regardless of presurgery employment status.

3. Two related factors contributed to employment status independently of disability compensation. As mentioned earlier, patients in higher status occupations were more likely to be employed prior to surgery, but those in physically demanding jobs were more likely to remain unemployed or to drop out of work after surgery ($P < 0.025$). Among patients working before surgery, 91% of the patients performing light physical work had returned to their jobs by follow-up, while approximately one-third of those performing moderate or heavy physical work had not. Given that we had few subjects performing physically heavy work, this finding suggests that even moderately demanding jobs inhibit work resumption.

Medical factors

Surprisingly few biologic or medical factors achieved significance in relation to work status.

1. Patient age was significantly related to presurgery employment status, but did not discriminate between those who did and those who did not return to work among the previously employed. Older patients were more likely to be retired before surgery and to remain so after surgery.
2. Postoperative left ventricular ejection fraction (LVEF) was not significantly related to presurgery employment status, and only modestly related to work resumption after surgery ($P < 0.10$). Patients who were working before surgery, but failed to resume work, had the lowest mean postoperative LVEF (50%). Patients who did resume work had a mean LVEF of 59%, which was similar to that (55%) of patients who were unemployed both before and after surgery.
3. Although our numbers are small, the data suggest that participation in a formal outpatient cardiac rehabilitation program facilitates return to work after surgery ($P < 0.10$). All 13 previously employed patients who were enrolled in a hospital-based outpatient cardiac rehabilitation program had returned to work by follow-up. None of the patients who failed to resume work after surgery had been in an outpatient rehabilitation program.
4. One additional finding was intriguing. Among the patients who were working before surgery, those who had known of their disease longer were less likely to resume work after surgery ($P < 0.005$). The average length of time between diagnosis of heart disease and CABS was 3.3 years for those who resumed work, and 6.4 years for those who did not. This could reflect more chronic disease, and/or a learning of illness behavior patterns.
5. Other medical factors such as length of hospital stay, rehospitalization after discharge, presence of symptoms, number of other chronic medical problems, and cardiovascular risk status were relatively insignificant in determining work status at follow-up.

Patient Perceptions and Behavior

Although objective measures of medical status were relatively unimportant in determining work status, patient perceptions and health behaviors were related to work resumption after surgery.

1. Patients who perceived an improvement in tolerance for physical activity as a result of surgery were significantly more likely to return to work ($P<0.005$). Over 45% of the patients who failed to resume work reported no change or a decrease in their physical tolerance after surgery, compared to 22% in the group that did return to work by follow-up. Although 77%–84% of the patients thought that surgery helped their heart function and reduced symptoms, neither of these items were related to postsurgery work status.
2. Self-ratings of depression during convalescence were also not predictive of work resumption. However, patients' self-reported compliance with medications and diet was related to work status at follow-up. The group as a whole reported fair compliance with medications, with most patients reporting fewer than four medication misses per week. However, patients who returned to work reported more medication misses than those who remained unemployed ($P<0.005$). Patients who resumed work were also more likely to attribute dietary failures to tension, while those who remained home attributed dietary problems to family eating patterns. Patients who returned to work were more knowledgeable about obesity as a cardiovascular risk factor, but actual weight loss after surgery was comparable in both groups (10–12 pounds). Thus, vocational outcome following CABS may influence health behaviors and attitudes in complex ways.

Summary

In summary, 20 or 15% of the previously employed patients in this subsample failed to resume work after CABS. Factors associated with failure to resume work after CABS include longer time off work before surgery, receipt of disability compensation, and moderately physically demanding jobs. Patients who had known of their disease longer, who had lower postoperative LVEF, and who had not participated in outpatient cardiac rehabilitation were more likely to drop out of work after surgery. Patients' perceptions of the benefits of surgery on physical activity tolerance were also predictive of work resumption at follow-up. A discriminant function analysis, using this combination of factors, correctly identified 75% of the patients who were working before surgery but failed to resume work after CABS. Clinically, this group is of greatest interest since interventions could be targeted for those who have a potential for returning to work but are at risk for dropping out after CABS. However, work resumption may adversely affect patient compliance with medications and dietary recommendations. Thus, precautions need to be taken in evaluating the total impact of returning the patient to work. An integrated approach to the biological, psychological, and social aspects of rehabilitation seems most effective for maximizing the benefits of CABS.

References

David P (1978) Contributing factors preventing return to work of cardiac surgery patients. Clev Clin Q 45:177–178

Davidson DM (1983) Return to work after cardiac events: A review. J Cardiac Rehabil 3:60–69

Gutmann MC, Knapp DN, Pollock ML, Schmidt DH, Simon K, Walcott G (1982) Coronary artery bypass patients and work status. Circulation [Suppl III] 66:33–42

Oberman A, Wayne JB, Kouchoukos NT, Charles ED, Russell RO, Rogers WJ (1982) Employment status after coronary artery bypass surgery. Circulation 65:115–119

Smith HC, Hammes LN, Gupta S (1982) Employment status after coronary artery bypass surgery. Circulation 65:120–125

Stanton BA, Jenkins CD, Denlinger P, Savageau JA, Weintraub RM, Goldstein RL (1983) Predictors of employment status after cardiac surgery. JAMA 249:907–911

Psychiatric Complications

A. E. Willner and C. J. Rabiner

The role of psychogenic and organic factors in the psychopathology associated with open heart surgery has been an extensive area of psychosomatic investigation [1–19]. Jenkins' role in elucidating behavioral factors in cardiovascular disease [20–21] is well known. Several research groups have investigated the relationship between neuropsychological measures and psychopathological and organic symptomatology [22–23].

Our previous studies [34–36] both within the hospital and over a 5-year period after the surgery confirmed some of our basic hypotheses but also raised puzzling questions. We found preoperative cognitive dysfunction in patients who would develop psychopathology after the surgery. This confirmed our prediction and supported the hypothesis that the psychopathology was related to preoperative brain dysfunction. But patients who had *preoperative psychopathology* (even years before the surgery) had even worse cognitive dysfunction than patients who had psychopathology only after the surgery. Why should that be?

We found that the frequently dramatic, disturbed behavior of delirious patients seen after open heart surgery was followed by a benign outcome as we observed them over the next 5 years. On the other hand, patients having much less dramatic depressions and/or organic brain syndromes had a very poor outcome. It is at first puzzling that one form of organic brain syndrome, delirium, should have such a better outcome than the other forms of organic brain syndrome.

We also found that time of onset of psychopathology was related to outcome. Patients whose psychopathology began before the surgery (preoperative onset) had a worse outcome than those who had psychopathology only after the surgery (postoperative onset).

We explained these findings by using a model of organic etiology for most of the psychopathology. Since patients who require open heart surgery have severely compromised cardiac functioning, many of them might also have severely compromised brain circulation. Meyendorf had earlier pointed out that the psychopathology associated with open heart surgery could be viewed as being *precipitated by,* rather than *caused by,* the surgery. He found descriptions of psychopathology very similar to postcardiotomy psychopathology in the German, French, and English medical literature as far back as the early 1800s, long before the advent of open heart surgery. He viewed open heart surgery as an "experimental procedure for precipitating psychopathology" in patients vulnerable because of preoperative organic damage. Those patients who had more severe organic damage could be expected to show psychopathology before the surgery.

Our method in this paper is to review the data which led us to our hypotheses, and to compare it with data from a current sample of 60 patients in which these hypotheses are tested prospectively. The original study had 83 open heart surgery patients, 27 of whom had psychopathology (33%). The current study has 60 open heart surgery patients, 34 of whom had psychopathology (57%).

Relationship of Cognitive Dysfunction and Psychopathology

The measure of cognitive dysfunction used here was a devastated score on the Conceptual Level Analogy Test (CLAT). The CLAT is an objectively scored multiple choice analogy test which is very sensitive to complex higher mental processes. A devastated score places the patient in the lowest one percent of the normal population and can be obtained by random answering. However, patients with devastated scores frequently seem unremarkable at interview.

In the original study, 59% (16/27) of patients having psychiatric symptoms had devastated CLAT scores, as compared with only 32% (18/56) of patients without psychopathology ($P<0.02$). In the replicating study, 65% (22/34) of patients with psychopathology had devastated CLAT scores as compared with 27% (7/26) of patients without psychopathology ($P<0.005$).

Relationship of Cognitive Dysfunction and Time of Onset of Psychopathology

Follow-up observation of our original sample of patients suggested that patients having *preoperative* psychopathology had greater cognitive dysfunction than patients who only had psychopathology *postoperatively*. We also assumed that preoperative psychopathology is more organically determined than psychopathology manifest postoperative only, because the former appears without the stress of open heart surgery. In the original study we found that the proportion of devastated CLAT scores increased in graded series as follows: no psychopathology, 32% (18/56); postoperative psychopathology only, 50% (9/18); and preoperative psychopathology, 78% (7/9); $P<0.01$. This finding was replicated in the current study thus: no psychopathology, 27% devastated CLAT scores (7/26); postoperative psychopathology only, 40% (4/10); and preoperative psychopathology, 75% (18/24); $P<0.001$.

Diagnosis and Outcome

We suggest that there is an organic basis for the differential outcome for patients with different types of psychopathology. In particular depression and/or organic brain syndrome are frequent sequelae of hypoxic brain damage. However, it was also evident that patients whose only psychopathology was delirium had a much better outcome than those who had other forms of organic brain damage (OBS) and/or depression. Tune et al. recently provided a rationale for our impression that postoperative delirium does not have organic etiology when they showed that the delirium is largely a function of the amount of anticholinergic medication taken by the patient.

Relationship Between Type of Psychopathology and Time of Onset of Psychopathology

In the original study, 78% (7/9) of the patients having depression and/or OBS had preoperative onset of psychopathology, as compared with 11% (2/18) of patients with other psychopathology ($P<0.005$). These results were replicated in the current study: 87% (20/23) of patients with depression and/or OBS had preoperative onset, and 36% (4/11) with other psychopathology ($P<0.005$). These findings are consistent with the hypothesis that depression and organic brain syndrome are more prevalent in patients with preoperative psychopathology, because both conditions have more of an organic component than postoperative psychopathology only or other psychopathology.

A further hypothesis is that delirium as the only psychopathology is a minimally organic type of postcardiotomy psychopathology, as suggested by Tune et al. Since preoperative psychopathology is assumed to be more organically determined than postoperative psychopathology only, the incidence of preoperative psychopathology is predicted to increase in graded series from delirium only, to other psychopathology, to depression and/or OBS. In the original study 0% (0/13) of the delirium only patients had preoperative psychopathology, as compared with 40% (2/5) of the other psychopathology group and 78% (7/9) of the depression and/or OBS group ($P<0.001$). The comparable figures for the replication sample were 0% (0.5) for delirium only, 67% (4/6) for other, and 87% (20/23) for depression and/or OBS ($P<0.001$).

Finally we focussed on just those patients who had delirium, contrasting those having delirium only with those who had delirium and other psychopathology. Our hypothesis was that delirium only does not reflect preoperative organic etiology, and that as Tune says it may well be an anticholinergic drug effect. In the original study we found that 0% (0/13) of the delirium only group had preoperative psychopathology, as compared with 75% (3/4) of those with delirium and other psychopathology ($P=0.006$). The comparable figures for the replicating study were 0% (0/5) for the delirium only group and 100% (8/8) for delirium plus other psychopathology ($P=0.001$).

Conclusion

We conclude that our replication study confirms the predictions generated by following our initial sample over a 5-year period. Specifically we found that:

1. Time of onset of psychopathology is related to degree of preoperative cognitive dysfunction; earlier onset is related to more severe cognitive dysfunction.

2. Time of onset of psychopathology is related to type of psychopathology. Depression and/or OBS have an earlier onset and delirium only has later onset.

In general these findings are related to our hypothesis that both preoperative onset and also depression and/or OBS are related to organic etiology.

References

1. Freyhan FA, Gianelli S Jr, O'Connell RA, Mayo JA (1971) Psychiatric complications following open heart surgery. Compr Psychiatry 12:181–195
2. Kimball CP (1972) The experience of open heart surgery: III. Toward a definition and understanding of postcardiotomy delirium. Arch Gen Psychiatry 27:57–63
3. Quinlan DM, Kimball CP, Osborne F (1974) The experience of open heart surgery: IV. Assessment of disorientation and dysphoria following cardiac surgery. Arch Gen Psychiatry 31:241–244
4. Heller SS, Frank KA, Malm JR, Bowman FO, Harris PD, Charlton MH, Kornfeld DS (1970) Psychiatric complications of open-heart surgery: A re-examination. N Engl J Med 283:1015–1020
5. Kornfeld DS, Heller SS, Frank KA, Moskowitz R (1974) Personality and psychological factors in postcardiotomy delirium. Arch Gen Psychiatry 31:249–253
6. Tufo HM, Ostfeld AM, Shekelle R (1970) Central nervous system dysfunction following open-heart surgery. JAMA 212:1333–1340
7. Blachly PH, Starr A (1964) Post-cardiotomy delirium. Am J Psychiatry 121:371–375
8. Ergerton N, Kay JH (1964) Psychological disturbances associated with open heart surgery. Br J Psychiatry 110:433–439
9. Gilman S (1965) Cerebral disorders after open-heart operations. N Engl J Med 272:489–498
10. Götze P, Dahme B (1980) Psychopathological syndromes and neurological disturbances before and after open-heart surgery. In: Speidel H, Rodewald G (eds) Psychic and neurological dysfunctions after open-heart surgery. Thieme, Stuttgart, pp 48–67
11. Meffert HJ, Flemming B (1980) Psychic and psychosocial stress before open-heart operations and their relationships with postoperative psychic disturbances. In: Speidel H, Rodewald G (eds) Psychic and neurological dysfunctions after open-heart surgery. Thieme, Stuttgart, pp 181–188
12. Flemming B, Meffert HJ (1980) The role of personality traits for psychic disturbances after open-heart surgery. In: Speidel H, Rodewald G (eds) Psychic and neurological dysfunctions after open-heart surgery. Thieme, Stuttgart, pp 169–180
13. Spehr W, Götze P (1980) Computerized encephalogram before and after open-heart surgery (preliminary results). In: Speidel H, Rodewald G (eds) Psychic and neurological dysfunctions after open-heart surgery. Thieme, Stuttgart, pp 67–73
14. Pokar H, Huse-Kleinstoll G (1980) Possible intraoperative influences by anesthesia and ECC on postoperative psychic dysfunctions. In: Speidel H, Rodewald G (eds) Psychic and neurological dysfunctions after open-heart surgery. Thieme, Stuttgart, pp 130–134
15. Longmore DB (1981) The value of prostacyclins in cardiopulmonary bypass. In: Longmore DB (ed) Towards safer cardiac surgery. GK Hall Medical, Boston, pp 355–377
16. Meyendorf R (1980) Psychopathology in heart disease aside from cardiac surgery: A historical perspective of cardiac psychosis. In: Speidel H, Rodewald G (eds) Psychic and neurological dysfunctions after open-heart surgery. Thieme, Stuttgart, pp 14–19
17. Meyendorf R (1979) Psychopathology in heart disease aside from cardiac surgery: A historical perspective of cardiac psychosis. Compr Psychiatry 30:326–331

18. Meyendorf R (1982) Psychopatho-ophthalmology, gnostic disorders, and psychosis in cardiac surgery: Visual disturbances after open heart surgery. Arch Psychiatr Nervenkr 232:119–135
19. Sotaniemi KA, Juolasmaa A, Hokkanen ET (1981) Neuropsychologic outcome after open-heart surgery. Arch Neurol 38:2–8
20. Jenkins CD (1981) Behavioral factors in the etiology and pathogenesis of cardiovascular diseases: Sudden death, hypertension, and myocardial infarction. In: Weiss S et al (eds) Perspectives of behavioral medicine. Academic press, New York, pp 41–54
21. Jenkins CD (1982) Psychosocial risk factors for coronary heart disease. Acta Med Scand [Suppl] 660:123–136
22. Åberg T, Kihlgren M (1974) Effect of open-heart surgery on intellectual function. Scand J Thorac Cardiovasc Surg [Suppl] 15:1–63
23. Åberg T, Kihlgren M (1976) Effect of open-heart surgery on intellectual function. Comments. Scand J Thorac Cardiovasc Surg 10:221
24. Åberg T, Kihlgren M (1977a) Cerebral protection during open-heart surgery: A comparison between a disk oxygenator and two bubble oxygenators. Thorax 25:146
25. Åberg T, Kihlgren M (1977b) Cerebral production during open-heart surgery. Thorax 32:525
26. Åberg T, Kihlgren M (1980) The use of psychometric testing as a quality criterion in open-heart surgery. In: Speidel H, Rodewald G (eds) Psychic and neurological dysfunctions after open-heart surgery. Thieme, Stuttgart, pp 107–111
27. Gilberstadt H, Sako Y (1967) Intellectual and personality changes following open-heart surgery. Arch Gen Psychiatry 16:210–214
28. Priest WS, Zaks MS, Yacorzynski GK, Boshes B (1957) The neurologic psychiatric, and psychologic aspects of cardiac surgery. Med Clin North Am 41:155–169
29. Zaks MS (1962) Longitudinal research studies of effects of heart disease and cardiac surgery on psychologic and neurologic functioning. In: Toulentes TT, Pollack SL, Himwich HE (eds) Research approaches to psychiatric problems. Grune and Strutton, New York, pp 164–178
30. Bethune DW (1980) The assessment of organic brain damage following open-heart surgery. In: Speidel H, Rodewald G (eds) Psychic and neurological dysfunctions after open-heart surgery. Thieme, Stuttgart, pp 100–106
31. Bethune DW (1981) Psychometric testing in the evaluation of the postoperative cardiac patient. In: Longmore DB (ed) Towards safer cardiac surgery. GK Hall Medical, Boston, pp 613–617
32. Savageau JA, Stanton B-A, Jenkins CD, Klein MD (1982) Neuropsychological dysfunction following elective cardiac operation. I. Early assessment. J Thorac Cardiovasc Surg 84:585–594
33. Savageau JA, Stanton B-A, Jenkins CD, Frater RWM (1982) Neuropsychological dysfunction following elective cardiac operation. II. A six-month reassessment. J Thorac Cardiovasc Surg 84:595–600
34. Willner AE, Rabiner CJ, Wisoff BG, Hartstein M, Struve FA, Klein DF (1976) Analogical reasoning and postoperative outcome. Arch Gen Psychiatry 33:255–259
35. Willner AE, Rabiner CJ, Wisoff BG, Fishman J, Rosen B, Hartstein M, Klein DF (1976) Analogy tests and psychopathology at follow-up after open heart surgery. Biol Psychiatry 11:687–696
36. Willner AE, Rabiner CJ (1979) Psychopathology and cognitive dysfunction five years after open heart surgery. Compr Psychiatry 20:409–418

Benefits and Psychological Problems of Aortocoronary Bypass and Valve Replacement Surgery

H.-J. Meffert, A. Boll, G. Huse-Kleinstoll, F. Lempp, G. Rodewald, and H. Speidel

The psychosocial outcome of heart surgery has not kept pace with its medical success. Thus while mortality has decreased from 30% to 2% over the last 30 years, the figures for psychic and vocational rehabilitation in the FRG remain as poor as years ago. Therefore describing the outcome of heart surgery means describing benefits and problems which reflect the discrepancy between the medical objective (from the surgeon's point of view) and the poor subjective outcome (from the patient's point of view) of heart surgery. But these are not only different ways of looking at the surgical outcome; they also represent a discrepancy between rationality and emotions that the patients discover in themselves: they see both aspects and suffer accordingly but are powerless to overcome the problem.

For about 25 years psychiatrists, psychosomaticists, and psychologists have been studying the influence of psychology in heart surgery. An impressive variety of factors contributing to patients' perioperative behavior have been identified (Speidel and Rodewald 1980; Becker et al. 1982), but introducing this knowledge into practical work as an aid to overcome the discrepancy between objective physical results and subjective feelings still seems a serious problem.

The intention of this article, therefore, is to throw more light on the discrepancies between objective and subjective success, the patients' expectations and their disappointments, and psychological knowledge and its practical insignificance.

The results and considerations are based on (a) 75 interviews (55 valve replacement and 20 bypass patients) which were performed 3–5 years after surgery and were part of an extensive study at the Hamburg University Hospital [DFG-SFB 115, Projekt A3/A20 (1974–1981)] designed to investigate the nature, conditional factors, and consequences of postoperative psychoses, following the patients through surgery until a couple of years later, and (b) practical psychological work in terms of ambulant and in-hospital counseling and psychotherapy at the Hamburg Cardiovascular Surgery Department. Since the subsamples are rather small, the results have a descriptive rather than a statistical character and value. But it is interesting that the results in valve patients and bypass patients concerning surgical success and the patients' later problems are on the whole quite similar.

The most reliable and therefore the best way to learn about the benefits and problems of surgery is to interview patients on the basis of a good long-term relationship. Asking them to compare their postoperative cardiac situation with their preoperative symptoms, 79% stated a definite success, which corresponded to the objective physical improvement as measured by surgeons and cardiologists. However, asking them to compare their present cardiac situation with their expectations, about 70% complained of unexpected cardiac problems. While doctors admitted that the patients' cardiac situation was not perfect but almost as good as could be expected, the patients mostly agreed that it was better than it had been but was still unsatisfactory.

The subjective complaints cast a shadow over the objective success of surgery. The discrepancy is striking. According to the cardiologists' rating, only 15% of the bypass patients showed serious symptoms of angina pectoris whereas 53% complained of severe symptoms under mild physical strain. Rhythm problems were objectively diagnosed in 33% but were reported by about 70% of patients. In the valve replacement group, cardiac insufficiency under heavy physical strain was objectively diagnosed in 38% of the patients but complained of by 45%. At 52%, the number of patients reporting anginose pain under physical strain is surprisingly high compared with the 10% in whom it was diagnosed by the cardiologists. These findings - together with additional bodily complaints in 65% of the patients which they themselves but not the physicians related to the heart and which therefore have to be regarded as functional psychosomatic symptoms - illustrate the psychological component of heart disease and surgery as well as its inadequate treatment.

But it is not only bodily complaints from which heart surgery patients suffer. Successful surgery and rehabilitation in the patients' eyes obviously mean much more than improvement of the cardiac situation and going back to work rather they involve a positive change in all facets of life. In fact, instead of enjoying their lives as would be expected from the objective positive outcome, many patients suffer from all sorts of problems which in their minds are mainly connected with the surgery.

Less than half of the patients (not including housewives, because they do not have a realistic chance of retiring) returned to work (47% of the bypass patients and 38% of the valve patients) but even about half of these complained of a vocational setback or too much stress, and of those who retired one-third had problems with this status. 21% of the bypass and 41% of the valve patients complained about partnership problems, 32% of the bypass and 15% of the valve patients suffered from memory disturbances and difficulties in concentrating, 47% of the bypass and 33% of the valve patients mentioned problems with sexuality in terms of impotence, lack of libido, fear of failure, or their own or their partner's fear of causing damage to the operated heart.

A number of serious problems which one can discover almost solely through interviews, and hardly by questionnaires, concern psychic alterations and, among these, ideas regarding death. 53% of the bypass and 41% of the valve patients stated that their character had changed, and most of them complained of a loss of self-esteem, depressive moods, psychic lability, hypersensitivity, irritability, and sometimes aggressive behavior. With 53% of the bypass but only 28% of the valve patients, death was a very affective idea: They complained about fears of death and failed to overcome the loss of relatives or friends (especially when death was related to heart disease) or even to endure suicidal ideas.

But psychic changes are not only experienced negatively; they can be positive as well. One-quarter of the patients felt emotionally stronger than before the surgery, appreciated their greater earnestness and sensitivity, and therefore estimated their life to be more valuable and richer.

Overall these results show that heart surgery patients, and especially bypass patients, form a group of psychically endangered individuals, who as a whole have not been psychically stable before surgery. Many patients needed psychopharmacological agents preoperatively, mostly tranquilizers and sleeping tablets during the last preoperative week, but more often and more intensively than any other group of heart surgery patients the coronary patients hold psychic reasons to be responsible for their basic illness and complain of decreased self-esteem. It is on this basis that the course through preparation, surgery, ICU, and recovery must be seen and understood. This course is routine for the doctors and the personnel, but an individual experience for the patients. For many of them it is a path that is full of contradictory experiences, expectations, and disappointments and for this reason often anticipates later problems.

The preoperative phase is marked by the patient's oscillation between fears of death and unrealistic expectations. From the doctor's information about surgery the patient learns that there is no reason to be anxious since the mortality risk of an uncomplicated bypass operation is about 2% (like that of a gallbladder operation), that his heart will be stopped during the surgical procedure, and that he can in all respects lead a normal life afterwards. For most patients, however, the operation is not a technical event; the heart is not an organ like the gallbladder but the center and motor of their life and emotions, and since a standstill of the heart means death, they experience this idea as a serious threat. Blacher (1983) came to the conclusion that most patients estimate a 50:50 chance of survival instead of the realistic 98% chance, and he discovered postoperatively a large number of rebirth and resurrection phantasies in his patients.

On the other hand there are the patients' unrealistic expectations about the surgery. There is the standing expression that after the operation everything will change for the better; even the solution of, for example, partnership problems is left to the future. The truth is, of course, that the operation usually does not solve this sort of emotional problem, and realizing that this hope was an illusion necessarily causes disappointment.

The early postoperative phase is marked by the patient's fluctuation between euphoric and depressive moods, physical pain and relief, mental clarity and cloudiness. More bypass patients than any other group of heart surgery patients, 58%, show psychopathological disorders (Götze 1981), but compared with valve patients (52% psychopathological disorders) the disorders are much more determined by psychological and psychosocial factors, especially in terms of suffering from anxiety and denying it at the same time (Meffert et al. 1983), which is further proof of the psychic lability of this group.

Neither before nor after the operation is the psychically labile patient the real master of his anxiety. But especially after the operation the patient becomes aware of the irrationality of his anxiety, when he experiences that despite the physician's assurance about the surgical success and despite his own confirmation that the number of his physical complaints has decreased, his intellect is not able to overcome his fears; in fact his anxiety and depression often increase after the surgery and are still stronger after 3 weeks than preoperatively.

Among the reasons for the poor subjective rehabilitation of bypass patients two external facts have to be discussed: the patients' psychosocial surroundings and the public subsidies for heart surgery patients in the FRG. Cardiac patients very often feel ashamed to talk about their emotional problems because they do not feel that they will be accepted. "Your heart has been successfully operated on, so why do you complain. But don't drink, don't smoke, don't carry heavy things, don't work too hard, don't get excited, just relax, feel fine and enjoy your life." In the name of caring for the patient, everybody else – partners, friends, and very often the family doctor – is convinced that they know better than the patient himself what is good for him. And as the patient can neither fulfil the paradoxical claims nor resist them (since he experiences them as others' worry about his life), he often resigns.

The second external reason concerns the legal regulations in our country, which grant every heart surgery patient the right to be treated as a disabled person and offer a number of, for example, financial privileges. This practice, of course, supports a sometimes admitted, sometimes unconscious secondary illness gain, and for quite a number of patients it is no longer attractive to become fully physically rehabilitated.

The poor subjective rehabilitation reflects the patients' perioperative experiences in terms of fear of death, depression, disappointments, and illness gain. The longlasting discrepancy between an objectively successful and a subjectively disappointing outcome reflects the biased rational behavior of the medical staff towards the patient's irrationality and its helplessness to handle and overcome the latter. The physician's rational explanations often help as little as the patient's own intellect to change emotions. What is necessary is at least to supplement the medical treatment of the physical condition with a psychological understanding of the patient's problems and feelings from his own subjective point of view. This empathic understanding must be a reliable escort through the surgery, sometimes lasting for a long time.

Only very slowly are the results and recommendations of 25 years of psychological research in heart surgery finding the respect they deserve and becoming integrated in daily clinical routine. One reason for this slow development is that during this period surgeons have concentrated solely on improving the surgical procedure in order to minimize mortality. Another quite different reason is that pure somatic medicine and psychosomatic or psychological medicine are based on two altogether different theoretical models concerning the localization and treatment of a defect which do not supplement but rather exclude each other (Uexküll 1979). Pure somatic medicine uses the basic model of an anatomic body and determines the position of a defect in the body. Psychosomatic or psychological medicine uses the model of a psychic system which is formed during an individual biography, and localization of a defect means identifying conflicts in this history. This discrepancy is supposedly still the most serious obstacle to a mutual acceptance of professional medical and psychological work and to more successful collaboration in many heart surgery centers.

References

Becker R, Katz J, Polonius M-J, Speidel H (eds) (1982) Psychopathological and neurological dysfunctions following open heart surgery. Springer, Berlin Heidelberg New York

Blacher RS (1983) Death, resurrection and rebirth: Observations in cardiac surgery. Psychoanal Q 52:56–72

Götze P (1981) Psychopathologie der Herzoperierten. Enke, Stuttgart

Meffert H-J, Boll A, Dahme B, Götze P, Huse-Kleinstoll G, Polonius M-J, Prüssmann K, Speidel H, Wessel M (1983) Der relative Anteil somatischer und psychischer Befunde an der Vorhersage psychopathologischer Auffälligkeiten nach Herzoperationen. In: Studt HH (ed) Psychosomatik in Forschung und Praxis. Urban & Schwarzenberg, Munich

Speidel H, Rodewald G (eds) (1980) Psychic and neurologic dysfunctions after open-heart-surgery. INA, vol 19, Thieme, Stuttgart

Uexküll T v (1979) Lehrbuch der psychosomatischen Medizin. Urban & Schwarzenberg, Vienna

Psychological and Behavioral Responses

D. S. Kornfeld, S. S. Heller, K. A. Frank, S. N. Wilson,
and J. R. Malm

Introduction

Coronary artery bypass surgery (CABS) has been shown to reduce angina, as well as to prolong life in some subsets of patients [1–4]. Studies of the postoperative quality of life are now considered important in further justifying the use of this costly procedure.

Several American studies have not shown sufficient improvement in postoperative employment rates to warrant surgery on that basis [5–9]. In fact, Lamendola and Pelligrini [8] and Gundle et al. [9] reported that employment actually decreased for all age groups in their samples. Noting that patients nevertheless were satisfied with the results of surgery and felt physically improved, the authors have suggested studying broader criteria of quality of life than merely return to work.

Long-term psychological and behavioral outcomes after cardiac valvular surgery have been studied [10–14] but have limited comparability to those after CABS, as the patients involved are substantially different both medically and psychologically. In general, coronary bypass patients are unburdened by the physical limitations and associated psychological adaptations produced by long-standing chronic cardiac illness. Indeed, many are typically hard-driving, competitive individuals showing the so-called type A behavior pattern. However, little is currently known about the persistence of these behaviors in the face of illness and surgical intervention.

The current study traced the postoperative psychological and behavioral courses of patients following CABS. Particular attention was paid to quality of life, compliance to medical regimens, and the postoperative stability of the type A coronary-prone behavior pattern. Medical outcome variables were concurrently examined.

Method

One hundred consecutive patients who underwent CABS at the Columbia Presbyterian Medical Center from December 1972 through February 1975 were evaluated at the time of surgery and then followed for as long as 4½ years in order to study their postoperative psychosocial and behavioral courses.

One death occurred within the first 30 postoperative days.

Fifty-four patients returned for a personal follow-up visit 9 months postoperatively. Fifty-seven patients, 30 of whom had been seen at 9 months, returned a follow-up questionnaire administered on average 3½ years after surgery. At approximately 4½ years, the medical outcomes for 92 patients were obtained by questionnaire or telephone follow-up.

Data were analyzed statistically by correlation analysis, with the criterion of statistical significance at the 0.05 level (two-tailed).

Sample

The mean age of the patients was 52.1 years; age ranged from 35 to 65 years (Table 1). Ninety-three percent were male and 91% married; half had attended college. The group was primarily middle-class, with 74% in social classes 3 and 4 [15]. Classes 1, 2, and 5 constituted 7%, 9%, and 11% of the group, respectively.

Table 1. Patient characteristics[a]

Characteristic	% of patients
Male	93
Married	91
Social class (3 and 4)	74
Angina	
Extreme	44
Mild to moderate	45

[a] The mean age of the patients was 52.1 ± 7.1 years; $n = 100$

Chest pain, the usual indication for surgery, was extreme in 44% and mild to moderate in 45% of patients. Only 11% had no preoperative anginal pain. Fifty-three percent had sustained at least one preoperative myocardial infarction and 13% more than one; 20% had a history of congestive heart failure. The mean New York Heart Association (NYHA) functional class was 3.2. At operation, 28% had one coronary artery bypassed, 56% two, and 16% three. Four patients had concomitant valvular surgery, and four had ventricular aneurysm repair. Nine percent sustained a perioperative myocardial infarction.

The patients evaluated at 9 months and 3½ years were statistically compared. They did not differ significantly from one another or from the overall sample in age, sex, marital status, or NYHA functional classification.

Types of Preoperative Data

Prior to surgery, semistructured psychiatric interviews lasting 1½ to 3 h were conducted, following which psychiatric and social data were recorded on a modified version of the Psychiatric Evaluation Form (PEF) [16]. Use of the PEF allowed current affect, behavior, and social role to be quantified.

To supplement the psychiatric assessment, the Cattell 16 Personality Factor (PF) Questionnaire [17], which permits comprehensive personality measurement in broad areas of functioning, was administered. In addition, the Rosenman-Friedman Standardized Interview to measure type A coronary-prone behavior was given, and ratings of overall type A behavior, as well as subratings of aggressive content, vocal stylistics, job commitment, and sense of time urgency, were made. The more extreme form of type A behavior is referred to as A1, the less extreme as A2. The absence of type A is termed type B, and is rated B3 and B4 according to degree.

Types of Postoperative Data

Interview (9 months). The semistructured psychiatric interview and the standardized interview for the coronary-prone behavior pattern were repeated. The presence and severity of angina and the occurrence of myocardial infarction and reoperation were coded.

Questionnaire (3½ years). Patients were given a questionnaire requesting demographic, psychosocial, behavioral, and medical data. They were asked to compare variables such as anginal pain and response to it, physical limitations, weight, smoking, exercise, and manifestations of coronary-prone behavior pre- and postoperatively. They also were requested to estimate their compliance with their doctors' advice with regard to smoking, diet, exercise, behavior, and medication.

Medical Follow-up (4½ years). The patients' postoperative medical courses were studied by contacting them, their physicians, or both. Among the data recorded were fatalities and cardiovascular events such as episodes of arrhythmia or congestive heart failure, myocardial infarctions, cerebrovascular accidents, and additional CABS. Severity of angina and extent to which activity was limited were quantified.

Results

Medical Outcome

After 3½ years, most patients were pleased that they had undergone the operation, 60% extremely so. Only 4% were displeased. Postoperatively, chest pain had been dramatically reduced. It was rated extreme by only 4%, moderate by 16%, and minimal by 28%, while 53% of patients were pain-free. Numbers of blocks walked and flights of stairs climbed had improved commensurately.

Twenty-eight percent had been hospitalized for cardiac disease at least once since surgery, and 11% had sustained a myocardial infarction. Sixteen percent had undergone repeat CABS.

At 4½ years, data were obtained on 92 patients (92%). Twenty-three were reported as deceased. Fifteen of the 23 deaths definitely resulted from cardiac causes, and in only three patients was a noncardiac cause known. Eighty-seven percent of the deaths were in individuals rated type A preoperatively, with 67% A1; the overall sample was 84% type A and 61% A1.

Data on angina assessment were available for 64 survivors. Thirty-five patients (55%) had no angina. Ten patients (16%) rated their angina as mild, 7 (11%) as moderate, and 12 (19%) as extreme.

Return to Work

Seventy-seven percent of the patients were working at the time of surgery, and 76% were working at the time of the 9-month evaluation. As would be expected, failure to return to work correlated with measures of cardiac disease severity. Patients who returned to work were significantly younger ($P<0.05$), showed more improvement in angina ($P<0.01$), and were more likely to be type A preoperatively ($P<0.05$) and postoperatively ($P<0.001$).

At the 3½ year follow-up, 65% were employed, with 6% having more than one job. Of those working, 62% worked full-time. Two-thirds of the patients reported improved satisfaction in their work.

Return to Sexual Activity

Sexual frequency preoperatively and nine months postoperatively were compared (Fig. 1). Prior to surgery, 67% were sexually active at least once a week, 22% were less active, and 11% had no sexual activity. Nine months postoperatively, only 38% were sexually active at least once a week, and 31% reported no sexual activity.

Postoperative increase in frequency of sexual activity correlated with preoperative cardiac impairment (NYHA functional class) ($P<0.001$), return to work ($P<0.01$), and pre- and postoperative type A ratings ($P<0.05$).

Patients' Subjective Report

According to a questionnaire administered 3½ years postoperatively, overall pleasure in life had improved substantially, with reduced overall nervousness, improved mood, and improved job, family, and sexual satisfaction. Pleasure in life improved in the most patients (77%), sexual satisfaction in the least (44%). Conversely, only a minority reported worsening in these areas, with family relations worsening in the least (4%) and sexual satisfaction in the most (23%) patients (Table 2).

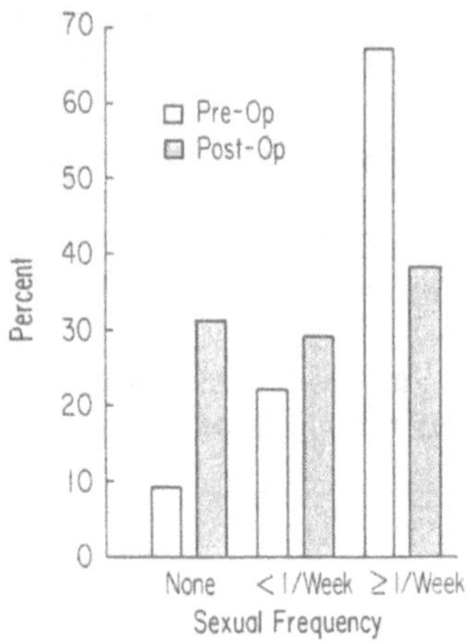

Fig. 1. Comparison of sexual frequency preoperatively and 9 months postoperatively

Table 2. Percentages of patients reporting various degrees of change in aspects of life adjustment ($n = 57$)

Aspect of adjustment	Status at 3½ years as compared to that before surgery (% change)				
	Much better	Slightly better	No change	Slightly worse	Much worse
Pleasure	65	12	12	9	2
Nervousness	30	23	32	11	4
Mood	42	24	24	5	5
Job satisfaction	41	21	22	10	6
Family relations	48	22	25	10	2
Sexual satisfaction	22	22	33	10	13

Behavioral Risk Factors

Smoking. At the time of surgery, 39% were smokers, with 30% consuming one pack or more per day. Nine months postoperatively, only 13% were smoking.

At 3½ years, 57% of the sample recalled being advised not to smoke. Sixty percent of these patients rated their compliance as full; 28% said they had complied fairly well, 9% poorly, and 3% not at all.

Weight and Diet. At nine months, weight generally differed little from that preoperatively; it had increased markedly in only 7% of patients. Weight gain was correlated inversely with smoking ($P < 0.05$).

At 3½ years, 62% of patients remembered being advised to change their diets, but only 22% of those had done so fully. Sixty-eight percent rated their compliance as fairly good and 11% as poor.

Exercise. At 3½ years, 67% had been advised to change their exercise pattern, primarily to increase it. Thirty-eight percent did so fully, 47% fairly well, and 15% poorly.

Compliance Regarding Medication. Compliance with advice related to cardiac medications generally was good, with 86% complying fully and 11% fairly well. Three percent did not comply at all.

Type A Behavior Pattern. Preoperatively, 64% of the patients were rated A1, 24% A2, 11% B3, and 2% B4. Postoperatively, 55% were A1, 29% A2, 15% B3, and 2% B4. Table 3 shows behavior type ratings preoperatively and 9 months postoperatively for the 54 patients reinterviewed and the changes within each type. In general, patients reported that their physicians had told them to slow down after surgery. Nine months after surgery, 41 (75%) were unchanged in overall A rating. Four patients (7%) had become more type A and ten patients (18%) less so. Only three patients (5%) changed from A to B. At 3½ years, 31% thought they had slowed down greatly, 21% somewhat, 25% a little, and 16% not at all; 7% pushed themselves more.

Table 3. Behavior type ratings ($n = 54$)

Preoperatively	At 9 months		
	Type	*n*	%
A1	A1	26	74
$n = 35$	A2	7	20
	B3	2	4
	B4	0	0
A2	A1	3	23
$n = 13$	A2	9	69
	B3	1	8
	B4	0	0
B	A1	1	17
$n = 6$	A2	0	0
	B3	5	83
	B4	0	0

Of the components of type A, vocal stylistics and aggressive content were extremely stable, whereas job commitment and time urgency showed some change. Less than half (12 of 27) of the patients showing type A1 job commitment remained A1 in this respect. Thirteen became A2, and one each became B3 and B4.

Preoperative A2 job commitment ratings were more stable. Nine (60%) of the 15 patients who were preoperatively A2 remained so, while four (27%) became A1 and two (13%) became B3. Six of the eight preoperative B3 patients were unchanged, while one each became A1 or B4. Again, few patients (only four) changed from A to B types. The results for time urgency were similar.

Postoperative angina correlated with persistence of type A behavior traits ($P<0.05$). However, it is not clear whether this association reflects a relationship between the behavior pattern and coronary heart disease or the extra demands placed on the myocardium by the behavior itself.

Ten patients who had died before the 4½ year follow-up had undergone the 9-month interview. Preoperatively seven had been rated A1 and one each A2, B3, and B4; this distribution is the same as for the sample as a whole. Nine had remained unchanged in overall type A score at 9 months.

All six patients who had extreme angina at the 4½ year follow-up and had been rated A1 preoperatively were still rated A1 at 9 months. Over time, however, severe angina apparently led to a change in behavior, for six of the eight patients who reported extreme angina on the 3½-year questionnaire stated that they had slowed down substantially since their surgery, although their type A status was not measured at 3½ years.

Discussion

Earlier studies of quality of life after CABS focused on return to work as a quantifiable variable [5–9]. In the Lamendola and Pellegrini study of 95 patients followed for 6–36 months, 60% of the sample was working before, but only 40% after, surgery. However, 79% of those who wanted to work were working, 97% of those who did not want to work were retired, and 50% of the retired group perceived themselves as without physical limits. These findings prompted the authors to point out that return to work cannot be used as the sole criterion for a successful outcome [8].

In our sample, 77% were working at the time of surgery and 76% 9 months postoperatively. Three-and-one-half years postoperatively, 65% were employed, an apparently very successful outcome. Yet Gundle et al., like Lamendola and Pellegrini, report very different findings: of 30 patients, only 17% were employed 12–24 months after surgery. However, only 22% had been employed at the time of surgery. The type A patients were more likely to be working. Their sample was heavily weighted with blue-collar workers, but they also found an inhibition to work among those in less strenuous jobs. Patients tended to continue to think of themselves as "damaged."

Gundle and his colleagues suggested that the prolonged period of unemployment prior to surgery in their group may have contributed to the failure to return to work. Indeed, most studies suggest that work status at the time of surgery is the best predictor of postoperative status. Although these patients, out of work preoperatively, might have been sicker at the time of surgery, with impaired ventricles with limited capacity for improvement, it is more likely that psychological or social factors determined whether they returned to work. For example, we must keep in mind that for some, the stress of working may have been perceived as contributing to coronary heart disease. How great a role this belief plays in the decision to retire or reduce one's workload remains unknown. For others, disability or retirement income may be adequate enough to justify giving up a larger income from a less than satisfactory job. We must therefore learn to distinguish between those patients who freely choose not to resume work and those who are prevented from working by a fear of working or by employers' policies or attitudes.

It is of interest that reports in the British literature more consistently show a high rate of return to work after surgery in both white-collar and heavy manual workers [18, 19], even in those with prolonged periods of unemployment [18]. It is not clear what there may be in British management of patients or social policy which accounts for these differences in outcome.

What of other outcome criteria? Most patients in our sample reported substantial improvement in angina and exercise capacity. The operation also led to substantial improvements in overall quality of life, including general pleasure; reduction of anxiety and depression; and improvement in job satisfaction and family relations.

Sexual adjustment improved less than other measures. In fact, at 9 months the frequency of sexual activity had declined for approximately one-third of the sample; and at 3½ years, one-fourth continued to report a worsened sexual adjustment.

The North Carolina group also found considerable impairment of sexual functioning postoperatively. Whereas 73% of their patients reported satisfactory sexual functioning before surgery, only 47% were satisfied with their sexual functioning afterward. Fifty-seven percent of the men were impotent. Yet, after surgery, 69% of their sample had been able to reach their predicted exercise tolerance on the treadmill. As in our group, the impairment of sexual functioning was most common in those patients who had been most symptomatic before surgery. Although the sicker patients thus appear to have less sexual activity after surgery, it is not clear whether this outcome is the result of persistent physical impairment or of persistent anxiety in the patient or spouse. It is of interest that in one British study, which shows an excellent rate of return to work, 96% of the patients reported restricted sexual activity prior to surgery but only 30% failed to improve postoperatively [19].

Our own findings of generally good overall psychological and social outcome following surgery, while essentially agreeing with those of Lamendola and Pellegrini [8], contrast with those of Gundle et al. [9], who report that considerable morbidity may persist despite correction of coronary insufficiency. In their sample, even the type A patients, who were more likely to be employed postoperatively, experienced an overall adaptation that was no better than that of the sample as a whole. These authors suggest that a prolonged period of symptoms and unemployment before surgery may yield a damaged self-image, which the surgery does not rectify. They also speculate that the discrepancy in outcome between their and other studies may reflect the lower socioeconomic status of their patients.

In contrast to cardiac-valve-repair patients, whose psychopathology tends to be in the direction of both pre- and postoperative passivity, a high percentage of CABS patients manifest the very active type A personality. The relatively large proportion of type A patients in this surgical sample probably reflects two factors: (1) the role of type A behavior in producing coronary heart disease and (2) the need of the type A patient to maintain his very active controlling way of life, which surgical treatment is expected to allow to continue.

At the consensus development conference held in December 1980, some participants stated that a significant number of patients may decide too quickly that surgery is the only acceptable way to improve their lives; such individuals find the limitations of a medical regimen unacceptable [21]. It was also suggested that it may be difficult for some physicians to find the time needed to manage these patients medically and encourage them to make significant changes in their way of life. Thus, the combination of a type A patient and a type A physician may be more likely to lead to a decision for surgical management of coronary artery disease.

Follow-up assessments revealed the persistence of the type A behavior pattern in a heavily type A group. Severe postoperative angina was associated with reduction of hard-driving behavior over time, while postoperative physical improvement typically allowed for resumption of such activity.

Prospective studies to determine whether persistent type A behavior is associated with arteriosclerosis in a grafted vessel are now needed. Type A behavior pattern has been associated with coronary artery disease recurrence in a post-myocardial infarction population [22]. Our own sample probably is too heavily weighted with the type A pattern to provide statistically significant data in a group of only 100 patients. It should be noted that the type A behavior pattern has a number of components: hostile competition, time urgency, job involvement, and a particular speech pattern. Perhaps modification of only some of them may be sufficient to reduce the progression of coronary heart disease [22].

Conclusion

Most studies of coronary artery bypass surgery patients demonstrate a substantial relief of pain and improvement in quality of life as measured by a variety of standards. Return to work as a criterion of successful outcome is a complex matter which should be examined further.

There appears to be a need for physicians to discuss postoperative sexual activity with their patients to relieve misconceptions and inhibitions, for this activity showed least improvement. Whereas compliance with medical recommendations regarding smoking and exercise was relatively good, little shift in the type A behavior pattern was found. The implications of this observation for recurrence of coronary heart disease should be studied.

Summary

One hundred consecutive patients who underwent coronary artery bypass surgery at the Columbia-Presbyterian Medical Center from December 1972 through February 1975 were evaluated at the time of their surgery and then followed for as long as 4½ years, to study their postoperative psychosocial and behavioral course. There was one death in the first 30 days. At 4½ years, 23 patients were reported as deceased, 15 from clearly cardiac causes. The majority of long-term survivors reported substantial improvement in angina and exercise capacity, although the surgery did not increase the number employed. The operation also led to substantial improvements in the quality of life, including general pleasure, reduction of anxiety and depression, and felt improvement in job and family roles. Sexual adjustment improved the least, with a tendency to decreased frequency. Compliance with their medical regimen was relatively good for smoking and exercise, but not for diet or hard-driving (type A) behavior, suggesting a need for psychological intervention.

Acknowledgement. This work was supported in part by Alcohol, Drug Abuse and Mental Health Administration Grant MH-12756 from the National Institute of Mental Health.

References

1. Braunwald E (1978) Evaluation of the efficacy of coronary bypass surgery II. Am J Cardiol 42:161
2. Loop FD, Proudjit WL, Sheldon WC (1978) Coronary bypass surgery weighted in the balance. Am J Cardiol 42:154
3. Huldgren HN, Taucaro T, Detrie KN, Murphy ML (1978) Evaluation of the efficacy of coronary artery bypass surgery I. Am J Cardiol 42:157
4. Coronary Artery Bypass Surgery (1981) Scientific and clinical aspects, NIH Consensus Development Conference Statement. N Engl J Med 304:680
5. Barnes G, Ray MJ, Oberman A, Kouchoukas NT (1977) Changes in working status of patients following coronary bypass surgery. JAMA 238:1259
6. Hammermeister KE, DeRouen TA, English MT, Dodge HT (1979) Effect of surgical versus medical therapy on return to work in patients with coronary artery disease. Am J Cardiol 44:105
7. Rimm AA, Barboriak JJ, Anderson AJ (1976) Changes in occupation after aorto-coronary vein-bypass graft surgery. JAMA 236:631
8. Lamendola WF, Pelligrini RV (1979) Quality of life and coronary artery bypass surgery patients. Soc Sci Med 134:457
9. Gundle MJ, Reeves BR, Tate S, Raft D, McLaurin LP (1980) Psychological outcome after coronary artery bypass surgery. Am J Psychiatry 137:1591
10. Heller SS, Frank KA, Kornfeld DS, Malm JR, Bowman FO Jr. (1974) Psychological outcome following open-heart surgery. Arch Intern Med 134:908
11. Frank KA, Heller SS, Kornfeld DS (1972) A survey of adjustment to cardiac surgery. Arch Intern Med 130:735
12. Kimball CP (1969) Psychological responses to the experience of open-heart surgery. Am J Psychiatry 126:348
13. Lucia W, McGuire LB (1970) Rehabilitation and functional status after surgery for valvular heart disease. Arch Intern Med 126:995

14. Blachly PH, Blachly BJ (1968) Vocational and emotional status of 263 patients after heart surgery. Circulation 38:524
15. Hollingshead A, Redlich FC (1978) Social class and mental illness. Wiley, New York
16. Spitzer R, Endicott J (1966) Progress report biometric research. NY. New York State Department of Mental Hygiene, Research Division, Washington Heights Community Service, New York State Psychiatric Institute, Department of Psychiatry
17. Cattell RB, Eber HW (1962) Handbook for the 16PF Questionnaire, Institute for Personality and Ability Testing, Urbana II, 1962 Edition
18. Wallwork J, Putter B, Caves PN (1978) Return to work after coronary artery bypass surgery. B Med J 12 (6153):1680
19. Westaby S, Sasford RN, Bentall HH (1978) Return to work and quality of life after surgery for coronary artery disease. Br Med J 2:1028
20. Jenkins CD, Zyzanski SJ, Rosenman RH (1976) Rise of new myocardial infarction in middle-aged men with manifest coronary heart disease. Circulation 53:352
21. Consensus of Bypass Surgery. Science 211:42
22. Frank KA, Heller SS, Kornfeld DS (1979) Psychological intervention in coronary heart disease: A review. Gen Hosp Psychiatry 1:18

Return to Work and Sexual Relations Among Patients Following Coronary Artery Bypass Grafting and Myocardial Infarction

M. Benyakar, S. Mibashan, L. Levinsky, C. Rosemberg, Y. Fuchs, and M. J. Levy

The terms "return to work" and "frequency of sexual relations" appear in the literature dealing with the rehabilitation of coronary patients. These terms are used as important measurements of the patients' rehabilitation. Most research work has dealt with the male patient and only rarely with the spouse of the male patient. Reports about the rate of return to work after the events of myocardial infarction (MI) or coronary artery bypass graft surgery (CABG) vary, and researchers point to a number of variables which are likely to explain the results of their work.

Concerning MI patients, a return to work rate ranging between 52% and 91% has been reported (Table 1) (Bar-On and Crystal 1981; Croog and Levine 1977; Kellerman et al. 1968; Kushnir et al. 1975; Osterman et al. 1981). Concerning patients who underwent CABG surgery, the literature points to a return to work rate ranging between 17% and 88% (Table 2) (Gundle et al. 1980; Jenkins et al. 1983; Oberman and Finklea 1982; Rosenfeldt et al. 1983). Researchers have explained their results on the basis of cultural background (Kellerman et al. 1968; Oberman and Finklea 1982), age (Rimm et al. 1976; Rosenfeldt et al. 1983), education (Croog and Levine 1977; De Backer et al. 1981), the type of work and effort involved in the work (Croog and Levine 1977; De Backer et al. 1981; Gundle et al. 1980; Jackson 1978; Rosenfeldt et al. 1983), psychological factors (Bar-On and Crystal 1981; Diedricks et al. 1981; Kellerman 1981), the patient/doctor and patient/employer relationship (Liddle et al. 1982), and the patients' participation in a rehabilitation program (Cody et al. 1981; Goble et al. 1981; Kushnir et al. 1975; Osterman et al. 1981).

Table 1. Return to work following MI – a comparison

Researchers	Year	Country	Rate of return to work (%)
Kellerman et al.	1968	Israel	91
Kushnir et al.	1975–7	England	60
Croog and Levine	1977	USA	62–79
Bar-On and Crystal	1981	Israel	52
Osterman et al.	1981	France	80
Present study	1984	Israel	82.6

Table 2. Return to work following CABG – a comparison

Researcher	Year	Country	Rate of return to work (%)
Gundle et al.	1980	USA	17
Oberman and Finklea	1982	USA	88
Rosenfeldt et al.	1983	Australia	68 (591 in sample) 78 (100 in sample)
Jenkins et al.	1983	USA	75
Present study	1984	Israel	85

Regarding the variable "frequency of sexual relations", which is the parameter most often investigated in coronary patients, the tendency in the literature is to report on a decrease in their frequency following the event (MI or CABG) (Table 3). Concerning MI patients, the percentage decrease in frequency of sexual relations ranges between 24% and 48% per month (Block 1975; Hellerstein and Friedman 1970; Johnston and Fletcher 1979; Lederman 1978). Concerning patients who underwent coronary artery bypass surgery, Johnston and Fletcher (1979) reported a decrease of 10% in the frequency of sexual relations following the surgery. Most researchers found a greater decrease in frequency of sexual relations in MI patients compared to CABG patients.

Table 3. Frequency of sexual relations among MI and CABG patients before and after the event. A comparison between the USA and Israel

Country	Research workers	MI patients			CABG patients		
		Before	After	Decrease	Before	After	Decrease
USA	Hellerstein and Friedman (1970)	8.4	6.4	24%			
USA	Bloch (1975)	5.2	2.7	48%			
USA	Johnston and Fletcher (1979)	6.4	4.6	28%	8.4	7.6	10%
Israel	Lederman (1978)	8.5	5.8	32%			
Israel	Present study	9.5	6.8	28.4%	9.6	9.0	6%

The present work, as in other studies, examines the variables "return to work" and "frequency of sexual relations" but also includes additional parameters such as "type of work," "effort involved at work," and a variable we call the "emotional involvement" at work.

The purpose of this study was to examine the changes occurring in 215 patients who suffered an MI or underwent CABG surgery. The variables studied included those associated with employment and those associated with sexual relations The relationship between work and sexual relation parameters was also studied, both from the viewpoint of the patient and his spouse.

Population Sample

Included in the sample were male and female patients after MI or CABG surgery, and their spouses. These patients were chosen out of those patients who underwent surgery at the department of cardiac surgery or were being followed up at the rehabilitation unit of Beilinson Hospital. They were chosen according to the following criteria:

1. Age between 35 and 60 years.
2. They were all married.
3. In the MI group, it was their first myocardial infarction. In the CABG group there was no previous myocardial infarction and they underwent surgery because of angina pectoris with or without congestive heart failure.
4. A period of 6 months to 3 years had passed since the event (MI or CABG).

Not included in the sample were:

1. Patients taking drugs likely to affect their sexual function
2. Patients suffering from illnesses likely to harm their sexual function, especially diabetes mellitus and hypertension among males, urogenital disorders, malignant diseases, valvular heart disease, collagen disorders, and neurological and psychiatric disorders
3. Illiterate patients

Research Methods

Collection of data in this work was done by the following methods:

1. A semistructured interview with the patient and spouse relating to the changes that had occurred since the event (MI or CABG) in the patients' life-style – particularly regarding sexual relations and emotional involvement at work.
2. A semistructured sexual questionnaire based on the Marriage Council of Philadelphia, I.N.C., Marriage Adjustment Schedule, 1B, Philadelphia, Pennsylvania. The questionnaire included questions meant to provide information on the patient's sex life and on the frequency of sexual relations (each partner answered about him or herself).

The process of research

The patients were invited to the hospital with their spouses for a medical examination and a conversation with the doctor. Upon their arrival the patients were separated from their spouses and interviewed separately, but at the same time so as not to permit exchange of information between themselves. The interviewers were a male and female doctor, and the male and female testees were divided equally between them. Concerning employment, the patient was asked to answer about himself and the spouse was asked to answer about him/herself and about the partner. Concerning the sexual questions each of the partners was asked to answer about him or herself.

Interpretation of Data

The statistical tests by means of which the data were interpreted were the chi-square and Student's *t*-tests.

Results

The population in question consisted of 430 examinees of whom half were patients and half their spouses. Of the 215 patients, 89 (41%) had had MI and 126 (59%) CABG. The majority were males. The percentage of females among the MI and CABG groups was 17% and 15% respectively (Table 4). The ages of the

Table 4. Research population[a]

	CABG	MI	Total
Male	107	74	181
Female	19	15	34
Total	126	89	215

[a] The research population included the 215 spouses of the above patients

patients ranged between 35 and 60 years, and on average the spouse (in most cases female) was younger (Table 5). Regarding education, more than half of the population under survey had had a high school or more advanced education, and only 3% had not had a formal education. Regarding employment, 83.7% of the patients were working after the event (MI or CABG). Fifty-five percent of these were working full-time. There was only a small difference between the MI and the CABG population in respect of the percentage working: 82.6% of the MI group compared to 85% of the CABG group. But there was a striking difference regarding full- or part-time work; 63.1% of the CABG patients were working full-time compared with 43.5% of the MI group (Table 6). Regarding the type of work and the physical effort involved at work, nearly 60% of the patients (CABG and MI) were working at a sedentary occupation or other light work, and nearly 40% were involved in light manual labor. This ratio was found separately in both groups (Table 7). However, a profound difference between the two population samples was that among the MI group 16.7% were salaried workers employed by the defence forces while not one of the CABG group was employed by the army (Table 8). 6.3% of the CABG group were pensioners while there were no pensioners in the MI group. 17.4% of the

MI group stopped working on account of their heart disease, compared to 5.6% among the CABG group (Table 6). According to this study, when comparing the two groups there was less tendency for the CABG patients to change from a physical to a less demanding occupation (Table 9).

Table 5. Population distribution by percentage according to age

	<30	30–34	35–39	40–44	45–49	50–54	55–59	60–64	65
MI patients	0	0	14	0	27	27	32	0	0
CABG patients	0	0	12	9	31	24	24	0	0
Total patients	0	0	13	5	30	25	27	0	0
MI spouses	10	0	0	21	11	26	21	0	11
CABG spouses	0	0	31	16	26	33	19	6	3
Total spouses	4	0	18	16	21	17	14	4	6
Total population	2	0	15	10	26	21	19	4	3

Table 6. Sample population distribution by percentage according to level of employment

Level of employment	MI		CABG	
	Patient	Spouse	Patient	Spouse
Full-time work	43.5	33.3	63.1	45.2
Part-time work	21.7	11.1	12.5	16.1
Housekeeper	17.4	38.9	9.4	38.7
Does not work on account of:				
a) Heart disease	17.4	0.0	5.6	0.0
b) Other medical reasons	0.0	0.0	3.1	0.0
c) Nonmedical reasons	0.0	0.0	0.0	0.0
Pensioner	0.0	16.7	6.3	0.0
Total	100.0	100.0	100.0	100.0

Table 7. Sample population distribution by percentage according to the amount of physical exertion at work

Type of work	MI		CABG	
	Patient	Spouse	Patient	Spouse
Sedentary	33.3	62.5	27.3	56.3
Light work (in shop)	16.7	12.5	31.8	25.0
Teacher	8.3	0.0	0.0	12.4
Postman/messenger	0.0	0.0	4.5	0.0
Dockworker/porter	8.3	0.0	0.0	0.0
Building/agricultural work	0.0	0.0	0.0	0.0
Worker in heavy industry	0.0	12.5	0.0	0.0
Light manual work	33.3	12.5	36.5	6.3
Total	100.0	100.0	100.0	100.0

Table 8. Sample population distribution by percentage - self-employed/salaried

Type of employment	MI		CABG	
	Patient	Spouse	Patient	Spouse
Defence forces employee	16.7	0.0	0.0	0.0
Salaried employee elsewhere	58.0	87.5	84.0	87.5
Self-employed	25.3	12.5	16.0	12.5

Table 9. Change in type of work (%) after MI or CABG according to patients and spouses

Change in type of work	MI		CABG	
	Patient	Spouse	Patient	Spouse
Less physical exertion	20.0	28.0	17.6	15.6
Less psychological strain	20.0	18.0	4.0	12.5
More physical exertion	12.0	0.0	7.0	11.0
More psychological strain	8.3	0.0	0.0	5.0
No change	27.0	35.0	49.0	46.0
Cessation of work on medical advice	6.0	14.0	11.8	3.1
Cessation of work own decision	6.0	5.0	8.8	6.3

Regarding "emotional involvement at work," there was no change in 62% of the MI group, while 19% increased and 19% decreased their emotional involvement. By contrast 50.6% of the CABG group did not change while 24.4% increased and 25% decreased their emotional involvement (Table 10). In the CABG group there was a difference in estimation by spouses and patients of emotional involvement at work.

Table 10. Change in emotional involvement at work following MI or CABG (in percentage) as reported by patients and spouses

Emotional involvement	MI		CABG	
	Patient	Spouse	Patient	Spouse
Less	19.0	11.8	25.0	11.1
Equal	62.0	76.4	50.6	70.4
Increase	19.0	11.8	24.4	18.5
Total	100.0	100.0	100.0	100.0

According to the results of this study it was not possible to draw conclusions about a possible connection between the frequency of sexual relations and the type (sedentary or physical) of employment (Table 11). There was, however, a significant increase in the rate of sexual relations in the MI group when a *change* was made to an occupation demanding less physical exertion ($P<0.01$) (Table 12). There was also a connection between the subjective parameter "emotional involvement at work" and the rate of sexual relations among the MI group of patients as follows (Table 13): Following the MI, when the emotional involvement of the patient at work increased, so the rate of sexual relations decreased (by 41% according to the patients and by 78% according to their marital partners). This change was significant ($P<0.001$) (Fig. 1). When there was no change in emotional involvement following the MI the decrease was 19% and 25% respectively. When the emotional involvement at work lessened, there was no change in frequency of sexual according to the patient, while the spouse reported on an increase of two and a half times in frequency. In the CABG group it was not possible to point to a connection between the subjective parameter "emotional involvement at work" and the frequency of sexual relations (Fig. 2).

Table 11. Physical exertion at work and the rate (per month) of sexual relations before and after MI or CABG

Type of work	MI patient		CABG patient	
	Before	After	Before	After
Sedentary	13.8	9.8	9.5	8.2
Light work (in shop)	–	–	14.1	12.6
Teacher	10.0	–	–	–
Postman/messenger	–	–	8.0	8.0
Dockworker/porter	16.0	16.0	–	–
Building/agricultural worker	–	–	–	–
Heavy industry	–	–	–	–
Light manual work	16.7	8.25	7.4	7.0

Table 12. Frequency of sexual relations (average/month) in relation to changes occurring at work (before and after MI or CABG)

Change in type of work	MI patient		CABG patient	
	Before	After	Before	After
Less physical exertion[a]	5.6	6.5	5.17	7.17
Less psychological strain	4.0	4.5	7.33	8.0
More physical exertion	7.0	6.0	–	–
More psychological strain	20.0	10.5	–	–
No change	11.3	8.0	10.56	8.53
Cessation of work on medical advice	16.0	6.0	8.5	7.0
Cessation of work own decision	12.0	2.0	17.3	19.0

[a] For MI group $P<0.01$

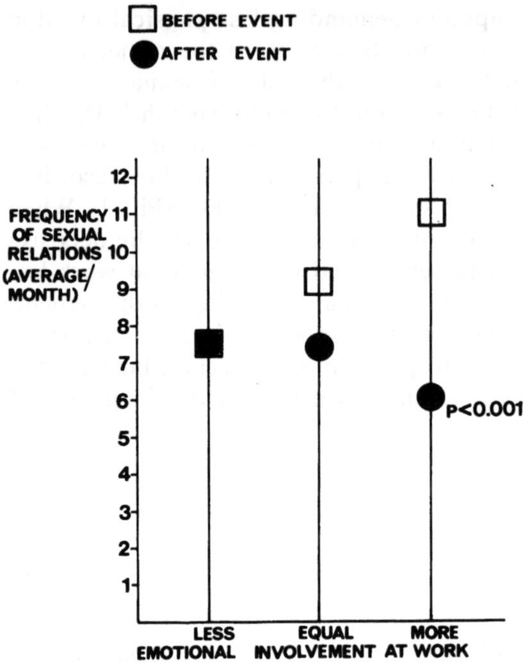

Fig. 1. The relationship between the level of emotional involvement at work and the frequency of sexual relations – MI patients

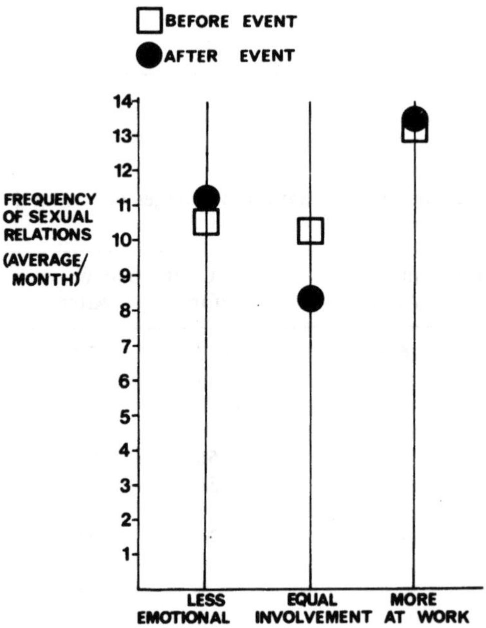

Fig. 2. The relationship between the level of emotional involvement at work and the frequency of sexual relations – CABG patients

Table 13. Frequency of sexual intercourse (average/month) in relation to the emotional involvement at work before and after MI or CABG

Emotional involvement	MI				CABG			
	Patient		Spouse		Patient		Spouse	
	Before	After	Before	After	Before	After	Before	After
Less	7.50	7.50	4.0	10.0	10.60	11.14	10.70	7.30
Equal	9.20	7.40	5.50	4.10	10.20	8.30	6.10	7.40
More[a]	11.00	6.00	11.50	2.50	13.20	13.40	8.40	10.20

[a] For MI group $P<0.001$

Discussion

This work deals with function after MI and CABG by examining two aspects: namely occupational and sexual factors and the possible connection between them.

Regarding employment, it was found that the rate of return to work of the MI patients was 82.6%. This is higher than that found in work done overseas, but lower than that found by Kellerman et al. (1968), who performed their study in Israel and found a return to work rate of 91%. It is possible that there are sociocultural reasons for these differences. In Israeli culture it is possible that the notion of the work ethic was more strongly developed at the time Kellerman et al. made their study (1968). However, in order to study the role of social and cultural factors both a national and international study would be necessary. Concerning the CABG population, the rate of their return to work (85% was higher than that found in most other studies except for that of Oberman and Finklea (1982) in the United States, whose work was done on a highly educated and motivated cultural group with a strongly developed work ethic. In our study the rate of return to work was also directly proportional to the patients' level of education.

Concerning any relationship between occupational and sexual parameters, there was a significant increase in the rate of sexual relations in the MI group when a change was made to an occupation demanding less physical exertion. It was not possible in this study to reach any conclusions about the rate of sexual intercourse and the level of, type of, and physical exertion involved in work in the CABG group. Bar-On and Crystal (1981) in Israel also found a direct relationship between the level of employment and the sexual rehabilitation in MI patients. A connection was also found in our study between the emotional involvement at work and the rate of sexual intercourse among the MI population sample. The rate of sexual intercourse was inversely proportional to the degree of emotional involvement at work. This connection between emotional involvement at work and rate of sexual intercourse was not found among the CABG patients. The reports of patients and spouses also did not tally in this regard. A possible explanation for this difference between the MI and CABG groups may lie in the sudden improvement in feelings of health and well-being found in this group after the surgery.

There is a misconception that the physical aspect plays the major role in determining a person's ability to perform a job. Technological advances have displaced this factor. The same misconception about physical ability exists in respect of sexual intercourse. There is a tendency to regard a "healthy person" as one who works hard, eats a lot, and performs frequent sexual intercourse. Our research shows that nowadays in western culture, return to work and the performance of sexual relations are not factors directly related to the physical ability of a person except when a pathological limitation is present, such as angina pectoris or congestive heart failure. There is no direct relationship between work and the frequency of sexual relations. Some other factors such as previous customs in sexual intercourse, the emotional involvement between the couple, and cultural and traditional factors may have more influence on sexual activity. However, the subjective aspect of work, namely the degree of emotional involvement of the person at work, may sometimes appear in inverse relationship to the frequency of sexual intercourse. This was shown significantly in the MI group of patients in our study.

Suitable guidance of coronary patients must take into account their customary practices in both work and sexual fields, which should be analyzed separately and not grouped together.

Summary

This study deals with the function of MI and CABG patients, in respect of employment and sexual function, from the viewpoints of both the patient and the spouse. The possible relationship between these parameters was also explored. The results show a high rate of employment in both population groups. There was a slight difference in type of work between the two groups. There was however, a significant increase in the rate of sexual relations in the MI group when a change was made to an occupation demanding less physical effort. The reports of both patients and spouses tallied in this respect. Furthermore, among the MI group an inverse relationship was found between the degree of emotional involvement at work and the frequency of sexual relations. Reports of both patients and spouses tallied in this regard also.

Acknowledgment. The authors would like to thank Professor Jacob Agmon and Dr. Samuel Friedman of the Department of Cardiology and Rehabilitation Center, Beilinson Hospital, for allowing us to interview patients under their care.

References

Bar-On D, Crystal N (1981) Return to work and sexual functioning after the first MI. The Beer Sheva Sample, II World Congress of Cardiac Rehabilitation, Jerusalem 1981

Bloch A (1975) Sexual problems after myocardial infarction. Am Heart J 90:536–537

Cody AV, Mammill A, Dunn E, Uther JB (1981) The effect of an integrated cardiac rehabilitation programme on return to work following myocardial infarction. II World Congress of Cardiac Rehabilitation, Jerusalem

Croog SH, Levine S (1977) The heart patient recovers. Human Science, New York, pp 315

De Baker G, Bran M, Unylsteek K, Denolin H, Pannier R (1981) Cardiac rehabilitation and return to work. II World Congress of Cardiac Rehabilitation, Jerusalem

Diedericks JPM, Weeda HWH, Schorbe MG (1981) Types of adaptation and outcome during recovery from myocardial infarction. II World Congress of Cardiac Rehabilitation, Jerusalem

Goble AJ, Bullen JF, Freer RA, Worcester MC (1981) Breakdown of employment following apparently successful cardiac rehabilitation. II World Congress of Cardiac Rehabilitation, Jerusalem

Gundle M, Reeves B, Tate S, Raft D, McLavrin LP (1980) Psychosocial outcome after coronary artery surgery. Am J Psychiatry 137:1591–1594

Hellerstein H, Friedman E (1970) Sexual activity and the postcoronary patient. Arch Intern Med 125:987–999

Jackson G (1978) Sexual intercourse and angina pectoris. Br Med J 1:7

Jenkins CD, Stanton BA, Savageau JA, Delinger P, Klein M (1983) Coronary artery bypass surgery - preliminary communication. JAMA 250:782–788

Johnston B, Fletcher G (1979) Dynamic electrocardiographic recording during sexual activity in recent post myocardial infarction and revascularization patients. Am Heart J 98:736–741

Kellerman JJ, Modan B, Levy M, Feldman S, Kariv J (1968) Return to work after myocardial infarction; comparative study of rehabilitated and non-rehabilitated patients. Geriatrics 3:151–156

Kellerman JJ (1981) Cardiac rehabilitation; reminiscences, international variations, experiences. Cardiovasc Rev Rep 1:43–49

Kushnir B, Fox KM, Tomkinson IW, Portal RW, Aber CP (1975) The influence of psychological factors and an early hospital follow up on return to work after first myocardial infarction. Scand J Rehabil Med 7:158–162

Kushnir B, Fox KM, Portal RW, Aber CP (1977) Factors influencing the resumption of work, sexual activity and driving following acute myocardial infarction. Am Heart J 93:261–262

Lederman N (1978) Sexual activity and coronary patient. PhD dissertation, University of Tel Aviv

Liddle H, Jensen R, Clayton P (1982) The rehabilitation of coronary surgical patients. Ann Thorac Surg 34:374–382

Oberman A, Finklea JF (1982) Return to work after coronary artery bypass. Ann Thorac Surg 34:353–382

Osterman G, Blaise C, Casette B, Elaeots J, Hardel B, Bajolet A (1981) Professional reinsertion after myocardial infarction. II World Congress of Cardiac Rehabilitation, Jerusalem

Rimm A, Barboriak JJ, Anderson AJ, Simon J (1976) Changes in occupation after aortocoronary vein-bypass operation. JAMA 236:361–363

Rosenfeldt FL, Lambert R, Burrows K, Stirling GR (1983) Hospital costs and return to work after coronary bypass surgery. Med J Aust 1:260–263

Sexual Relations and the Perception of Health and Happiness Among Patients Following Coronary Artery Bypass Grafting and Myocardial Infarction

M. J. Levy, M. Benyakar, S. Mibashan, L. Levinsky, C. Rosemberg, and Y. Fuchs

Myocardial infarction (MI) and coronary artery bypass graft surgery (CABG) are two acute but contrasting events for the patient. From the patients' perspective these events differ in that MI presents as a sudden pathophysiological event as a result of which the patient is categorized as chronically ill with a potential threat to his life. Coronary artery surgery, on the other hand, can be categorized as a surgical intervention which may prevent a pathophysiological development and may represent for the patient a potential turning point from a state of illness to one of health. Researchers who have examined the implications of MI and CABG for the patient's life-style have emphasized those parameters directly concerned with the disease which are related to the pathophysiological event and the symptomatology. Psychological parameters have been referred to less commonly. Most of the research has involved male coronary patients and rarely their spouses.

The purpose of this work is to examine the changes that occur in the patient after MI or CABG from his and his spouse's viewpoint at three levels:

1. At the symptomatological level expressed as the frequency and degree of anginal pain
2. At the sexual level expressed as the frequency of sexual relations
3. At the psychological level expressed as the subjective feelings of health and happiness

"Health and happiness" as evaluated in this study are subjective parameters expressed as the feeling of the patient at a certain point in time. Cantril and Loyds (1962), who asked patients to grade themselves according to variables such as state of health, family life, social life, and happiness, found that "happiness" and "health" were very important indicators of the state of satisfaction of the participants with their lives. This is the reason why we chose to include these variables in our research and to evaluate them according to Cantril's test.

Population Sample

Included in the sample were male and female patients after MI or CABG surgery and their spouses. They were among the group of patients who underwent surgery at the Department of Cardiac Surgery or were being followed up at the rehabilitation unit of Beilinson Hospital. They were chosen according to the following criteria:

1. Age between 35 and 60 years
2. They were all married
3. In the MI group, it was their first myocardial infarction. In the CABG group there was no previous myocardial infarction and they underwent surgery because of angina pectoris with or without congestive heart failure
4. A period of 6 months to 3 years had passed since the event (MI or CABG)

Not included in the sample were:

1. Patients taking drugs capable of affecting their sexual function
2. Patients suffering from illnesses likely to harm their sexual function, especially diabetes mellitus and hypertension among males, congenital disorders, malignant diseases, valvular heart disease, collagen disorders, neurological and psychiatric disorders
3. Illiterate patients

Research Methods

Collection of data in this work was done by the following methods:

1. A semistructured interview with the patient and spouse, relating to the patient's state of health. The severity of angina pectoris was graded as follows:
   Grade 1. No pain
   Grade 2. Mild. Slight functional limitation; normal physical activity does not cause chest pain
   Grade 3. Moderate. Considerable functional limitation; light physical activity or excitement may cause chest pain
   Grade 4. Severe. Rest pain; pain during the night, after meals, or during excitement
   Grade 5. Intractable pain
2. A semistructured sexual questionnaire, based on the Marriage Council of Philadelphia, I.N.C., Marriage Adjustment Schedule 1B, Philadelphia, Pennsylvania. The questionnaire included questions meant to provide information on the patient's sex life and on the frequency of sexual relations (each partner answered about him or herself).
3. Cantril's test, by means of which the variables "happiness" and "health" were evaluated. In this test the patient was shown a diagram of a ladder with ten steps. With regard to "happiness," the topmost step represents "man at his happiest" while the lowermost step represents "man at his unhappiest." With regard to the variable "health," the topmost step represents "man at his healthiest" while the lowermost step represents "man at his sickest." The testee was asked to indicate with a pencil the position he saw himself in relation to the variables happiness and health. The testee was

asked about his feelings before and after MI or CABG. The patient was asked about himself and the spouse was asked about the patient.

The Process of Research

The patients were invited to the hospital with their spouses for a medical examination and a conversation with the doctor. Upon their arrival the patients were separated from their spouses and interviewed separately but at the same time so as not to permit exchange of information between them. The interviewers were a male and female doctor and the male and female testees were divided equally between these two doctors.

Interpretation of the Data

The statistical tests by means of which the data were interpreted were the chi-square and Student's *t*-test.

Results

The population in question consisted of 430 examinees of whom half were patients and half their spouses. Of the 215 patients 89 (41%) had had MI and 126 (59%) CABG. The majority were males (83% males and 17% females among the MI patients and 85% males and 15% females among the CABG patients) (Table 1).

Table 1. Research population[a]

	CABG	MI	Total
Male	107	74	181
Female	19	15	34
Total	126	89	215

[a] The research population included the 215 spouses of the above patients

Table 2. Population distribution by percentage according to age

	<30	30–34	35–39	40–44	45–49	50–54	55–59	60–64	65
MI patients	0	0	14	0	27	27	32	0	0
CABG patients	0	0	12	9	31	24	24	0	0
Total patients	0	0	13	5	30	25	27	0	0
MI spouses	10	0	0	21	11	26	21	0	11
CABG spouses	0	0	31	16	26	33	19	6	3
Total spouses	4	0	18	16	21	17	14	4	6
Total population	2	0	15	10	26	21	19	4	3

The age of the patients ranged between 35 and 50 years and usually the spouse (in most cases female) was younger (Table 2). Regarding country of origin, the population was fairly mixed but by chance half were of eastern and half of western (Ashkenazi) origin (Table 3). This was also true of the spouses. Regarding education, more than half of the patients under survey had a high school or more advanced education and only 3% had not had a formal education (Table 4). Regarding employment at the time of the survey, 83.7% of the patients were working after the event (CABG or MI). Fifty-five percent of these were working full-time. There was only a small difference between the MI and the CABG population in this regard: 82.6% of the MI group compared to 85% of the CABG group. But there was a striking difference regarding full- or part-time work: 63.1% of the CABG patients were working full-time compared with 43.5% of the MI group (Table 5). Regarding the type of work and the physical effort involved, the distribution between the two groups (CABG and MI) was quite similar: however, none of the patients were involved in

Table 3. Population distribution by percentage according to region of origin

Israel	20.5
Europe/USA	43.4
Africa/Asia	36.1
	100.0

Table 4. Population distribution according to level of education

	No formal	Primary	Religous	High school	Technical	Academic
Patients (percentage)	3	20	16	25.8	13.2	22
Spouses (percentage)	6	39	1.6	35	4.6	13.8

Table 5. Sample population distribution by percentage according to level of employment

Level of employment	MI		CABG	
	Patient	Spouse	Patient	Spouse
Full-time work	43.5	33.3	63.1	45.2
Part-time work	21.7	11.1	12.5	16.1
Housekeeper	17.4	38.9	9.4	38.7
Does not work on account of:				
a) Heart disease	17.4	0.0	5.6	0.0
b) Other medical reasons	0.0	0.0	3.1	0.0
c) Nonmedical reasons	0.0	0.0	0.0	0.0
Pensioner	0.0	16.7	6.3	0.0
Total	100.0	100.0	100.0	100.0

heavy manual work while 12.5% of the MI spouses were involved in such labor (Table 6). In Table 7 the distribution between salaried and self-employed is shown. This was similar in the two groups.

Table 6. Sample population distribution by percentage according to the amount of physical exertion at work

Type of work	MI		CABG	
	Patient	Spouse	Patient	Spouse
Sedentary	33.5	62.5	27.3	56.3
Light manual	33.5	12.5	36.5	6.3
Light nonmanual	33.0	12.5	36.2	37.4
Heavy manual	0.0	12.5	0.0	0.0

Table 7. Sample population distribution by percentage – self-employed/salaried

Type of employment	MI		CABG	
	Patient	Spouse	Patient	Spouse
Salaried employee	74.4	87.5	84.0	87.5
Self-employed	25.3	12.5	16.0	12.5
Total	100.0	100.0	100.0	100.0

Regarding the presence of anginal pain after the event (CABG and MI) compared with the period before, analysis of the results related to two parameters:

1. A static measurement; namely a recording of the presence of anginal pain before and after the event
2. A dynamic measurement which compared the type and intensity of anginal pain before and after the event

According to this study, in the MI group following the event there was a significant increase in the intensity and occurrence of anginal pain ($P=0.0332$) (Fig. 1). Regarding the CABG population, following surgery there was a marked improvement both in frequency and in intensity of pain (Fig. 1). Seventy-one of the patients (56%) were completely free from angina following surgery. Thirty-nine patients (31%) had mild pain. Eight patients (6%) had moderate pain (grade III) and another eight had severe pain. The greatest improvement was seen in those patients suffering from intractable pain (grade V) prior to surgery. There were 26 patients in this group and 22 of them were angina-free following surgery, while four suffered from mild angina. These changes in intensity of angina were significant ($P<0.001$) (Fig. 1).

Regarding the frequency of sexual relations in the two groups, examination of the results related to three time periods:

I. The asymptomatic period, namely the period before the disease
II. The symptomatic period, namely the period in which the symptoms of coronary artery disease appeared, before the event
III. The period following the event (MI or CABG)

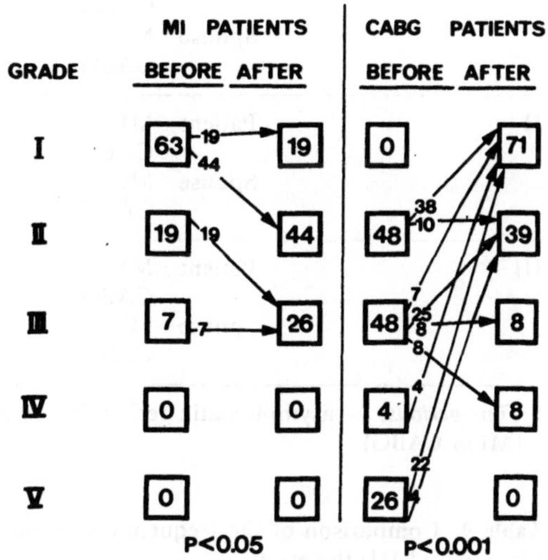

Fig. 1. Change in the level of anginal pain before and after MI or CABG

According to information from patients and spouses, the frequency of sexual relations among the CABG group in the three time periods is higher than among the MI group (Table 8). In the first period, the asymptomatic period, the frequency of sexual relations in the CABG group was 1.55 times higher than in the MI group according to patient information and 1.43 times higher according to spouse information. In the second period, the symptomatic period, the frequency of sexual relations was 1.05 times higher in the CABG group than in the MI group according to patient information and 1.39 times higher according to spouse information. In the third time period, the period after the event, the frequency of sexual relations in the CABG group was 1.33 times higher than in the MI group according to patient information and 1.63 times higher according to spouse information. These differences were not statistically significant. It is not possible to explain the differences in frequency of sexual relations by means of variables such as age or sex as their scatter was similar throughout both groups.

Regarding the connection between the event (MI and CABG) (Table 9) and the frequency of sexual relations, following MI the patients reported a decrease in the frequency of sexual relations from 9.47 to 6.78 times, namely a decrease in frequency of 28.4%, and this difference is statistically significant ($P = 0.01$). The spouses of the MI group reported a decrease in frequency from 4.58 to 4.28 times a month, namely a decrease of 9.04%.

In the CABG group following surgery the patients reported a decrease of frequency from 9.64 times a month before to 9.00 times after surgery. The

Table 8. Frequency of sexual relations – a comparison between MI and CABG patients according to time periods I, II, and III as related by the patient and separately by his spouse

Time period[a]	Population group		Frequency of sexual relations (average/month)	
I	Patient	MI	9.17	NS
		CABG	14.32	
	Spouse	MI	7.78	NS
		CABG	11.06	
II	Patient	MI	9.47	NS
		CABG	9.64	
	Spouse	MI	4.58	NS
		CABG	6.41	
III	Patient	MI	6.78	NS
		CABG	9.00	
	Spouse	MI	4.28	NS
		CABG	7.00	

[a] *Time periods,* I – asymptomatic period, II – symptomatic period, III – period after the event (MI or CABG)

Table 9. Comparison of the frequency of sexual relations before (time period II) and after (time period III) the event

Population	Status	Time period[a]	Frequency of sexual relations (average/month)	
MI	Patients	II	9.47	$P = 0.01$
		III	6.78	
	Spouses	II	4.58	NS
		III	4.28	
CABG	Patients	II	9.64	NS
		III	9.00	
	Spouses	II	6.41	NS
		III	7.00	

[a] Time period II – symptomatic period, Time period III – period after the event

spouses reported on an increase in frequency from 6.40 to 7.00 times a month, namely an increase in frequency of 9.4%. These changes were not significant.

Regarding the subjective parameters "feeling of health" and "feeling of happiness" as examined according to Cantril's test (Cantril and Loyds 1962), here the maximum score attainable was 10 (Tables 10, 11). Among the MI group, following the infarction the patients reported a decrease in their feelings of health from 8.05 to 5.00 and this change is statistically significant ($P = 0.0001$). The spouses reported on a decrease from 7.44 to 4.72 and this change is also statistically significant ($P = 0.001$).

Regarding the "feeling of happiness," following MI there was a tendency toward a decrease in the score for this parameter both as reported by the pa-

Table 10. Feelings of health and happiness as reported by the patients

Population group	Subjective feelings	Average	
MI group	Feeling of health before	8.05	$P=0.0001$
	Feeling of health after	5.00	
	Feeling of happiness before	8.21	NS
	Feeling of happiness after	7.37	
CABG group	Feeling of health before	4.66	$P<0.02$
	Feeling of health after	6.69	
	Feeling of happiness before	6.68	$P<0.01$
	Feeling of happiness after	8.13	

Table 11. Feelings of health and happiness among the patients as perceived by their spouses

Population group	Subjective feeling	Average	
MI group	Feeling of health before	7.44	$P=0.001$
	Feeling of health after	4.72	
	Feeling of happiness before	7.82	NS
	Feeling of happiness after	6.47	
CABG group	Feeling of health before	4.32	$P=0.001$
	Feeling of health after	7.13	
	Feeling of happiness before	5.66	$P=0.0001$
	Feeling of happiness after	8.38	

tients and by their spouses but these changes were not statistically significant. Among the CABG group, the patients reported an increase in their "feeling of health" from 4.66 to 6.69, and this change was statistically significant ($P=0.013$). The spouses reported an increase from 4.32 to 7.13 and this change was also statistically significant ($P=0.001$). In this group the patients also reported an increase in their "feeling of happiness" from 6.68 to 8.13, which was again statistically significant ($P=0.008$). Their spouses reported an increase from 5.66 to 8.38, and this, too, was statistically significant ($P=0.0001$).

Discussion

According to the results of our research the state of patients who underwent CABG improved following surgery as regards the frequency and severity of anginal pains, and also regarding the patients' feeling of health and happiness. This was also emphasized by the marital partners of these patients. Regarding the frequency of sexual relations, according to the patients there was a slight decrease in frequency, while according to the spouses there was a slight increase. By contrast, in the MI group following the infarct there was a deterioration in all three aspects examined in this work (symptomatology, sexual performance, and psychological aspects). The version given by patients and spouses tallied.

Results of research performed in different parts of the world on the influence of CABG on the state of patients following surgery indicate that the surgery is beneficial pathophysiologically (Croog and Levine 1977; Jenkins et al. 1983; Kellerman 1975; Kolodny et al. 1979; Lane 1973). On the other hand the researchers are divided as to the contribution surgery makes to the patients' quality of life and day-to-day function. While some workers point to an improvement (Jenkins et al. 1983; Kolodny et al. 1979; Ross et al. 1981), others point to problems, especially in the fields of sex and employment (Croog and Levine 1977; Gundle et al. 1980; Johnston and Fletcher 1979; Rimm et al. 1976). Gotze et al. (1980), Heller et al. (1974), and Lane (1973) point to the psychological problems associated with the operation.

Regarding specifically those parameters examined in our study, we see that many workers have reported beneficial effects of the operation in improving anginal pain (Gundle et al. 1980; Jenkins et al. 1983; Lane 1973). In our study, in addition to the presence and frequency of pain we examined its severity, something which in our opinion is likely to give a more exact picture of the state of the patient. This parameter is not only theoretical but is also of prognostic importance.

Regarding the frequency of sexual relations, the tendency in the literature is to report a reduction in frequency following both MI and CABG in comparison to the period before the onset of coronary disease. According to the literature the decrease in frequency among the MI patients ranges from 24% (a drop in frequency from 8.8 to 6.4 times a month) to 48% (a drop in frequency from 5.2 to 2.7 a month) (Block 1975; Johnston and Fletcher 1979; Hellerstein and Friedman 1970; Lederman 1978). Johnston and Fletcher (1979) reported a decrease in frequency of 10% in sexual relations following CABG (a decrease from 8.4 to 7.6 times a month). According to our study the decrease in frequency of sexual relations among the CABG patients according to the patients themselves was 7.2%, compared with 28.4% among the MI patients. Frequency of sexual relations before and after the event was higher in our groups than in the groups of other comparative studies (Table 12).

Table 12. Frequency of sexual relations among MI and CABG patients before and after the event. A comparison between the USA and Israel

Country	Research workers	MI patients			CABG patients		
		Before	After	Decrease	Before	After	Decrease
USA	Hellerstein and Friedman (1970)	8.4	6.4	24%			
USA	Bloch (1975)	5.2	2.7	48%			
USA	Johnston and Fletcher (1979)	6.4	4.6	28%	8.4	7.6	10%
Israel	Lederman (1978)	8.5	5.8	32%			
Israel	Present study	9.5	6.8	28.4%	9.6	9.0	6%

We saw fit to include the parameters "feeling of health" and "feeling of happiness" in this work because of their importance as a measurement of man's satisfaction with his life and because of their actual influence on the behavior of man as shown by previous studies (Cantril and Loyds 1962, Kilpatrick and Cantril 1960). This study shows that surgical intervention drastically reverses the deterioration in the patient's subjective feelings of health and happiness which occurs if the natural history of coronary artery disease is not reversed. It has been shown in this study that the frequency of sexual relations is not the only important parameter indicating the state of well-being of the patient. It is possible to conclude that there are quantitative and qualitative benefits to the patients following CABG surgery.

Summary

This research work examined the influence of MI and CABG on the function of the patient at three levels:

1. At the symptomatological level as expressed by the frequency and severity of anginal pain
2. At the sexual level as expressed by the frequency of sexual relations
3. At the psychological level as expressed by the feelings of health and happiness

An estimate of the state of the patient in these fields was made both from his and from his spouse's viewpoint.

According to the results of this study, CABG contributes to an alleviation of symptoms and also to an improvement in the subjective feelings of health and happiness. According to the patients these is a decrease in the frequency of sexual relations, but according to the spouses there is a slight increase after CABG surgery.

By contrast, there is a deterioration in the state of the MI group in all parameters examined both from the point of view of the patients and from that of their spouses.

In conclusion, CABG is not only beneficial in the alleviation of symptoms but also has a positive action in improving the quality of life of the patient.

Acknowledgment. The authors would like to thank Professor Jacob Agmon and Dr. Shmuel Friedman of the Department of Cardiology and Rehabilitation Center, Beilinson Hospital, for allowing us to interview patients under their care.

References

Bloch A (1975) Sexual problems after myocardial infarction. Am Heart J 90:536–537

Cantril H, Loyds AF (1962) Hopes and fears for self and country. Am Behav Sci 6:361–368

Croog SH, Levine S (1977) The heart patient recovers. Human Science, New York, p 315

Götze G, Huse-Kleinstoll G, Speidel H (1980) Psychic and neurological dysfunction after open heart surgery: a review of the present state of research. In: Speidel H, Rodewald G (eds) Psychic and neurological dysfunction after open heart surgery. Thieme, Stratton, New York

Gundle M, Reeves B, Tate S, Raft D, McLawrin LP (1980) Psychosocial outcome after coronary artery surgery. Am J Psychiatry 137:1591–1594

Heller S, Frank K, Kornfeld DS, Malm I, Bowman FJ (1974 Psychological outcome following open heart surgery. Arch Intern Med 134:908–914

Hellerstein H, Friedman E (1970) Sexual activity and the post coronary patient. Arch Intern Med 125:987–999

Jenkins CD, Stanton BA, Savageau JA, Denlinger P, Klein M (1983) Coronary artery bypass surgery - preliminary communication. JAMA 251:782–788

Johnston B, Fletcher G (1979) Dynamic electrocardiographic recording during sexual activity in recent post myocardial infarction and revascularization patients. Am Heart J 98:736–741

Kellerman JJ (1975) Rehabilitation of patients with coronary heart disease. Prog cardiovasc Dis 17:303–327

Kilpatrick FP, Cantril H (1960) Self anchoring scaling, a measure of individuals' unique and reality world. J Indiv Psychol 16

Kolodny R, Masters W, Johnson V (1979) Sex and cardiovascular disease. Textbook of sexual medicine. Little Brown & Co, Boston, pp 169–179

Lane FM (1973) Mental mechanisms and the pain of angina pectoris. Am Heart J 85:563–568

Lederman N (1978) Sexual activity and the coronary patient. Phd dissertation, University of Tel Aviv

Rimm A, Barboriak J, Anderson A, Simon J (1976) Changes in occupation after aortocoronary vein bypass operation. JAMA 236:361–363

Ross JK, Monro JL, Diwell AE, et al (1981) The quality of life after cardiac surgery. Br Med J 282:451–453

Psychosocial Aspects

G. Bergmann, M. Welsch, W. Saggau, and H. Ferner

This randomized collaborative study shows that coronary bypass graft surgery improves the quality of life as manifested by relief of chest pain, improvement of both subjective and objective measurements of functional status, and a diminished requirement for drug therapy. However, no significant effect on employment or recreational status was observed. [1] (CASS)

Starting from this observation, which has also been made by other authors [2–6], the question arises as to which objective and subjective conditions prevent return to work. In dealing with this question, an exact documentation of clinical findings, especially of the successful transplantation rate, is necessary. Conditions resulting from the actual socioeconomic situation, the current unemployment rate, and aspects of premature retirement because of a higher age should play a minor role in investigations concerning psychological factors [7]. Such factors are probably of minor importance in patients under 50 years of age, and it can be suggested that these patients are particularly motivated to return to work.

Selection of Patients and Methods

Between February 1981 and April 1983, 268 patients whose surgical results were documented by postoperative coronary angiography underwent coronary bypass surgery (CBS). For further data on this subject, see also the contribution by M. Welsch et al. in this volume. The CBS was carried out at the Thoracic Surgery Department of the Surgical Clinic of Heidelberg University. At the time of operation 67 of the patients were 50 years of age or younger (mean 44.5 years; SD 4.32). The cardiac condition was documented by angina pectoris symptoms according to the New York Heart Association classification (I–IV), by left ventricular function, and by coronary angiography pre- and postoperatively.

Sixty-seven patients were followed up 12–36 months after operation. Twenty patients refused the interview, were unattainable, or had moved in the meantime. Semistructured interviews were conducted with the remaining 47 patients and used to examine those conditions which – in the patients' opinion – prevented their return to work. The complaints at the time of the interviews were documented by the Giessener Beschwerdebogen (GBB – Giessen Complaint List) [8]. The Freiburg Personality Inventory (FPI) was used to describe personality characteristics [9].

The aim of the research was to answer the following questions:

1. What is the working status of the men under 50 who underwent CBS and in whom the postoperative conditions of the grafts were documented by coronary angiography?
2. Is there any connection between clinical data (LV function, AP symptoms, and number of open bypasses) and return to work?
3. Are there any physical noncardiac complaints at the time of the interview that are connected with return to work?
4. Do the patients who have returned to work show any differences in personality from those who have not?
5. Which conditions, according to the patients' own opinion, have hindered their return to work?

Results

The working status of patients under 50 years of age who underwent CBS and in whom the postoperative condition of the grafts was documented by coronary angiography is shown in Table 1.

In Table 2, the patency rate and the ventricular function are listed. The patency rate shows no significant difference for the two groups. Therefore, the return to work cannot depend on the outcome of CBS. Ventricular function in relation to work status in this sample is significant at $P=0.041$. The sample of 47 patients in whom this semistructured interview was conducted is representative for the sample of patients under 50 years of age with regard to the somatic variables (except ventricular function).

It seems (Table 3) that preoperative AP symptoms are indicative of the later working status. Patients who did not return to work had more AP symptoms ($P=0.0001$) at the time of the interview (12–36 months after operation) than the rest of the sample. Thus, the improvement in AP symptoms is an important factor in the return to work.

The results of the GBB are listed in Tables 4 and 5. General complaints without heart pain were listed significantly more often by the nonworkers.

Table 6 shows the results of the FPI, with the correlation between work status and personality characteristics.

Conditions which, in the patient's opinion, hinder or promote return to work are shown in Tables 7 and 8 respectively.

Table 1. Working status of patients under 50 years after CBS and postoperative coronary angiography

Work	No work	Died	Total
34	32	1	67

Table 2. Relationship between work status and patency rate and ventricular function (from Lienert [23])

Variable	Statistical method	Description of connections/differences	Significance
Patency rate	*t*-test	$\bar{x}_{yes} = 91.4\%$ $\bar{x}_{no} = 80.5\%$	NS
Ventricular function	Contingency table Chi-square	Cont. coeff. = 0.247 Corr. coeff. = 0.349	0.041

Table 3. Relationship between work status and angina pectoris (from Lienert [23])

Variable	Statistical method	Description of connections/differences	Significance
Angina pectoris preoperatively	Contingency table Chi-square	Cont. Coeff. = 0.316 Corr. Coeff. = 0.446	0.0069
Angina pectoris at interview	Contingency table Chi-square	Cont. coeff. = 0.422 Corr. coeff. = 0.625	0.0001

Table 4. Relationship between work status and certain scales of the GBB (exhaustion, stomachache, limb pain, heart pain)

Variable	Contingency coefficient	Correlation coefficient	Significance
Exhaustion	0.339	0.479	0.02
Stomachache	0.076	0.107	NS
Limb pain	0.289	0.408	0.05
Heart pain	0.328	0.463	0.03

Statistical analysis by contingency tables

Table 5. Relationship between work status and certain scales of the GBB (general complaints with and without heart pain)

Variable	Contingency coefficient	Correlation coefficient	Significance
General complaints (with heart pain)	0.415	0.586	0.004
General complaints (without heart pain)	0.372	0.526	0.01

Statistical analysis by contingency tables

Table 6. Freiburg Personality Inventory (FPI): correlation between work status and personality

	Work ($\bar{x}$)	No work ($\bar{x}$)	*t*-test
Nervousness	5.55	7.47	0.0006
Depression	4.25	5.95	0.01
Emotional instability	4.15	5.80	0.001
Feminine self-description	4.80	3.23	0.003

Table 7. Conditions which, according to the patient's own opinion, have hindered his return to work

1) CHD and heart pain
2) Difficulties in terms of assurance, opinions, and conditions of public service
3) General restriction of efficiency

Table 8. Conditions which, according to the patient's own opinion, have promoted his return to work

1) Success of the operation and good physical condition
2) Will to work, pleasure at work
3) Self-confirmation, preservation of self-awareness
4) Financial necessity to take care of family

Discussion

Influence of the Individual Context

On the basis of the presented results there is no doubt that improvement in the AP symptoms is a decisive factor for the return to work [10]. Furthermore, there is a correlation between left ventricular function and return to work. This correlation, however, is lower than expected for the corrected contingency coefficient explains only 12.2% of the variance. As 87.8% of the variance remains unexplained, these results imply that it is necessary to look for additional psychological parameters which may exert some influence. The patency rate (n.s.) does not permit prediction of whether or not the patients may return to work.

Psychological factors played an important role in why these men under 50 years did not return to work. At the time of the interview, i.e., between 12 and 36 months after the operation, a lot of noncardiac complaints were reported. The nonworkers differed significantly from the workers in some personality characteristics: They were more nervous, depressive, and emotionally unstable and showed a more feminine self-description. At the moment it is not clear whether the reported complaints and the personality characteristics already existed before the operation or whether they arose afterwards as a reaction. The results, however, underline the fact that rehabilitative measures after CBS must include not only clinical and efficiency-oriented aspects, but psychotherapeutic aims as well. Only then can it be expected that an increased number of patients will return to work. Especially for the age group examined here, return to work is part of the quality of life. Because of their personality structure, the loss of work creates for these patients a situation to which they respond with depression, nervousness, and general complaints. The loss becomes more severe because they feel highly responsible for their families and place great emphasis on family bonds.

Coustry-Degree [11] distinguishes impulsive patients from adapted and regressive ones. The prognosis was best for the adapted patients and most unfavorable for the regressive ones. The longer the patients wait to return to work, the more their attitude changes from an impulsive to an adapted and to a regressive reaction. A very early return to work is often observed in impulsive subjects. Furthermore, it was noted that all patients who died before returning to work belonged to the regressive group. 36% of the regressive patients did not go back to work for purely psychological reasons. In 64% of these the regressive behavior seemed to be partly related to their unstable medical condition or their physical capacity being insufficient for them to resume their previous jobs.

Cay [12] observed in infarct patients that psychological factors were important. The severity of infarct or residual angina had no influence on the return to work, but emotional problems, especially anxiety and depression, were noted to be influencing factors.

Croog and Levine [13] found that the return to work was mostly determined by the medical assessment of the patient's condition. Our investigations with young patients with CBS confirm the results of Croog and Levine, who described psychological changes in patients aged 30–60 years after a myocardial infarction: In this study it was shown that the variable "depression" correlated positively with the number of physical complaints, and that depressive symptoms were negatively associated with unemployment, with subjective evaluation of the achieved health improvement, and with satisfaction with the actual life situation.

Mayou et al. [14] found symptoms like anxiety and depression and further disturbances such as feelings of exhaustion, lack of concentration, and irritability following myocardial infarction. The physical complaints showed no correlation with the evaluation of the cardiac status.

Langosch [15, 16] also found in psychological studies in patients with myocardial infarction that psychological variables are of great significance in respect of the rehabilitative process and its outcome: While the whole duration of illness, the time of rehabilitation, and the number of lost working days are influenced by the impairment of well-being, the individually experienced degree of physical or intellectual efficiency is exclusively predictable by psychological variables. He points out that particularly those patients who are psychologically conspicuous during hospitalization should be elected for psychotherapeutic measures. As can be concluded from continuous observation, a spontaneous remission of psychological symptoms cannot be expected in these patients.

These observations complete the findings of our group in patients after myocardial infarction [17]. We were able to differentiate between the sociable patients who are adapted and efficiency oriented, the impulsive-aggressive ones, and the regressive-anxious ones. We also found a difference between the impulsive-aggressive and the anxious-regressive patients: The regressive ones were more motivated to improve their health condition, whereas the impulsive patients were not interested in such therapeutic measures.

From these findings therapeutic recommendations result which can also be used for the regressive patients after CBS. Patients with general complaints and regressive reactions are more motivated as regards therapy. However, it is more likely that the resistance energies of these patients may be exhausted and that the somatic-oriented general complaints may persist. It should be the aim of the rehabilitative process to accept the patients in their regression. In a second phase, resources which are set free enable the patients to find a constructive way out of their dependence. It may then be possible that they are able to detach themselves from an efficiency-oriented society.

Influence of the Familial Context

In our investigation we tried to gain a conception of family bonds and family support - according to the patients' point of view. The evaluation in the interview was carried out according to the following criteria [18, 19]: a reciprocal emotional relationship between the married couple and the other family members; degree of dependence of the conjugal coalition; time spent together; feeling of responsibility for the material and general prosperity of the wife and offspring; decisions made with regard to the family. This self-estimation and observation is related to the manifest and not the latent experiences. During the interview situation, we were surprised that family-related conflicts were often talked about. This seems to contradict the more extensive tendencies of denial and, at first glance, does not correspond to the image we have of the so-called psychosomatic family.

The self-estimation of the patient represents the idea of strong family bonds. It cannot be directly concluded that this is a good precondition and support for the management of the disease, but it underlines the special meaning the family has for the patient's experience and thus the necessity to include the family in the coping process. To the patient, the family is the greatest potential of resources. This subjective feeling and experience has a high significance and should be included in further therapeutic and rehabilitative planning.

If we prefer a family-oriented mode of consideration, we must ask to what degree the patient's behavior depends on his individual development and to what degree on his context of dynamic relations.

For further research the following questions can be formulated:

1. How important are general complaints within the family context of coronary or bypass patients?
2. How does the family system react to the patient's regression after CBS and to the fact that he does not return to work?
3. What is the potential of development for family systems where one member falls sick with CHD?

In a patient report [20] of ambulant coronary groups the patients emphasized the difficulties they encountered when they had to redefine themselves in their own social background. Patients expected not only physical treatment but also a certain degree of psychological support.

Windner and Kellermann [21] established that family structures and relations between the couple have multidirectional influences on rehabilitative progress. Discouragement by the family has been reckoned to be one of the principal reasons for failure no return to work [22].

Conclusions

Rehabilitative measures for patients after CBS have to take into account psychological developments in the patient as they result from the patient's individual situation and from his position in the family. In this way one can activate the individual capabilities which were present before CHD and which had, at that time, given the patient a high level of self-confidence.

Furthermore, the resources, which are – according to our investigations – very considerable, must be reactivated during the rehabilitation process. Thus, the regressive development will remain transitional. We conclude that:

1. After CBS nonworkers have more non-cardiac-related complaints than workers.
2. Nervousness, depression, emotional instability, and feminine self-description in nonworkers indicate a disturbance of the psychodynamic equilibrium.
3. Family bonds play a considerable role in determining the patient's self-perception.

These findings demand both individual and family-oriented psychosomatic measures. It could then be expected that the patients would be able to return to work, which for them is an element of the quality of life. CBS would then show better long-term results than are achieved at the moment by means of mere improvement in cardiac functions.

References

1. Cass Principal Investigators and Their Associates (1983) Coronary artery surgery study (CASS): A randomized trial of coronary artery bypass surgery. Circulation 68/5:951-960
2. Barnes GK, Ray MJ, Oberman A, Kouchoukos NT (1977) Changes in work status of patients following coronary bypass surgery. JAMA 238:1259
3. Oberman A, Kouchoukos NT (1979) Working status of patients following coronary bypass surgery. Am Heart J 98:132
4. David P (1979) Contributing factors preventing return to work of cardiac surgery patients. In: Roskamm H, Schmuziger M (eds) Coronary heart surgery - A rehabilitation measure. Springer, Berlin Heidelberg New York, p 370
5. Blümchen G, Scharf-Bronhofen E, Brabdt D, van den Bergh, Bierck G (1979) Clinical results and social implications in patients after coronary bypass surgery. In: Roskamm H, Schmuziger M (eds) Coronary heart surgery - A rehabilitation measure. Springer, Berlin Heidelberg New York, p 375
6. Lichtlen P, Liese W, Leitz K, Borst HG (1978) Postoperative Klinik nach aorto-koronarem Venenbypass in Relation zum Ausmaß der Revaskularisation. Z Kardiol 67:83
7. Weiß B (1983) Wiederaufnahme der Arbeit nach erstem Herzinfarkt. Dtsch Med Wochenschr 108:1872-1875
8. Brähler E, Scheer JW (1979) Skalierung psychosomatischer Beschwerdekomplexe mit dem Gießener Beschwerdebogen (GBB). Psychother Med Psychol 29:14-27
9. Fahrenberg J (1970) Das Freiburger Persönlichkeitsinventar (FPI). Hogrefe, Göttingen
10. Council of Scientific Affairs (1979) Indications for aortocoronary bypass graft surgery. JAMA 242:2709
11. Coustry-Degree MD (1976) Psychological problems in rehabilitation programmes. In: Stocksmeier U (ed) Psychological approach to the rehabilitation of coronary patients. Springer, Berlin Heidelberg New York
12. Cay EL (1982) Psychological problems in patients after myocardial infarction. Adv Cardiol 29:108-112
13. Croog SH, Levine S (1977) The heart patient recovers. Human Sciences, New York
14. Mayou R, Williamson B, Foster A (1978) Psychosocial adjustment in patients one year after myocardial infarction. J Psychosom Res 22:447-453
15. Langosch W (1976) Personality structure and actual condition of patients with heart diseases. In: Stocksmeier U (ed) Psychological approach to the rehabilitation of coronary patients. Springer, Berlin Heidelberg New York
16. Langosch W (1980) Ergebnisse psychologischer Verlaufsstudien bei Herzinfarktpatienten. In: Langosch W (ed) Psychosoziale Probleme und psychotherapeutische Interventionsmöglichkeiten bei Herzinfarktpatienten. Minerva, Munich
17. Altmann-Herz U, Reindell A, Petzold E, Ferner H (1983) Zur psychosomatischen Differenzierung von Patienten nach Herzinfarkt. Z Psychosom Med 29:234-252
18. Wirsching M, Stierlin H (1982) Krankheit und Familie: Konzepte, Forschungsergebnisse, Therapie. Klett-Cotta, Stuttgart
19. Boszormeny-Nagy I, Spark GM (1981) Unsichtbare Bindungen: Die Dynamik familiärer Systeme. Klett-Cotta, Stuttgart
20. Mohn E (1981) Die Infarktnachsorge aus der Sicht des Patienten. In: Halhuber C (ed) Ambulante Koronargruppen. PeriMed-Fachbuch, Erlangen
21. Wintner J, Kellermann JJ (1976) Psychological factors involved in cardiac rehabilitation. In: Stocksmeier U (ed) Psychological approach to the rehabilitation of coronary patients. Springer, Berlin Heidelberg New York, pp 156-172
22. Mulcahy R, Hickey N (1970) The rehabilitation of patients with coronary heart disease. Scand J Rehabil Med 2:108
23. Lienert GA (1969) Testaufbau und Testanalyse, 3. Aufl. Beltz, Weinheim, p 291ff

Psychological Adaptation of Patients in the Early Rehabilitative Phase After Heart Surgery*

A. Boll, J. Koch, A. Sheikhzadeh, P. Thoran, and A.-F. Langbehn

Introduction

About 10 years ago psychosomatic studies of patients who had had heart surgery were mainly oriented toward the measurement, the frequency, and the causes of the psychopathological disturbances which occurred in the early postoperative period – impressing the onlooker by their dramatic symptoms [2, 14, 16]. Comparisons with other surgery patients made these remarkable psychopathological disturbances in the intensive care unit appear as if they were specific to heart surgery patients [5].

We are today witnessing a widening of the time range to which attention is directed in this field of study. Long-term medical and occupational rehabilitation [3, 13, 19] as well as psychological and psychosocial adaptation [6, 9, 18] have become focal points of interest.

Closest in time to the operation, fears and anxiety and the way of coping with these feelings [4, 8] are of special psychological significance; long-range postoperatively, general difficulties in dealing with physical incapacity and chronic illness are more typical problems.

The results of Heller et al. [7] indicate that 38% of patients experience remarkable psychological problems during their long-term postoperative course. The outhors judged the recovery process of 21% to be severely hindered by emotional disturbances. Kimball [12] reports on 20% of patients after heart surgery who need psychological and/or psychiatric treatment. Kimball [11] as well as Möhlen et al. [15] found that a patient's emotional condition prior to the operation and the way preoperative stress was dealt with influenced the postoperative course. Kimball shows that patients who preoperatively were symbiotic-dependent, as well as those who were depressive or denying their anxiety, had in their long-range postoperative course physical as well as considerable emotional difficulties.

The conclusions of Möhlen et al. confirm the importance of ego functions, especially defense mechanisms. Patients who preoperatively were able to divert their psychic energy away from objects and toward their own self showed the fewest symptoms of depression postoperatively.

The prognostic value of preoperative psychological adaptation for the emotional overcoming of the intensive care unit is reported by Huse-Kleinstoll et al. [8]. Increased preoperative trait anxiety, emotional lability, and negative

* Translated from German by Dr. Peter Thoran

emotional changes due to the illness are risk factors. Stable object relationships as well as an optimistic and realistic attitude toward the future are supportive elements.

Questions

The primary objective of this study is to describe the psychological adjustment of patients who have undergone heart surgery 6–8 weeks after the operation. Specifically the following questions are to be answered:

1. Which general emotional and psychosomatic adjustment do patients show in the postoperative period?
2. Which problems caused by their illness or inherent in the situation do patients experience during this time?
3. Which opportunities do patients utilize to overcome postoperative stress?
4. In which way are the nature and extent of subjective stress as well as the nature and extent of coping opportunities related to general postoperative emotional and psychosomatic adjustment?

Sample

The randomized sample contained 89 patients, 73 men and 16 women. The mean age was 53.8 years, range 38–70 years. Seventy-eight patients had had coronary bypass surgery, 11 open-heart surgery for other ailments. For 95% of patients this was the first time their heart had been operated on. Of the coronary patients, 90% had had one or more heart attacks prior to their operation.

Methods

These 89 patients were examined 6–8 weeks after their operation with the following standardized psychological tests, during their stay at the rehabilitation center:

- The German version of the Spielberger State-Trait-Anxiety Inventory [17]. The two scales developed by Spielberger discern state anxiety and trait anxiety. State anxiety signifies momentarily present feelings of fear and anxiety; trait anxiety signifies an underlying disposition, independent of momentary situations, to react with anxiety.
- The Giessen test scale "Basic Mood" [1]. This bipolar scale measures the extent of an underlying depressive attitude, independent of the momentary situation on the one hand and hypomanic tendencies on the other.
- The Hamburg-Heidelberg-München list of complaints [10]. The sum total of complaints permits an assessment of the extent of plaintiveness concerning physical and psychic symptoms.

Patients also received two questionnaires developed by ourselves to assess stress in this specific postoperative situation as well as ways of dealing with it. Patients were asked to assess the extent of subjectively felt stress as well as the extent of subjectively experienced support for each of the alternatives given, on a three-point scale.

Results

First of all differences between patients with coronary artery bypass surgery and patients with open-heart surgery for other ailments were tested. No statistically significant differences could be found concerning the psychological variables included in this study.

To describe the general emotional and psychosomatic adjustment the patients' data from standardized psychological tests were taken. Using cluster analysis we could classify patients in groups differing widely in the extent to which the psychological variables were manifested. Four different patient groups could be identified this way. Figure 1 shows mean values (after z-transformation) of the different variables for the various groups.

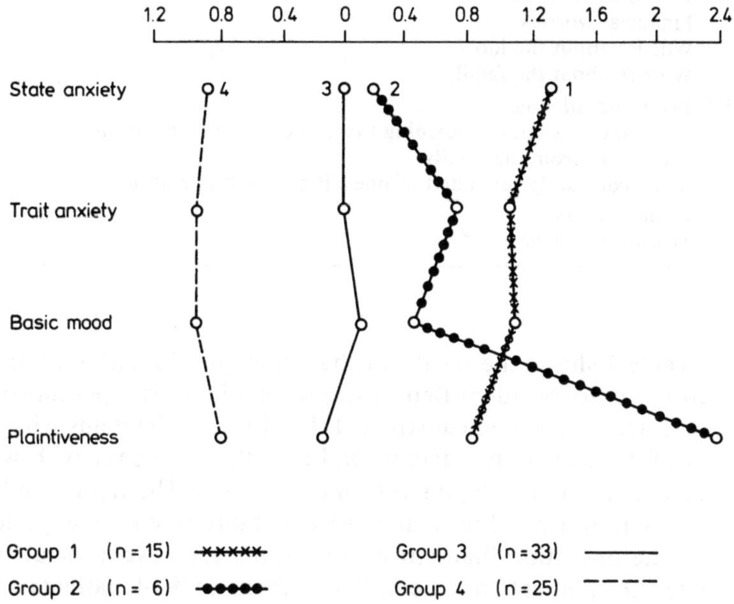

Fig. 1. Four groups characterizing the general emotional and psychosomatic adaptation of patients 6–8 weeks after the operation

Group 1 consists of 15 patients characterized by high levels of state and trait anxiety, by depression, and by a high number of emotional and physical complaints. These patients are quite unstable emotionally and in their vegetative functions.

Group 2 is a special one containing only 6 patients, showing increased trait anxiety and a maximum rate of complaints.

Group 3 consists of 33 patients showing medium values for all variables.

Group 4 consists of 25 patients characterized by very low values for the psychological variables. They seem particularly stable in their vegetative functions, and they have neither state or trait anxiety nor depression. They are marked by hypomanic tendencies.

To be able to put the items of the questionnaires developed by ourselves into scales they were subjected to factor analysis.

Table 1. Stress factors specific to the patients' situation in the early rehabilitative phase

Factors	"Medium or high stress"
I *Psychosomatic stress*	
Somatic condition	77%
Emotional condition	58%
Lack of concentration and/or memory	50%
II *Psychosocial stress*	
Financial worries	33%
Worries about the job	33%
Worries about the family	31%
III *Psychological stress*	
Fears and anxieties concerning the success of the operation	66%
Separation from the family	73%
Being constantly reminded of one's illness and operation	55%
IV *Medical stress*	
Medical treatment	46%

Table 1 shows the results of the stress questionnaire. Four significant stress factors could be identified: psychosomatic stress, psychosocial stress, emotional stress, and medical stress. Table 1 shows the items with the highest loadings of each respective factor, and also the frequency with which patients assigned a medium or high stress value to them. The figures indicate that overall emotional and psychosomatic stress is more intensely experienced 6–8 weeks after the operation than stress concerning the psychosocial situation or stress related to medical treatment. Thus about 58% of patients feel oppressed by emotional instability and depressive moods. Two-thirds of patients suffer from fears and anxiety concerning the success of the operation. The general physical condition constitutes a problem for 77%. 50% complain of lack of concentration and memory capacity.

Financial as well as job- and family-related problems, on the other hand, are judged burdensome by only about 30%. It therefore appears that patients in this postoperative period are still mainly concerned with themselves, that their own emotional and somatic condition is the focal point of interest.

Table 2 shows three factors, each marking a different coping pattern. The items with the highest loadings are also added, as well as the frequencies with which patients found different ways of coping helpful.

Table 2. Coping factors to manage postoperative stress

Factors	"Very helpful"
I *Dependent, rather passive, not specific to the clinical situation*	
Support of the family	83%
Resting and recuperating	50%
Religious faith	14%
II *Independent of others, active*	
General improvement of the somatic condition	69%
Improvement in physical capacity	55%
Optimistic view of life	68%
III *Dependent, rather passive, specific to the clinical situation*	
Care by hospital staff	65%
Medical care and treatment	49%
Taking tranquilizers	10%

Factor I ("Dependent, rather passive, not specific to the clinical situation") comprises a coping pattern characterized by the patient's capacity to derive strength from his own reserves not connected with the hospital: family support, books as well as his personal religious faith. Passive tendencies predominate.

Factor II ("Independent of others, active") is a coping pattern marked by independence of other people. The patient deals with his stress factors on his own strength, by a optimistic view of life as well as by physical activity.

Factor III ("Dependent, rather passive, specific to the clinical situation") is equal to the first factor except for the fact that this coping pattern is closely related to hospital conditions. There are important relations with doctors, nurses, and therapists. Here, too, passive aspects predominate.

The percentage figures show that human relationships are highly important in this postoperative period. Close family ties and support by family members are felt to be very helpful by 80% of the patients. Contact with the doctor recedes behind this, perhaps because he can devote only a fraction of his time to each patient.

Two-thirds of patients find the general improvement of their physical well-being, the improvement in their physical performance, as well as an optimistic view of life very helpful in overcoming postoperative stress. The small importance attached by patients to tranquilizer medication is striking.

Using a one-way analysis of variance we checked for differences between the groups of emotional and psychosomatic adjustment (Fig. 1) concerning stressing and supporting factors. Table 3 shows that the four groups have significantly differing mean values for three stress factors and one coping factor. The more pronounced the emotional and psychosomatic instability of patients, the higher is their susceptibility to stress caused by their illness or by the situa-

Table 3. Significant differences between the four patient groups of psychological adaptation related to the stressing and supporting factors

Stressing or supporting factors	$\bar{x}_{group\ 1}$	$\bar{x}_{group\ 2}$	$\bar{x}_{group\ 3}$	$\bar{x}_{group\ 4}$
Psychosomatic stress	6.1	5.8	4.2	1.6
Psychosocial stress	2.9	2.0	1.4	0.9
Emotional stress	4.8	4.5	3.9	1.5
Coping factor II	4.3	4.5	4.9	5.5

tion. Apparently the emotionally less stable patients cannot adequately cope with the actual stresses.

Concerning the supportive factors, the groups of postoperative adaptation differ insofar as emotionally and in their vegetative functions more stable patients can more easily cope with actual stress on their own resources, without depending on other people's help. No differences were found in coping factors I and III (Table 2). In this postoperative phase all groups felt equally dependent on human support from their families as well as doctors, nursing staff, and therapists.

Discussion

Comparing the results of general psychological adjustment during the early postoperative rehabilitative period with that during later postoperative phases, the similarity of the percentage figures is striking. Patients of group 1 characterized by the high degree of their emotional lability and psychosomatic disturbance plus group 2 with attention focussed on their complaints (Fig. 1) together make up 24% of the sample; this corresponds to the findings of Heller et al. [7] and Kimball [12]: About 20% of patients who underwent heart surgery have considerable emotional problems in their long-range postoperative course. The patients of groups 1 and 2 suffer most from stress arising from the specific postoperative situation or from their illness, and have few independent and active coping possibilities; this seems to mark them as risk patients also for the later course. Momentary stress not adequately coped with can induce further emotional lability in these patients.

All patients consider interpersonal contacts with their families as well as with hospital staff very important in dealing with postoperative stress. This corresponds to the importance of object relations for emotionally overcoming the time spent on ICU, as reported by Huse-Kleinstoll [8].

Patients in groups 1 and 2 with lesser ability for independent, active coping seem to be in danger of having their contacts with other people influenced by symbiotic tendencies and dependency needs; this adversely affects their long-range prospects [11].

Patients of group 4 have the lowest anxiety and depression; they are relatively immune to postoperative stress (Table 3). They emphasize help on the basis of independent, active coping possibilities. This finding can be assumed to mean that these patients have relatively intact defenses which protect them from stressing emotions. The data shown allow us to conclude that denial is the preferred defense mechanism of these patients.

This underlines at first glance the importance of stable defenses as postulated by Möhlen et al. [15]; one should note, however, that this study does not detail the extent of denial. If it concerns the illness generally, risk factors, and physical limitations, these defenses surely cannot have only positive effects in the long run.

From the therapeutic point of view the following conclusions can be drawn from the results:

1. During the early rehabilitative phase interest should be focussed on patients' interpersonal relations.
   Intensifying contacts with the family may have a stabilizing effect for the stressed patient.
2. Patients with a relatively stable psychological adaptation but with fears and anxiety concerning the success of the operation should receive thorough medical information together with psychological counseling.
3. For patients with a high degree of emotional lability and with psychosomatic disturbances, psychotherapeutic treatment should be available during their stay at the rehabilitation center and also after discharge.
4. Attention of doctors and psychologists should also be directed towards the intensively denying patients. It should be clarified whether they are only denying the emotional impact of the actual situation or whether they are also denying the impact of the illness in general, with its risk factors and physical limits.

References

1. Beckmann D, Richter HE (1972) Gießen-Test (GT). Huber, Bern
2. Dahme B, Götze P, Wessel M (1983) Brief psychiatric inventory for assessment of psychopathological disorders after open-heart surgery. In: Becker R, Katz J, Polonius M-J, Speidel H (eds) Psychopathological and neurological dysfunctions following open-heart surgery. Springer, Berlin Heidelberg New York, pp 77–83
3. Davies-Osterkamp S, Siefen G, Möhlen K, Müller H, Schlepper M (1983) Psychosocial situation of the open-heart surgery patient one year after operation. In: Becker R, Katz J, Polonius M-J, Speidel H (eds) Psychopathological and neurological dysfunctions following open-heart surgery. Springer, Berlin Heidelberg New York, pp 227–231
4. Flemming B, Dahme B, Götze P, Huse-Kleinstoll G, Meffert H-J, Müller L, Reimer C, Speidel H (1983) Patients' fear of cardiosurgery and its significance for the pre- and postoperative state. In: Becker R, Katz J, Polonius M-J, Speidel H (eds) Psychopathological and neurological dysfunctions following open-heart surgery. Springer, Berlin Heidelberg New York, pp 281–287
5. Götze P (1980) Psychopathologie der Herzoperierten. Enke, Stuttgart
6. Heller SS, Frank KA, Kornfeld DS, Wilson SN, Malm JR (1983) Psychological and behavioral responses following coronary artery bypass surgery. In: Becker R, Katz J, Polonius M-J, Speidel H (eds) Psychopathological and neurological dysfunctions following open-heart surgery. Springer, Berlin Heidelberg New York, pp 238–245

7. Heller SS, Frank KA, Kornfeld DS, Malm JR, Bowman FO Jr (1974) Psychological outcome following open-heart surgery. Arch Intern Med 134:908–914
8. Huse-Kleinstoll G, Boll A, Dahme B, Flemming B, Götze P, Meffert H-J, Priebe K, Speidel H (1982) Die psychische Belastung kardiochirurgischer Intensivpatienten. Presented at the congress of the society for medical psychology, Hannover
9. Jenkins DC, Stanton BA, Savageau JA, Denlinger P, Klein MD (1984) Die koronare Bypass-Chirurgie - die physische, psychische, soziale und wirtschaftliche Situation nach sechs Monaten. JAMA - D 3 (2):99–106
10. v Kerekjarto M, Meyer AE, v Zerssen D (1972) Die HHM-Beschwerdenliste bei Patienten einer internistischen Ambulanz. Psychosom Med Psychoanalyse 18:1–16
11. Kimball CP (1969) A predictive study of adjustment to cardiac surgery. J Thorac Cardiovasc Surg 88:891–896
12. Kimball CP (1976) The experience of cardiac surgery and cardiac transplant. In: Howells JG (ed) Modern perspectives in the psychiatric aspects of surgery. Brunner-Mazel, New York, pp 243–266
13. LaMendola WF, Pellegrini RV (1979) Quality of life and coronary artery bypass surgery patients. Soc Sci Med 13 A:457–461
14. Meffert H-J, Boll A, Dahme B, Götze P, Huse-Kleinstoll G, Polonius M-J, Prüssmann K, Speidel H, Wessel M (1983) Der relative Anteil somatischer und psychischer Befunde an der Vorhersage psychopathologischer Auffälligkeiten nach Herzoperationen. In: Studt HH (ed) Psychosomatik in Forschung und Praxis. Urban and Schwarzenberg, Munich, pp 505–520
15. Möhlen K, Davies-Osterkamp S, Müller H, Scheld H, Siefen G (1983) Relationship between preoperative coping styles, immediate postoperative reactions and some aspects of the psychosocial situation of open-heart surgery patients one year after the operation. In: Becker R, Katz J, Polonius M-J, Speidel H (eds) Psychopathological and neurological dysfunctions following open-heart surgery. Springer, Berlin Heidelberg New York, pp 232–237
16. Speidel H, Rodewald G (eds) (1980) Psychic and neurological dysfunctions after open-heart surgery. Thieme, Stuttgart
17. Spielberger CD (1975) Anxiety: State-trait process. In: Spielberger CD, Sarason IG (eds) Stress and anxiety. vol 1. Halsted, New York, pp 117–132
18. Stanton BA, Zyzanski SJ, Jenkins CD, Klein MD (1983) Recovery after major heart surgery: Medical, psychological, and work outcomes. In: Becker R, Katz J, Polonius M-J, Speidel H (eds) Psychopathological and neurological dysfunctions following open-heart surgery. Springer, Berlin Heidelberg New York, pp 217–226
19. Walter P, Thies B, Gerhardt U (1983) Wie viele Patienten nehmen nach einer Koronaroperation ihre Arbeit wieder auf? Med Klin 78:276–280

Some Questions and Remarks

M. Halhuber

I have no statistics and I do not want to repeat what has been written elsewhere in this symposium. I will try only to pose some questions and propose some hypotheses as consequences of this symposium and the personal experience of a retired medical director of a rehabilitation hospital in West Germany.

Are we asking the right questions (not only during this symposium)?
From elsewhere in this book we learn that for many patients psychosocial factors (and not only socioeconomic factors) are equally or even more important than physiological factors for return to work after bypass surgery.

How should we cope with these results of interdisciplinary research in the daily practice of rehabilitation after bypass surgery?
For me as a senior clinician it is a really wonderful experience to listen to cardiac surgeons and psychiatrists and psychologists during the same meeting and to understand them, because they today speak nearly the same scientific language. When I remember the situation 10 years ago it was quite different. During this symposium I have learnt to hope that in the future we will establish really *comprehensive coronary care* and management before and after bypass surgery. For this task psychiatrists, psychologists, nurses, social workers, and others have to be really integrated in the therapeutic team, even in the surgical department and in the rehabilitation program.

Our colleague H. C. Smith from the Mayo Clinic has elsewhere in this symposium discussed the definition of the "quality of life" – that it is the sum of satisfaction that makes life worthwhile. More and more cardiac surgeons accept this soft endpoint as an important goal of bypass surgery. I think they are right to do so, but *now do we measure the quality of life for scientific purposes?* I think it is possible for the present and the coming generation of clinical psychologists: They are able to quantify some psychological factors: anxiety, depression, denial, overmotivation, the changes of coronary-prone behavior, satisfaction and working capacity, change of life-style after counseling and exercise, etc. We have to encourage an interdisciplinary comprehensive program of practice, research, and education, measuring the quality of life before and after bypass surgery.

My *first hypothesis* at the end of this symposium is that the psychosocial aspects of coronary heart disease before and after bypass surgery are as important as after acute myocardial infarction. The words of the Dutch cardiologist Hands Weeda, "After a heart attack there are more problems in the mind than in the heart," may be adapted to heart surgery too. A quotation by T. P. Hackett, J. F. Rosenbaum, and C. P. Kimball serves as an example: "The highest incidence of postoperative mortality and morbidity occurs in patients who are depressed before the operation or who deny anxiety, even though they are obviously apprehensive." After many discussions with patients after bypass surgery it seems to me that we underestimate the special anxiety of the patient concerning the occlusion of the grafts during the first weeks and months after the operation (also after PTCA).

Generally speaking: The patient's philosophy of life (how he is able to anticipate and to see his own future) is an important factor for his quality of life after bypass surgery. The self-experience gained in a therapeutic group guided by an experienced therapeutic team seems to me a good method of secondary prevention. Counseling during this phase is as important as exercise and changes in life-style, o.g., "learning by doing" in a rehabilitation center. But we need more interdisciplinary research in this field.

My *second hypothesis* as a result of all I have learnt during this symposium is that the long-term success of bypass surgery depends on really comprehensive, interdisciplinary residential and outpatient care and management.

Practical consequences that can be expected from this important symposium seem to me to be more and better communication between the different members of the medical community, the real integration of the psychiatrist and psychologist in the medical and surgical team, and new methods of research in this interdisciplinary field.

I do not know after the experiences with recent studies – I am thinking of the MRFIT study – whether controlled or randomized studies are really feasible; perhaps we need new methods of evaluation in this field. Nevertheless, this meeting seems an important step in the right direction. Personally, I therefore wish to thank Doctor Walter and his committee for this symposium.

Summary of the Discussion

D. S. Kornfeld

Like any good scientific conference, this one ends with more questions than answers. What research questions emerged from these proceedings?

Many of our speakers have talked about the problems associated with the failure to return to work. We must first establish if the failure to return to work is caused by the fact that these individuals are physically more impaired than those who do return to work, or we are dealing with the effects of psychological and social factors. That issue can only be examined in prospective studies where the medical factors are controlled. This must be done.

A number of people have commented on the impact of rehabilitation programs, but as a number of individuals have commented from the floor, the flaw in these observations is that they are, for the most part, retrospective studies often carried out in volunteer populations. As Dr. Gutmann has told us, she has begun a study with patients assigned in a prospective randomly assigned manner. Such a study will allow us to determine whether it is the rehabilitation program which has the effect, or the self-selection process. Other such studies are needed, since rehabilitation programs differ.

A number of investigators have told us about the harmful effects of the extended waiting period prior to surgery. The longer a patient is out of work, the less likely he is to return to work. Assuming we can no nothing, at least for now, to shorten the waiting period, then perhaps some kind of psychotherapeutic intervention during the waiting period might be attempted in order to influence return to work. A prospective randomized trial would be necessary.

A number of individuals have commented that some patients complain postoperatively of symptoms which are not "physical," i.e., they are anxious, depressed, etc. What effect would psychotherapeutic intervention have in such patients if it were commenced immediately following surgery? Could we reduce these complaints if we made an effort to intervene immediately postop? A prospective randomized trial could answer that question.

As you know, I am particularly interested in the Type A behavior pattern (Coronary Prone Behavior Pattern). I would therefore urge us to move forward in an effort to determine if it, or any of its components, contribute to the reatherosclerosis process after coronary artery bypass grafting.

I believe one of Dr. Halhuber's statements best summarizes my feelings. He said he was impressed with the fact that such a multidisciplinary and multinational group had come together for 2 days and identified so many common problems. I agree. We have managed to talk a common language, and I do not mean English, but rather the language of science. It was this which bound us together in our effort to identify problems and potential solutions. I therefore leave this conference optimistic regarding the prognosis for the ultimate resolution of these issues.

Economic Considerations: Costs of Coronary Artery Bypass Surgery

Comparison of Costs for Medical and Surgical Treatment of Coronary Obstructive Disease

J. J. Collins, Jr.

A comparison of costs for medical and surgical management of patients with coronary heart disease is not easy. Carefully studied groups frequently include primarily patients with chronic stable angina pectoris who have a relatively low rate of hospitalization for medical management. Thus, the impact of hospitalization costs for coronary bypass surgery becomes extremely great relative to the overall cost of management. For patients with unstable angina pectoris or multiple myocardial infarction, the costs of hospitalization become more significant. In a previously reported analysis, we found that hospitalization after coronary bypass surgery was substantially reduced in a group of patients undergoing coronary bypass operations. Other studies of patients with more chronic angina have shown no significant difference in postoperative hospitalization for surgical patients as compared to those followed medically.

In addition to the direct cost of coronary bypass surgery, the possibility of return to a productive existence may be justification for the higher initial cost of operation. Numerous studies have come to divergent conclusions as to the utility of coronary surgery in promoting employment. We have examined patterns of employment in patients following coronary bypass surgery in an attempt to discover whether patterns of preoperative disability may be significantly predictive for postoperative employment.

Data Acquisition

Between 1 January 1970 and 31 December 1980, 2004 patients underwent coronary artery bypass graft at the Peter Bent Brigham Hospital and Brigham and Women's Hospital without additional procedures such as valve replacement or aneurysm resection. Data concerning preoperative condition, risk factors, operative variables, and postoperative status were gathered in an organized fashion and entered into a computerized patient file. During 1978, a consecutive series of 100 patients were subjected to analysis of hospitalization for 2 years before and 2 years subsequent to coronary bypass surgery in order to obtain an accurate assessment of pre- and postoperative medical costs. These patients were included in the overall analysis of the group of 2004 patients.

Among these, 1761 patients provided data concerning their working status in 1982 at a mean follow-up time of 4.8 ± 2.7 years after coronary bypass surgery. Attempts to obtain specific information on the prevalence of disability insurance, disability compensation, and economic incentives for return to work were met with resistance on the part of many patients, and because of the doubtful accuracy of the data obtained, these attempts were abandoned and that information considered not useable. Selected risk factors were then examined as to their influence on the probability of postoperative patients being employed, unemployed, or disabled. Simple categorization as working or not working did not appear adequate to describe productive activity.

Results

In Table 1, the postoperative working status of males is shown. Male patients under 65 years of age showed a 24% probability of considering themselves disabled, with 54% actively employed and 22% not employed although considering themselves capable of employment. Among male patients over 65 years of age, only 9% (36 patients) considered themselves disabled while only 29% were working and 62% were not working but considered themselves employable. The data for females are shown in Table 2. There is a similar discrepancy among patients considering themselves disabled between the younger and the more elderly. Among women under 60 years of age, 29% considered themselves disabled (48 patients) while only 7% (9 patients) among those older than 60 years of age at the time of operation considered themselves disabled at the time of follow-up. Only 26% of females in the younger group were working, and 5% in the older group. There were 88% not working in the older group and 45% not working in the younger group.

Table 1. BWH surgical series, 1970–1980: working status of males

	<60 years % (*n*)	>60 years % (*n*)
Disabled	24 (261)	9 (36)
Working	54 (575)	29 (114)
Not working	22 (230)	62 (243)
	100% 1066	100% 393

Table 2. BWH surgical series, 1970–1980: working status of females

	<60 years % (*n*)	>60 years % (*n*)
Disabled	29 (48)	7 (9)
Working	26 (44)	5 (7)
Not working	45 (76)	88 (118)
	100% 168	100% 134

The influence of the severity of coronary artery disease on the reported working status at the time of follow-up in these patients is shown in Table 3.

Table 3. Quantity of CAD vs working status ($n = 1760$)

	One-vessel	Two-vessel	Three-vessel	LM
Working	41% ($n = 65$)	43% ($n = 191$)	42% ($n = 360$)	40% ($n = 123$)
Not working	36% ($n = 57$)	37% ($n = 161$)	38% ($n = 322$)	41% ($n = 127$)
Disabled	23% ($n = 37$)	20% ($n = 89$)	20% ($n = 171$)	19% ($n = 57$)
Total	100% ($n = 159$)	100% ($n = 441$)	100% ($n = 853$)	100% ($n = 307$)

There was a significant difference in the probability of working, not working, or being disabled among patients with one-, two- or three-vessel coronary artery disease or obstruction of the left main coronary artery. A history of myocardial infarction did exert a deleterious effect on the probability of patients being gainfully employed (Table 4). Patients who had had no previous myocardial infarction had a 45% chance of being employed, those with one previous myocardial infarction had a 42% chance of being employed, and those with more than one previous myocardial infarction only a 34% chance of being employed. In this group, the probability of disability also increased significantly with the presence of one or more myocardial infarctions. Severity of symptoms of angina pectoris as judged by the New York Heart Association classification also affected probability of subsequent employment (Table 5). The probability of being employed diminished progressively with increasing severity of anginal symptoms, while the probability of patients considering themselves disabled

Table 4. BWH surgical series, 1970–1980: history of MI vs working status ($n = 1761$)

	0	1	>1
Working	45% ($n = 333$)	42% ($n = 309$)	34% ($n = 98$)
Not Working	40% ($n = 295$)	36% ($n = 263$)	38% ($n = 109$)
Disabled	15% ($n = 116$)	22% ($n = 159$)	28% ($n = 79$)
Total	100% ($n = 744$)	100% ($n = 731$)	100% ($n = 286$)

was not significantly different in any group having active angina pectoris at the time of operation. Various indices of left ventricular contractile capability, including analysis of ejection fraction, necessity of intraaortic balloon counterpulsation, and presence of symptoms of congestive heart failure, all had an effect on the probability of subsequent employment as shown in Tables 6–8. Be-

Table 5. BWH surgical series, 1970–1980: NYHA vs working status ($n=1761$)

	I	II	III	IV
Working	62.5% ($n=55$)	52% ($n=232$)	39% ($n=307$)	32% ($n=146$)
Not working	25% ($n=22$)	30% ($n=133$)	39% ($n=305$)	46% ($n=207$)
Disabled	12.5% ($n=11$)	18% ($n=78$)	22% ($n=167$)	22% ($n=98$)
Total	100% ($n=88$)	100% ($n=443$)	100% ($n=779$)	100% ($n=451$)

Table 6. Ejection fraction vs working status ($n=1491$)

	<50	≥ 50
Working	36% ($n=112$)	43% ($n=507$)
Not working	38% ($n=117$)	38% ($n=455$)
Disabled	26% ($n=80$)	19% ($n=220$)
Total	100% ($n=309$)	100% ($n=1182$)

Table 7. Working status vs intraaortic balloon utilization ($n=1761$)

	No balloon	Balloon
Working	42% ($n=718$)	38% ($n=22$)
Not working	38% ($n=649$)	31% ($n=18$)
Disabled	20% ($n=336$)	31% ($n=18$)
Total	100% ($n=1703$)	100% ($n=58$)

Table 8. Congestive heart failure (CHF) vs working status ($n = 1758$)

	No CHF	CHF
Working	44% ($n = 698$)	25% ($n = 42$)
Not working	36% ($n = 578$)	51% ($n = 87$)
Disabled	20% ($n = 313$)	24% ($n = 40$)
Total	100% ($n = 1589$)	100% ($n = 169$)

cause of the small number of patients involved, the data concerning balloon counterpulsation as a deleterious effect do not achieve statistical significance.

Discussion

The true cost of medical treatment of patients with coronary artery disease is not easily definable. Among the variety of studies which have addressed the question of employment status after coronary artery surgery, there has been no general agreement as to the influence of preoperative risk factors. In most studies, the strongest determinant of postoperative employment status has been preoperative employment status. Some studies have suggested that the level of education, preoperative income, and possibly the presence of workmen's compensation or disability insurance exert a substantial influence on the probability of subsequent employment. While these data do not appear easily acquired, it seems likely that some factors other than physical capability are involved in the determination of disability, employment, or absence of employment. This is strongly suggested by our observation that the probability of disability is substantially less in patients not needing disability to explain lack of employment. Thus, older men and older women have a substantially and significantly reduced probability of considering themselves disabled at follow-up after coronary surgery. Also, patients with impaired left ventricular function are substantially less likely to become employed.

Assessment of our data suggests that the overall cost of coronary artery surgery may vary according to the degree of disability of patients in the surgical sample. Patients having a major preoperative probability of hospitalization may be more economically treated surgically than those having a relatively small need for hospitalization during medical management programs. Those having a significant number of previous myocardial infarctions, congestive heart failure, and severe angina pectoris have not only a higher probability of preoperative hospitalization, but a lower probability of return to postoperative employment.

Summary

There are a variety of factors which may alter the cost-benefit relationship in coronary surgery patients, making comparison with medically treated patients difficult or unreliable. In particular, there is an apparent tendency for patients in preretirement age to have a higher chance of disability than older patients. While some preoperative factors influence later productive employment, the direction of influence suggests that those who are unemployed may also be those who would otherwise require more frequent hospitalization.

Costs of Open Heart Surgery: ACVB Surgery vs Valve Replacement

P. Kalmár, M.-J. Polonius, K.-J. Hahn, I. Radtke, and G. Rodewald

In recent years it has become fashionable to criticize the so-called explosion of costs in the medical field. Three main reasons are usually given for this explosion:

1. The pharmaceutical industry sets excessively high prices for their products.
2. Physicians use too many and too expensive apparatus, and do so too uncritically.
3. Patients demand the use of such apparatus because they want to benefit from all the modern trends in medicine.

These critics forget, however, that many diseases which were untreatable in the past can nowadays not only be dramatically improved but even cured. This is certainly true for some procedures in cardiac surgery, which have undergone incredible development over the last 3 decades. For congenital cardiac defects and valve and coronary heart diseases one calculates 550 operative open-heart procedures per 1 million of the population and year. Unfortunately we do not know what these patients cost if they are not treated surgically but we can calculate – in the last few years with increasing accuracy – what the operative treatment costs.

The financing system of most of the general nonprivate hospitals in Europe, however, enables only the gross calculation of supply and personnel costs. If a department carries out only or mainly open-heart procedures, one may calculate from the total costs the average for a single procedure. Therefore at the University Hospital Hamburg-Eppendorf we tried to investigate the different costs which ensue during the surgical treatment of heart patients. We present our data comparing the three most common procedures.

1. Aortocoronary bypass procedures
2. Single valve replacement (aorta and mitral)
3. Double valve replacement

The prospective study was carried out over a period of 4 months in 50 patients after an ACVB procedure and in 40 patients after valve replacement. All costs were listed or calculated. Patients with extremely long postoperative intensive care treatment were excluded. However, in all groups there were a few cases involving technical or biological difficulties, which resulted in a prolonged operating time as well as the need for additional procedures in ICU.

Table 1 shows the duration of treatment and monitoring during the different phases of treatment in the cardiac surgery unit. We intentionally avoided the usual graphic distribution of age, sex, and the preoperative clinical grading. Our patients are just as severely ill as those anywhere else, and in terms of age and sex there are no differences worthy of mention, at least not in matters relating to finances. As intimated above a group of 50 patients who underwent surgery for aortocoronary bypass grafts were compared to a collective of 40 patients, of whom 15 received aortic valve replacements, 15 mitral valves, and 10 double prosthetic valve replacements. The average duration of surgery was between 4 and 6 h. The duration of extracorporeal circulation (ECC) during mitral valve replacement averaged 1.3 h and was maximally 2.5 h during aortic valve replacement. The postoperative phase of intensive care lasted between 45 and 53.6 h. The patients then spent another 118–158 h, i.e., 6–8 days, on the normal ward, after which time they were transferred to the referring cardiologic clinics. The manner in which the costs are derived is shown by Table 2.

Table 1. Duration (mean values in hours) of treatment and care during the different phases of stay in the cardiac surgery department

Phase	Type of procedure			
	ACVB ($n=50$)	AVR ($n=15$)	MVR ($n=15$)	A/MVR ($n=10$)
Operation	4.84 (1.75–9.2)	5.96 (3.23–14.0)	3.94 (2.4–6.0)	4.48 (3.25–7.8)
ECC	2.12 (0.62–4.4)	2.50 (0.9–8.9)	1.29 (0.5–2.3)	2.22 (1.35–5.3)
Recovery room	1.91 (1–4.5)	1.77 (0.5–6.0)	2.3 (0.75–3.7)	2.17 (0.75–5.0)
ICU	51.77 (18–138)	49.44 (3–116)	42.75 (19–83)	47.08 (20–118)
Intermediate care	158 (96–312)	134 (0–360)	118 (0–192)	146 (24–264)

( ) min-max
Abbreviations: n, number of patients; *ACVB*, aortocoronary vein bypass; *AVR*, aortic valve replacement; *MVR*, mitral valve replacement; *A/MVR*, double valve replacement

The activities of all personnel involved in the surgical phase, including preoperative enlightenment of the patients and preparations for and induction of anesthesia, were meticulously registered on an hourly basis. The costs were then computed from the tables of standard wage costs. The costs of postoperative nursing care were calculated from the available nursing staff performing the maximal duties of the unit as would be expected if all nursing positions were filled. The allotment of part of the nursing capacity to the patients studied was also calculated according to the occupied beds in the unit. The physicians' activities in the surgical unit, that is, the actual time spent in treating patients,

Table 2. Investigation of costs

Personnel[a]	Op:	calculated from the actual hours worked with patients
	ICU + ward:	working hours, including all activities
	Not included:	teaching, research, conferences, out patient clinic, administration
Material[a]	All material, including drugs and infusion	
	Not included:	investments and amortization
Laboratory tests[b] Blood Transfusion X-ray Histological and bacteriological tests	Official tariff of City of Hamburg	
Accommodation[b]	Official tariff of University of Hamburg	

[a] Paid for from the budget of the department
[b] Paid for from the budget of the University Hospital, but charged to the account of the department

were recorded in *net* time of work, while postoperative patient care was calculated in *gross* time of work. This also includes activities not directly involving patient care. The work load of the surgical staff - including teaching, research, conferences, the care of ambulatory patients, and administrative activities - and the share of the costs of personnel per individual patient are the objectives of a new study now being done which has not been considered here.

The cost of materials covers such items as drugs and infusions. Materials which were used directly during surgery could be exactly recorded by means of a checklist. Such articles and drugs whose use was necessary during the employment of the heart-lung machine are also included. Empty packages of used materials, ampules after use, empty containers of infusions etc. were collected in a plastic bag and counted at the end of the treatment period. Parallel to this, attempts were made at estimating the costs. The probable estimations were mostly in the order of 30%–50% of the actual costs. The result is that the only possible means remaining for the exact determination of costs is the time-consuming and organizationally problematic method of meticulous collection of materials. Mixed expenditures which involve materials as well as personnel ensued during registration of laboratory tests, blood transfusions, X-ray examinations, histology, and bacteriology. These costs, which have been determined by other agencies, are included in the itemized table of costs of the City of Hamburg.

Finally one must add to these the hotel accommodation costs, which are revised each budget year by the university hospital administration. As far as costs of investments and amortization are calculated, they are included under mixed expenditures and not under materials and hotels.

The average costs (Table 3) for the various surgical patient groups are as follows: 15700 DM for a coronary bypass graft operation, 21700 DM for aortic valve replacement, 18500 DM for mitral valve replacement, and 23700 DM for double prosthetic valves.

Table 3. Cost of various typical open-heart procedures (in DM)

	Type of procedure			
	ACVB ($n=50$)	AVR ($n=15$)	MVR ($n=15$)	A/MVR ($n=10$)
Min–max	11545–31324	16990–38070	15592–26772	19400–30651
Mean	15736	21703	18505	23711

The cost differences between valvular and coronary heart patients could partially be explained by the fact that the expensive prosthetic valves cost on average 4000 DM. The relatively higher costs of aortic valve surgery arose partially the above-average utilization of blood transfusions in this group, and partially because two of these patients had complications intraoperatively which necessitated excessive blood transfusion and the use of expensive drugs.

Table 4 gives detailed information on the costs of the various groups. The expenditure on personnel ranged from 4800 DM for mitral valve patients to 6000 DM for patients undergoing bypass surgery and aortic valve replacement. The cost of materials, including prosthetic valves, was 4700 DM in the coronary group, 8800 DM in the mitral group, 9400 DM in the group with aortic valve replacement, and finally 12600 in the group receiving double prosthetic valves. "Other expenditures," in which laboratory tests, blood transfusions, X-rays, histology, bacteriology, and hotel accommodation costs are included, ranged between 4900 and 6300 DM. The overall expenditures have already been shown (Table 3). It remains to be noted that, in this table and in those which follow, the amounts have been rounded up.

Table 4. Cost of diverse areas of expenditure during various typical open-heart procedures (in DM in round figures)

Type of cost	Type of procedure			
	ACVB	AVR	MVR	A/MVR
Personnel	5500	6000	4800	5700
Materials (incl. valve prostheses)	4700	9400	8800	12600
Others[a]	5500	6300	4900	5400
Total	15700	21700	18500	23700

[a] Laboratory tests, X-rays, histological and bacteriological tests, blood transfusions, accommodation costs (food, laundry, energy, etc.)

In Table 5 the costs are itemized for the aortocoronary bypass patients and compared to those for the entire group of valvular patients. Differences in the personnel costs in the order of 10% were somewhat offset by similar costs in the categories of materials and drugs and blood transfusions. Thus after deducting the costs of the prosthetic valves, the overall expenditure in the two groups was almost identical. In such case then, the distribution of the diagnosis within the group of valvular patients in the ratio of 1.5:1.5:1 between aortic, mitral and double valvular replacements corresponds to the fundamental figures of this analysis, which, however, do not correspond to the reality, at least not in our clinic.

Table 6 shows the resultant sum of the costs and the itemized costs after subdivisions according to the varying valve diseased.

Table 5. Amount of different types of cost incurred during the two chief forms of open-heart procedure (in DM in round figures)

Type of cost	Type of procedure	
	ACVB	VR[a]
Personnel	5500	4900
Prosthetic valve	–	4300
Materials and drugs	4700	4600
Laboratory tests	2100	1900
Blood transfusions	1200	1300
X-ray, histological and bacteriological tests	400	300
Accommodation	1800	1400
Total	15700	18700[b]

[a] Valve replacement (AVR:MVR:A/MVR = 1.5:1.5:1.0)
[b] 14400 DM without prosthetic valve

Table 6. Amount of different types of cost incurred during various typical open-heart procedures (in DM in round figures)

Type of cost	Type of procedure			
	ACVB	AVR	MVR	A/MVR
Personnel	5500	6000	4800	5700
Prosthetic valve	–	5400	4100	7800
Material and drugs	4700	4000	4700	4800
Laboratory tests	2100	2300	1900	2100
Blood transfusions	1200	2000	1200	1200
X-ray, histological and bacteriological tests	400	400	400	400
Accommodation	1800	1700	1400	1700
Total	15700	21700	18500	23700
Without prosthetic valves	15700	16300	14400	15900

The next step was the analysis of the distribution of expenditure in the various phases of treatment. Table 7 demonstrates that 41% of the overall costs in the coronary group arise during the period of surgery, 38% during the period of intensive care (which lasts on average a little over 2 days), and only 11% during the period of intermediate care. In the group of patients with valve replacement the surgical costs account for 55%–60% of the overall costs owing to the expenditure on prosthetic valves; the phase of intensive care costs between 28% and 30%, and the phase on normal ward between 12% and 16%.

If the expenditure incurred during the different phases of the treatment of a single patient is divided by the total number of hours spent by the patient in each phase, we obtain the costs per 24 hours.

Table 7. Costs according to the different time periods (in % of total costs)

Time period	Type of procedure			
	ACVB	AVR	MVR	A/MVR
Operation	41	55	56	60
ICU	38	29	30	28
Ward	11	16	14	12

Table 8. Total costs per day according to ICU and ward

Time period	Type of procedure			
	ACVB	AVR	MVR	A/MVR
ICU	2690	3090	2990	2850
Ward	490	570	520	530

Table 8 demonstrates the calculated daily costs, which cover personnel, materials, laboratory tests, blood transfusions, and such other costs as X-rays, histology, bacteriology, and hotel accommodation. The results show that the most economical group is that of the coronary bypass patients, with an average cost of 2690 DM per day on the ICU; by contrast the patient with valve replacement costs between 2850 and 3090 DM per day on the ICU. The normal ward care costs between 490 and 570 DM per day.

Innumerable check lists with data on the cost of items used by the various centers enable even more detailed analyses which certainly may supersede the framework of this paper. Nevertheless, I believe that we have succeeded in carrying out a patient-related expenditure analysis with a relatively high degree of precision, even if this discourse considers only the net costs of personnel and could not take into consideration the costs of investment and amortization.

The accuracy of this expenditure analysis could and must be improved by means of further studies. Nevertheless, the findings enable a higher degree of price calculation and assessment of expected costs during the procurement of materials. Furthermore, they may be of help in discussions relating to problems of costs.

The Costing of Coronary Artery Bypass Surgery

W. J. Keon, S. C. Menzies, and C. M. Lay

Introduction

The high cost of health care is causing increasing concern to the public, government, and health care professionals. Coronary artery disease and particularly its surgical treatment is an enormous health care burden. The University of Ottawa Heart Institute, in conjunction with the Health Administration Program of the Faculty of Administration, has embarked on studies to determine the cost and cost-effectiveness of coronary artery bypass grafting (CABG). The first step of this has been an investigation to determine the overall episode cost and cost variability for patients undergoing CABG. This is the first time an analysis of this type and detail has been undertaken in a Canadian institution.

The Canadian health care system is "public," with hospitals being reimbursed by provincial governments on a global budget basis. The question of the cost of heart surgery is currently of interest in Canada because we lack the basic data for public decision-making about funding for increases and/or changes in this area. The lack of data is common to the whole health care system in all provinces and specifically impacts on cardiovascular disease, Canada's number one health care problem.

The University of Ottawa Heart Institute at the Ottawa Civic Hospital is a free-standing structure devoted to the prevention, investigation, treatment (both medical and surgical), and rehabilitation of patients with cardiovascular disease. It has 125 set-up beds, including eight surgical and eight medical intensive care beds with an additional six recovery room, eight day care, and four emergency resuscitation beds. We perform in excess of 1000 operative procedures per year, of which 750 are bypass grafting. There are 290.5 staff assigned to the Institute; 36.5 medical, 157 nursing and orderly staff, 34.5 technical, 9 allied health professionals, i.e., physiotherapists, pharmacists, etc., 44 clerical and administrative, and 9.5 research staff. The current operating budget for the Institute for the year 1984–85 is 15 million dollars.

Methodology

Costs for services provided for CABG patients were determined through the use of accepted disease costing methodology [1]. The first step in determining costs was to design a cost center matrix that integrated six arbitrary stages of the patient's hospital stay into admission, preoperative, ward, operating room, recovery room - surgical intensive care, postoperative ward, and discharge. With the hospital cost centers defined in previous research at the Ottawa Civic Hospital [5], these cost centers were divided into three categories: support departments, diagnostic and therapeutic departments, and patient care departments. All hospital operating costs and treatment elements applicable to the CABG procedure were identified and classified as either direct, indirect, or overhead. Costs were assigned to an individual patient and aggregated to obtain the cost of an episode of illness for CABG (Fig. 1) [8]. The cost of labor on the wards pre- and postoperatively was determined using a 7-day work sampling ratio delay study [2–6]. The hospital charts of 50 randomly selected coronary artery bypass patients were reviewed in detail to determine the actual cost for patients' admissions for catheterization and/or separate admission for surgical procedures. Professional fees were determined by recording the actual amounts reimbursed by the provincial government plans to the medical staff involved in the treatment: surgeon, anesthetists, surgical assistants, cardiologists, and radiologists.

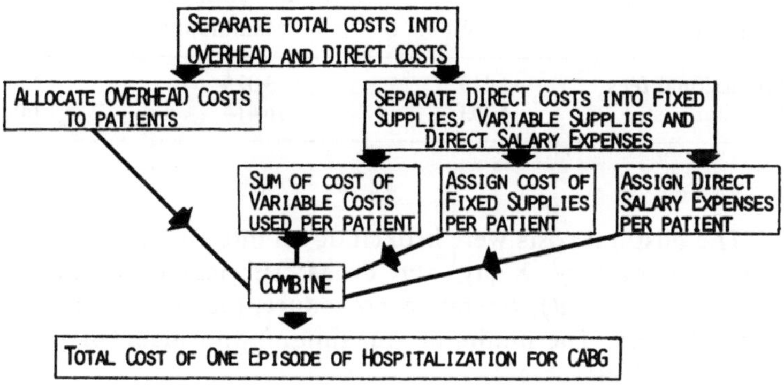

Fig. 1. Method of ascertaining the total cost of one episode of hospitalization for CABG ($n = 50$)

Results

Clinical Profile of Patients

We reviewed charts of 50 patients who underwent CABG surgery between April and September 1983, excluding patients undergoing reoperation or those who died in hospital. There were 42 males and 8 females with a mean age of 55.3 years (range 39–73 years). This is representative of the male-female ratio and age range of our total patient population. Four had single vessel disease, 12 double vessel, and 34 triple vessel. Seven had received surgery on an emergency basis and 43 as elective cases. Thirteen had poor ventricular function (class III or IV) [3], and the remaining 37 had normal to mild impairment. Seven patients underwent additional procedures - six coronary endarterectomies and one left ventricular aneurysm resection – and two patients required intraaortic balloon assist early postoperatively. The total length of stay averaged 16.54 days, with a range of 8–43 days.

Total Episode Cost

An episode of illness for this costing study if defined as a patient stay in hospital for the surgical procedure, including separate admissions for the cardiac catheterization procedure. Twenty-five patients had catheterization procedures done on the same admission as surgery, three done as outpatients, and one done at a different hospital (therefore, that single procedure was not costed). The episode costs are the total costs for all treatment elements to patients during their stay. The total costs for CABG patients varied from $ 6387.00 to $ 18415.00 (Canadian 1983 dollars), with an average cost of $ 9595.00. This is composed of two areas: professional fees and hospital costs (Table 1).

Table 1. Episode cost

Category	Minimum $	Maximum $	Mean $	%
Professional fees	1419	3025	2254	23.5
Hospital costs	4703	16414	7345	76.5

The hospital costs were broken down into five categories: cardiac catheterization; laboratory, X-ray, and drugs; surgical ward (including preoperative coronary care unit); operative procedure, recovery room, and CSU; and professional fees. The minimum, maximum, and mean of these subcategories is summarized in Table 2.

The total episode cost, not surprisingly, was directly related to length of stay (Table 3). It was also found to be directly related to the number of diseased vessels, secondary diagnoses, left ventricular dysfunction, and age (Table 4). It was not related to sex, emergency category of a patient, number of bypass grafts, or auxiliary procedures performed.

Table 2. Hospital costs

Category	Minimum $	Maximum $	Mean $
Catheterization	–	–	409
X-ray, drugs, lab	349	1621	555
Surgical ward + CCU	1205	11828	2750
CCU, pre-op	474	9006	1828
OR, RR-CSU	2332	8894	3629
OR alone	1700	1943	1817

Abbreviations: CCU, coronary care unit; *OR,* operating room; *RR,* recovery room

Table 3. Episode cost vs length of stay (LOS)

LOS (days)	*n*	Range	Mean cost ($)
9	5	6389– 8143	7584
10–12	15	6949–16183	9319
14–16	6	8458–10363	9702
17–19	7	7568–10804	9126
20–29	10	8931–18415	13067
30–43	3	10872–14997	13159

Table 4. Variables affecting episode cost

Variable	*n*	Range of cost ($)	Mean cost
Age (yrs)			
37–49	15	6387–16183	8616
50–59	17	7329–16224	9603
60–73	18	7317–18415	10404
Number of diseased vessels			
Single	4	6387– 8143	7624
Double	12	7329–18415	9319
Triple	34	6949–16224	9702
Secondary diagnoses			
Diabetes	6	6387–13174	11059
Hypertension	5	7979–14999	10599
Other atherosclerosis			
PVD	5	7317– 8885	7905
TIA	2	8303– 9154	8728
COPD	2	16225–18415	17320
Subtotal 2° diagnosis	20	6387–18415	10549
CAD alone	30	6949–16412	8495
Left ventricular function			
Poor	13	7341–14998	10196
Good	37	6387–18415	9383

Abbreviations: PVD, peripheral vascular disease; *TIA,* transient ischemic attacks; *COPD,* chronic obstructive pulmonary disease; *CAD,* coronary artery disease

Discussion

In the academic year 1983–84 the Heart Institute and the Program in Health Administration at the University of Ottawa have carried out a detailed study of the cost of treating 50 patients undergoing coronary artery bypass surgery. Figure 2 shows the distribution of total costs ranging from the lowest to the highest for each of these 50 patients. For the first time in Canada we know the actual costs of treating a group of heart surgery patients. To do this we studied the treatment process for CABG patients, carrying out a detailed cost analysis in every department of the hospital participating in their treatment. We studied their cost patterns and developed unit costs for every identifiable component of patient care that could be related to the patients' medical charts and others such as administration, overhead, and capital equipment that were not recorded in the charts. We covered all direct and indirect aspects of care. These costs were then used in conjunction with a detailed review of the charts to develop a pseudo "bill" for each patient.

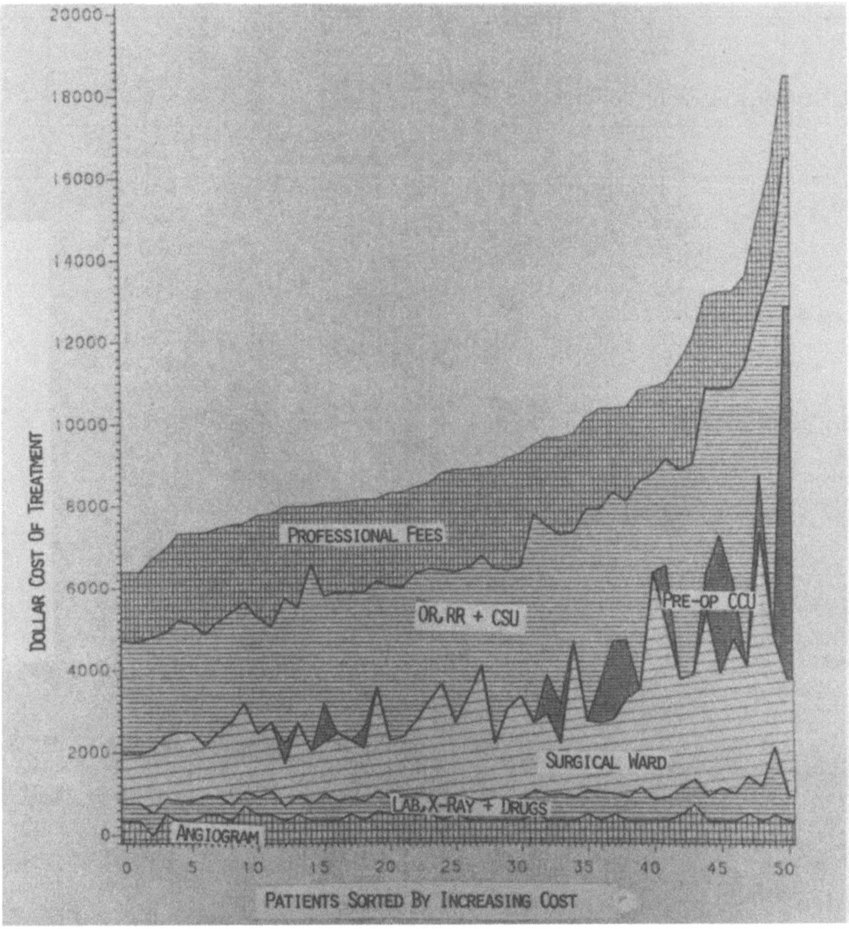

Fig. 2. Distribution of total costs in the 50 patients who underwent coronary artery bypass surgery ($n = 50$ patients)

There have been two other detailed costing studies done in North America, in the United States; one was published in 1978 [7] and one in 1979 [4]. Although the method of costing and reimbursement for patient's services were different among the three institutions, a comparison is possible after adding an annual inflationary factor and converting U.S. dollars to 1983 Canadian dollars. Despite the differences between the institutions and the methodology, the percentage of the total hospital cost versus that of professional fees remains fairly constant (Table 5), with professional fees representing 20%–30% of total costs and hospital charges 70%–80%. Stoney and his colleagues, reporting on Vanderbilt University School of Medicine in Nashville, show a considerable difference in hospital costs when they are subdivided. Most notably, nursing costs on the ward are half that of our nursing costs, operating room expenses twice the amount, catheterization procedures three times, and blood sixteen times the amount at our Institute. It must be noted, however, that the costs of $ 21.00 per patient for blood in the Institute refer only to the charges for cross-matching, since all blood transfusions per se are free of charge.

Table 5. Comparison of hospital costs in CABG studies (1983 Canadian dollars)

	Nashville [7]	Birmingham [4]	Ottawa
Ward	1268	–	2749
ICU/day	684	–	474
ECG	254	–	46
OR	3729	–	1800
Catheterization	1151	–	408
Blood	324	–	21
X-ray	160	–	117
Pharmacy	–	800 (4.4%)	144 (1.5%)
Prof. fees	6344 (30%)	3860 (20.6%)	2254 (23.5%)
Total in hosp.	14983 (70%)	14104 (75%)	7345 (76.5%)
Total/episode	21332	18764	9595

This pilot study is our first step toward dealing with disease costing and cost-effectiveness analysis at the Institute. We expect to further refine the costing components of care and develop a patient care information system which will generate data for medical peer review. This will be of use to both medical and "economic" grand rounds and will eventually lead to studying the cost-effectiveness of alternative forms of treatment for coronary artery disease.

Hospital information systems in Canada are in their infancy in the area of clinical patient information systems. With the development of cost data, physicians and surgeons will not only be able to routinely present clinical cases, they will have the precise cost data with which to judge the economic implications of their decisions to utilize one form of investigation and treatment as opposed to another. An example of the potential for such a system is to develop an "estimated day of discharge" system focusing on the expeditious treatment and discharge of patients and thus reducing unnecessary lengthy stays, to which cost is directly related. This frees beds to allow flexibility in the patient flow through the course of treatment. Other alternatives to investigate are to have cardiac catheterizations routinely performed on an outpatient basis and have step-down (and consequently less expensive) "hostel" inpatient care areas for patients from out of town or for those with minor complications who do not require "full inpatient" treatment.

One area of continuing concern is whether the particular courses of treatment have long-term cost benefits for the patients and for society as a whole. Up to this point we have simply addressed the cost of one mode of treatment. However, the proposed research will address the broader questions. The objective, of course, is to continue to treat patients as effectively but also as economically as possible. The added bonus of a clinical information system would be for administrative use in planning patient load and work loads, both by department and institution and as a tool in budgeting and forecasting.

The days of open-ended financial attitudes when planning health care have passed. Improvements must come from within the system and be initiated by the physicians and surgeons concerned rather than be imposed by the funding bodies. Accurate and responsible disease costing studies are a prerequisite for this intelligent planning.

Acknowledgments. The authors wish to thank Jann Darlington, David Kay, John MacIntyre, Janie Reed, and Melissa Sonberg, Masters students in the Health Administration Program, and Mrs. Katrin Smith, Research Assistant, University of Ottawa Heart Institute, for their assistance in this study.

References

1. Babson JL, Heidemann EG, Lay CM (1975) Disease costing applied to measuring the cost of treating patients undergoing surgical removal of the gall bladder (cholecystectomy). Master of Health Administration Programme, University of Ottawa
2. Barnes RM (1963) Work sampling. In: Motion and time study, design and measurement of work. Wiley, New York, p 517
3. Keon WJ (1978) Expectations of myocardial revascularization. CMA J 118:408
4. Kronenfeld JJ, Charles ED Jr, Wayne JB, Oberman A, Kouchoukos NT, Rogers WJ, Mantle JA, Rackley CE, Russell RO (1978) Unstable angina pectoris, an examination of modes and costs of therapy. Circulation [Suppl I] 60:I 16
5. Lay CM, Lowry E (1982) Programme expense reporting project. Ottawa Civic Hospital, Ottawa
6. Roche JF (1965) Work sampling of nursing activities. Smalley HE, Freeman JR (ed) Hospital industrial engineering. Reinhold Corp., New York, p 247
7. Stoney WS, Alford WC, Burrus GR, First RA, Thomas CS (1978) The cost of coronary bypass procedures. JAMA 240:2278
8. Williams SV, Finkler SA, Murphy CM, Murphy JM (1982) Improved cost allocation in case-mix accounting. Med Care 20 (5):452

Cost-Effectiveness of Coronary Artery Bypass Surgery

W. B. Stason and M. C. Weinstein

Coronary artery bypass graft surgery (CABG) has become the mainstay of treatment for patients with severe refractory angina and extensive coronary artery disease (CAD). Approximately 170,000 operations were performed in 1983 in the United States at a cost of $ 20,000 to $ 25,000 per operation for a total cost of between 3 and 4 billion dollars. Hence, CABG contributes significantly to total health care costs and requires special scrutiny to determine whether these costs are justified by the added health benefits enjoyed by recipients.

Additional reasons to focus attention on CABG are the dynamic changes that are occurring in other cardiac diagnostic and treatment technologies. These technologies undoubtedly will have important influences on the future use of CABG. Percutaneous transluminal coronary angioplasty (PTCA), a less invasive and less expensive procedure, may substitute for surgery in patients with proximal and localized disease in their coronary arteries. Some estimates suggest that as many as 10%–15% of patients with coronary artery disease are potential candidates for this procedure. Improved medical treatment of angina pectoris also may reduce the need for surgery. Long-acting nitrates, beta-blockers, and calcium channel blockers, alone or in combination, have proven to be very effective in controlling the symptoms of angina in many patients, and the recently released results of the Coronary Artery Surgery Study (CASS 1983) suggest that better medical treatment may also improve survival.

Conversely, the trend toward early surgery in the patients who have recently suffered myocardial infarctions may increase the use of CABG. Coronary arteriography, in conjunction with the use of intracoronary streptokinase or tissue plasminogen activator, will identify residual coronary artery stenoses and provide the impetus for early surgery. Similarly, concern over the high risk of mortality in the first year following myocardial infarction provides a rationale for performing coronary arteriography and surgery soon after myocardial infarctions, especially in view of the low and declining operative mortality of CABG.

We cannot be sure of the net effects that these factors will have on the future use of CABG, but the confluence of the dynamic nature of these technological changes, escalating medical care costs, and the perception that medical care resources are limited indicates the need to evaluate the benefits of alternative treatments for coronary artery disease in relation to their costs. This paper addresses this issue by comparing CABG to medical management. Our goals are to identify the characteristics of patients for whom CABG appears to represent the best use of medical care resources and then to compare the cost-effectiveness of CABG to that of hypertension treatment and the use of diagnostic strategies for coronary artery disease. The analysis applies only to patients with stable angina and not to those who have recently suffered myocardial infarctions or who have unstable angina.

Principles of Cost-Effectiveness Analysis

Cost-effectiveness analysis is a technique which allows one to compare treatment strategies, both in terms of the health benefits and in terms of the medical care costs involved. If medical care resources are limited, the strategy that provides the least expensive way to purchase a given level of health benefits is preferred.

Cost-effectiveness analysis begins with a careful assessment of the expected health benefits of each treatment and an effort to balance these benefits against corresponding risks. Patient characteristics, such as age, sex, the extent of coronary artery disease, and left ventricular ejection fraction can be considered explicitly. Health outcomes are expressed as differences in patient survival, disability, or quality of life, or in a combined measure termed "quality-adjusted life years." These outcome measures serve as a risk–benefit analysis for those who are not concerned with costs.

The costs of surgical and medical management are then determined. When assessing costs, one cannot focus solely on the costs of the initial treatment episodes. Instead, the time stream of costs over a defined period or the lifetime of the patient must be examined. For a patient treated surgically, costs include not only those of surgery, but also those of any required medical treatment, any subsequent hospitalizations related to cardiac events, and any future cardiac diagnostic or treatment procedures. For patients managed medically, costs include those of any surgery that may be required at a later date, as well as the costs of medical management and hospitalizations. The difference in net costs over time between a patient treated initially by surgery and one treated medically is the measure used in our cost-effectiveness analysis.

Both health benefits and costs are discounted (at 5% per annum) to account for the fact that future benefits and costs are subjectively, and in terms of real opportunity costs, less valuable.

The ratio of net costs to net benefits is the measure of cost-effectiveness and is expressed as dollars per year of life or per quality-adjusted year of life. This ratio provides a basis for evaluating the use of CABG in different types of patients and also permits comparison between resources devoted to CABG and those devoted to the treatment of other health problems.

Cost-Effectiveness of CABG and Medical Management

Information for our analysis was taken broadly from the medical literature. This information, though imperfect, provides a reasonable basis for making judgements about the use of CABG in the individual patient and about allocating health care resources to this procedure. As new evidence accumulates, policies based on this analysis can be revised.

Target Population

Our analysis applies to 55-year-old males with stable angina and coronary artery disease which has been considered to be operable on the basis of the patients' clinical characteristics and coronary arteriography results. Criteria include 50% or more obstruction of one, two, or three coronary arteries or the left main coronary artery and good ventricular function as defined by an ejection fraction of at least 40%.

Life Expectancy with Surgical and Medical Management

Operative mortality rates were obtained from the pooled results from major surgical centers, including the European Coronary Surgery Study group (Table 1). Operative mortality rates from the VA Cooperative Study performed in the early 1970s are presented for their historical interest.

Table 1. Operative mortality for coronary artery bypass surgery

	1 VD	2 VD	3 VD	LMD
Pooled studies	1.0%	1.5%	2.0%	3.0%
VA cooperative study	2.8%	3.4%	4.0%	6.0%

1 VD, one-vessel disease; *2 VD*, two-vessel disease; *3 VD*, three-vessel disease; *LMD*, left main disease

Pooled results of survival after surgery and with medical management were derived from the Veterans' Administration and European trials, from nonrandomized studies represented by the Duke and Seattle data banks, and from several other surgical series (Table 2). The recently reported Coronary Artery Surgery Study (CASS 1983) results are shown for comparative purposes. All surgical results exclude operative mortality.

Annual mortality rates from pooled studies were converted to life expectancies by assuming that the mortality rates for medical and surgical treatment were identical after 6 years and corresponded to those obtained from U.S. life tables for males of the same age. Estimated life expectancies are shown in Table 3. For one-vessel disease, survival on medical management is better than that on surgical treatment, while for other disease levels surgical results are better.

Table 2. Annual mortality rates for coronary artery bypass surgery excluding operative mortality

	1 VD[a]	2 VD	3 VD	LMD
Pooled studies				
Surgical	1.3%	1.6%	1.4%	2.0%
Medical	1.3%	2.4%	4.9%	10.5%
Coronary artery surgery study (CASS)[b]				
Surgical	0.4%	0.7%	1.8%	-
Medical	1.4%	1.2%	2.1%	-

[a] For definitions of 1 VD, 2 VD, 3 VD, and LMD, see Table 1
[b] 5-year follow-up data. Assumes that the average operative mortality of 1.4% was independent of the number of coronary arteries with 70% or greater stenosis

Table 3. Estimated life expectancies in years for surgical and medical management from pooled study results

Treatment	1 VD[a]	2 VD	3 VD	LMD
Surgical	20.7	20.3	20.4	19.5
Medical	20.9	19.7	17.2	12.6
Difference	−0.2	+0.6	+3.2	+6.9

[a] For definitions of 1 VD, 2 VD, 3 VD, and LMD, see Table 1

Quality-Adjusted Life Expectancy with Surgery and Medical Management

Few would argue that the quality of life is better without angina pectoris than with it. How much better will depend upon the severity of the angina, its psychological effects, and the preferred life-style of the individual. For many patients, in fact, the superior ability of CABG to relieve angina is the principal reason for the procedure.

We use information on the relative success of surgical and medical management in relieving angina pectoris and rely upon the concepts of preference theory to obtain a range of estimates for benefits related to improved quality of life after surgery. Our time-tradeoff approach seeks a balance between a number of years with angina and some fraction, Q, of those years that a patient would accept to be free of angina (Fig. 1). In the absence of empirical data, we assume that a patient who is severely burdened by angina would be willing to trade 10 years with his symptoms for 7 years with no symptoms. Hence, the Q factor is 0.7. Similarly, for a patient with mild angina, we assume a Q of 0.9. Combining these weights with the demonstrated evidence of surgery's superiority in relieving symptoms, we adjust the life expectancies shown in Table 3 to obtain comparisons between surgical and medical treatment on quality-adjusted life expectancy (Table 4). These figures assume severe angina and a Q of 0.7. When severe symptoms are present, surgical treatment becomes preferable

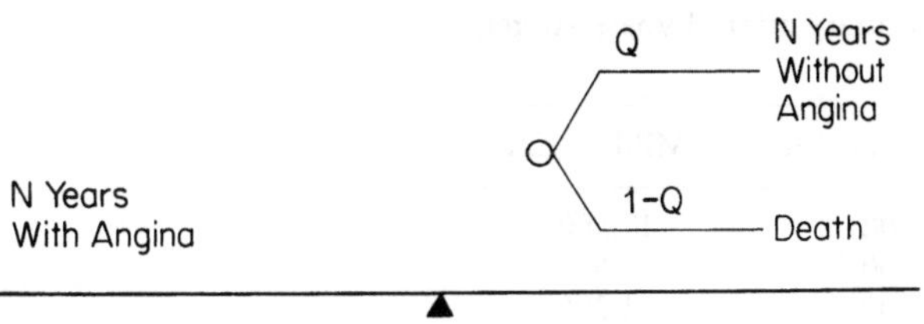

Fig. 1. Time-tradeoff approach to valuing the effects of angina on the quality of life

Table 4. Estimated quality-adjusted life expectancies in years for surgical and medical management in patients with severe angina (*Q*, 0.7)

Treatment	1 VD[a]	2 VD	3 VD	LMD
Surgical	17.1	16.8	16.9	16.2
Medical	16.6	15.7	13.7	10.0
Difference	+0.5	+1.1	+3.2	+6.2

[a] For definitions of 1 VD, 2 VD, 3 VD, and LMD, see Table 1

to medical treatment, even for one-vessel disease and more strikingly so for two-vessel disease. Results are not appreciably affected for three-vessel or left main disease because of the predominant effects of enhanced survival in these patients.

The important point is that symptom relief does need to be factored in to any meaningful risk-benefit evaluation of surgical compared to medical treatment. The weights we apply are arbitrary, though we believe reasonable, but would be individualized to the patient when clinical treatment decisions are actually made.

Costs

Our cost comparison of surgical to medical treatment is shown in Table 5. Prices are in 1981 U.S. dollars. We estimate that the average cost of surgery in 1981 was $ 17,500 and that the average annual costs of medical management were $ 716, $ 343, and $ 170 for patients with severe, mild, or no angina, respectively. The differences in expected lifetime costs of medical management between surgical and medical treatment strategies are about $2,300 for a patient with severe angina and about $ 600 for a patient with mild angina.

Differences in costs due to a lower incidence of acute myocardial infarctions after surgery were estimated from the results of two small randomized trials and a projected unit cost for treating a myocardial infarction and its lifetime sequelae of $ 7,500. These two studies indicated that the average annual rates of myocardial infarction are 4.5% per year for surgery and 6.8% per year for medical management. Using these figures, lifetime cost savings from myo-

Table 5. Net resource costs of coronary artery bypass surgery (in 1981 dollars)

Cost component	Severe angina	Mild angina
Surgery	$ 17,500	$ 17,500
Medical management	−2,300	− 600
Myocardial infarctions	−1,300	−1,300
Subsequent surgery[a]	0	0
Totals	$ 13,900	$ 15,600

[a] Costs of late surgery in medically treated patients and repeat surgery in patients treated initially by surgery are assumed to cancel

cardial infarctions prevented in surgically treated patients are about $ 1,300. Recent results from the European study and CASS, which show no difference in rates of myocardial infarction in medically and surgically treated patients, suggest that these estimates are too favorable to CABG.

Finally, the expected costs of repeated surgery in patients treated initially with CABG and later surgery in the medical group were assumed to be equal and, therefore, to cancel. We include this factor, however, to emphasize the appreciable crossover rate from medical management to surgery, on the one hand, and the fact that the benefits of surgery are not permanent and that subsequent surgery will be necessary in a significant number of patients, on the other.

Summing up components, we estimate the expected net resource costs of surgical treatment to be $ 13,900 for patients with severe angina and $ 15,600 for patients with mild angina. The higher figure for patients who present mild angina reflects the decreased savings realized in the costs of medical management.

Cost-Effectiveness

The ratio of the differences in net costs to the difference in quality-adjusted life years between surgical and medical management becomes the cost-effectiveness ratio. The lower the ratio, the more attractive is surgery as a use of medical resources. Our results for 55-year-old males with severe angina are shown in Fig. 2. The cost per year of quality-adjusted life expectancy ranges from $ 30,000 for patients with one-vessel disease to $ 3,800 for those with left main disease. Patients with two-vessel disease and three-vessel disease have intermediate values of $ 17,500 and $ 7,200 per quality-adjusted life year respectively.

A sensitivity analysis in which the quality of life factor, Q, varies is shown in Fig. 3. Most important is the dramatic increase in the cost-effectiveness ratio in patients with one-vessel disease and mild angina to $ 470,000 per quality-adjusted life year. The ratio, in fact, becomes undefined in one-vessel disease and no symptoms. Similarly, surgical treatment of two-vessel disease becomes

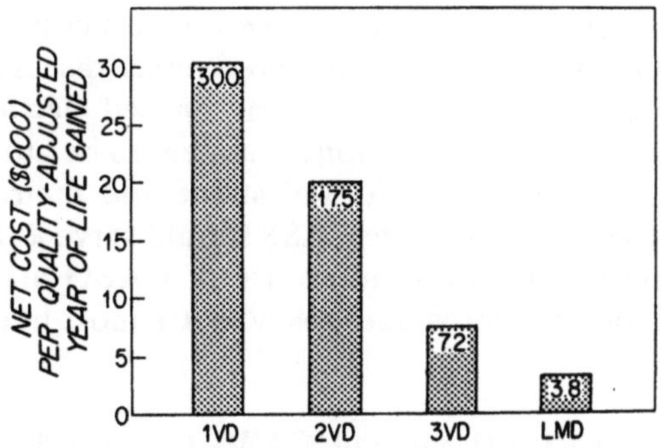

Fig. 2. Cost-effectiveness of CABG in relation to medical management for 55-year-old males with severe angina (Q, 0.7)

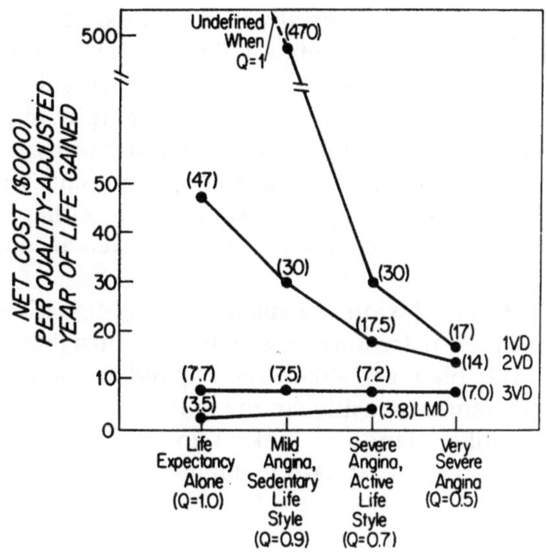

Fig. 3. Cost-effectiveness of CABG as a function of the perceived severity of angina

much less attractive if the symptoms are mild or nonexistent. For patients with three-vessel disease or left main disease, the results are only minimally affected by the weight assigned to symptoms. The value attached to relief of symptoms is absolutely critical in patients with one- or two-vessel disease from the point of view of the cost-effectiveness of treatment.

Insights from the Coronary Artery Surgery Study (CASS 1983) shed important new light on the effectiveness of CABG and on its cost-effectiveness in patients with mild stable angina.

The essential findings of this study are the extremely low mortality in the medically treated group (annual mortality 1.6% compared with 3.3% in the European study) and the fact that differences in annual mortality between the surgically and medically treated groups were confined to patients with left ventricular ejection fractions of less than 50%. Essentially no differences in survival were noted in patients with ejection fractions above 50%.

Using these results, we estimate a cost-effectiveness ratio of $ 77,500 per life-year for patients with three-vessel disease but normal ejection fractions and $ 5,000 for those with compromised ejection fractions. Patients with three-vessel disease thus no longer appear to be attractive candidates for surgery if their symptoms are mild and stable and their left ventricular function is normal. These results of the CASS should serve as an impetus for us to reevaluate criteria for the appropriate use of CABG and to increase our efforts to identify those patient subgroups who are most likely to benefit.

Cost-Effectiveness of CABG Compared with Other Medical Treatments

CABG appears to be a relatively cost-effective use of resources in patients with severe angina, especially if three-vessel disease or left main disease is present. These results are comparable to those obtained for the treatment of hypertension and better than for the vigorous pursuit of the diagnosis of CAD with non-invasive tests and coronary arteriography in patients who have atypical symptoms or are asymptomatic. In the case of hypertension, the cost-effectiveness of treatment is relatively favorable in patients with severe hypertension, less so in those with mild hypertension and, in either case, is severely compromised by the failures in compliance that so often accompany treatment of a chronic disease.

In conclusion, we suggest that systematic analysis of the costs and benefits of medical treatments can provide insights of importance to physicians and health planners alike. The expanded use of these techniques, particularly if they remain sensitive to the real needs of patients, physicians, and policy makers alike, stands to make important contributions to our efforts to contain health care costs while maintaining and enhancing the quality of patient care.

References

1. Weinstein MC, Stason WB (1982) Cost-effectiveness of coronary artery bypass surgery. Circulation 66:III56–III66
2. CASS Principal Investigators and their associates (1983) Coronary artery surgery study (CASS): a randomized trial of coronary artery bypass surgery. Survival data. Circulation 68:939–950

Cost-Effectiveness in Coronary Artery Surgery: In Relation to the Gross National Product

F. Unger

Introduction

General health care in Europe has been hit by an explosion of costs which has begun to be critical in view of the large state deficits. As a consequence it is necessary to evaluate different forms of therapy in regard to their outcome and costs. This will have an impact on quality control too.

Before examining the effectiveness of coronary artery surgery, we must be aware that everybody has a right to adequate medical treatment and good health in their old age [1].

Coronary artery surgery has developed drastically within the past 7 years. The last WHO report shows an incidence of coronary artery bypasses in the USA of 396 operations per million population; today this incidence has increased to almost 1000 per million. In comparison, in West Germany the increase has been from 20 to 200 operated patients per million population. Due to the positive outcome of coronary artery surgery, waiting lists are growing rapidly, though they, might be reduced with new cardiac surgery centers.

In medicine, a cost-benefit analysis is per definitionem not possible. A strict cost-benefit analysis implies that the evaluated objects can be assessed in monetary terms. In medicine, the cost of a form of therapeutic management can be calculated, but the benefit cannot be assessed in the same way; rather it is expressed in the improvement in the quality of life: It is nevertheless the aim of this study to quantify to what extent the costs justify the effective results.

The results in coronary artery surgery are very impressive in terms of the excellent relief of pain and the fact that patients with lesions of the left main coronary artery have an increased life expectancy [4–6]. The improved quality of life allows us to calculate the cost-effectiveness of coronary artery surgery, for healthy people earn and spend money, contributing toward the gross national product (GNP).

Coronary artery surgery is a means through which relief of pain and improvement in the quality of life can be achieved dramatically with minor complications and risks (Table 1), [4, 5, 6]. Thus the operative mortality is 0.74%, the incidence of perioperative myocardial infarction is 5%, patent grafts occur in 86%, relief of pain occurs in 90%, and the rate of reoperation is only 1%.

Table 1. Risks and benefits in coronary artery surgery

Risks	Rahimtoola	Own experience
Operative mortality	0.6–3%	0.74%
Perioperative myocardial infarction	≧10%	5%
Vein graft occlusion	15%	14%
No patent grafts	12%	6%
No relief of pain	15%	10%
Relief not longlasting	15%	4%
Reoperation	8%	1%

Benefits	
LM - CAD	Prolongs life
CAD	Better symptomatic relief of pain than medical therapy; life prolongation possible, depending on the degree of CAD

Costs

In a cost-effectiveness analysis both fixed costs and variable costs must be considered. For this calculation, the costs have been evaluated which would exist in a unit dealing with 300 patients per year.

Fixed Costs

The fixed costs (A1) are: the extracorporeal circulation laboratory analysis, X-rays, physical therapy, medication, blood, and food. These costs vary somewhat from country to country and are estimated at ÖS 40000.

Variable Costs

The variable costs (A2) consist mainly in personnel costs, maintenance costs, investment funds, and documentation. The variable costs decrease directly with the quantity of operations, and the relative load per patient decreases (Fig. 1). At a rate of 100 patients/year, the variable costs are ÖS 80000 (0.6% of the total annual costs, 40% of a mean annual income). At a rate of 300 patients/year, the variable costs decrease to ÖS 26666 (0.3% of the total annual costs, or 22% of a mean income (Table 2).

Patients

The effectiveness of an operation is given when the patient can walk and spend or earn money after the operation. This implies that every surviving patient participates in the gross national product. The nature of this participation depends, of course, on his professional status. There is a big difference between employed patients and patients who are self-employed or employers. For our calculation, the mean annual income is based on ÖS 300000 for employed people.

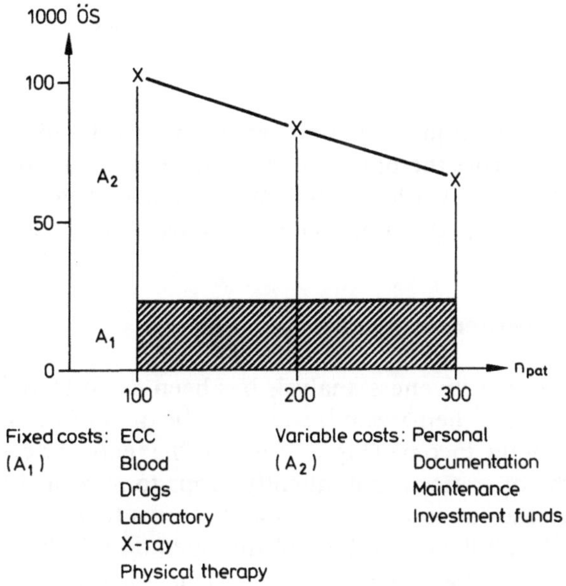

Fig. 1. Decrease in variable costs according to number of patients (*shaded area,* fixed costs)

Table 2. Fixed and variable costs for 100 and 300 patients

(A_1)	Fixed costs:	ÖS 40000	(0.2% of TC)	
(A_2)	Variable costs:			
	for 100 patients/year	ÖS 80000	(0.4% of TC)	
	for 300 patients/year	ÖS 26666	(0.2% of TC)	
Total	(A_1+A_2)		MI	TC
	100 patients/year	ÖS 120000	40%	0.6%
	300 patients/year	ÖS 66666	22%	0.3%

Abbreviations: MI, mean annual income; TC, total annual costs

Among our patients three groups were to be observed (Fig. 2):

Group A represents patients (29%) who had retired at the time of the operation.

Group B represents patients who were working at the time of the operation (43%) and remained so afterwards.

Group C represents patients (28%) who retired after their operation, having been working beforehand.

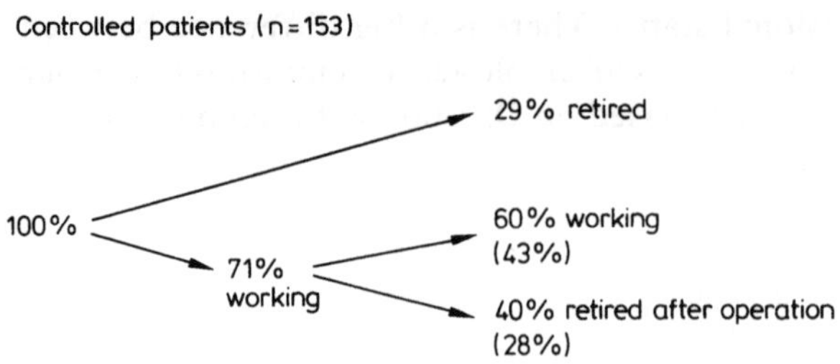

Fig. 2. Working status before and after operation

Examination of the numbers in groups B and C shows that 60% of those working before the operation continued to do so afterwards, while 40% retired. The reason why a lot of patients retire is that most of them are aged over 60 years and the prevailing socioecconomic policy makes retirement easy.

Effectiveness Analysis

The effectiveness analysis has been performed for patients who are employed, because their mean income can be quantified. In an employed patient with an average income (Fig. 3, Table 3) the income decreases on average 1 year before the operation, subsequently drops to 30% of the original income, and then increases as soon as the patient returns to work. The cost curve shows a peak of ÖS 120000 at the time of the operation (Table 4).

Is a patient–entrepreneur (Fig. 4), income drops more drastically. Before the operation, the estimated curve drops to below 0 and usually recovers 3 months postoperatively to a higher level than before the operation. The peak of the costs is the same, at ÖS 120000.

A nonoperated patient who has the same pain experiences the same reduction in his income, which drops within 5 years to 66% of his original income, the costs of treatment increasing to ÖS 100000 (Fig. 5). The cost curve increases especially significantly if the patient suffers a myocardial infaction in the meantime (Table 5).

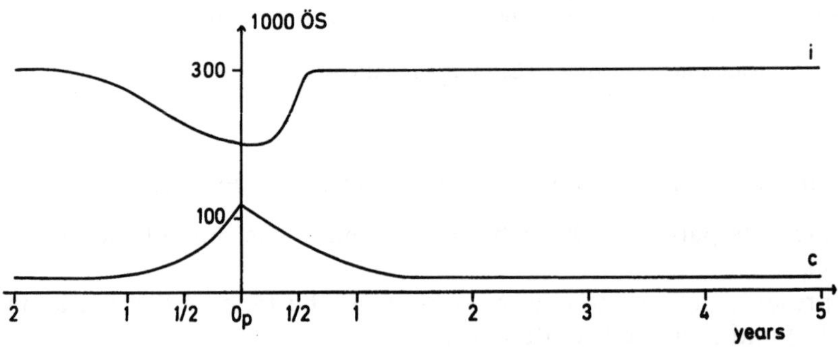

Fig. 3. Cost *(c)* and income *(i)* curves for an employed patient with optimal outcome after coronary artery bypass surgery

Table 3. Income (i) of an operated and a nonoperated patient

$$\sum i = i_0 + i_1 + i_2 + i_3 + i_4 + i_5 \qquad (1)$$

$\sum i$ for an operated patient

$$= \begin{pmatrix} 300 + 300 + 300 + 300 + 300 + 300 \\ \quad\; 24 \quad\; 48 \quad\; 72 \quad\; 96 \quad 120 \end{pmatrix} \cdot \underset{\text{interest}}{1000}$$

$$\sum i_{op} = 2.16 \text{ mill. ÖS}$$

$$n = 1$$

$\sum i$ for a nonoperated patient

$$= \begin{pmatrix} 250 + 240 + 230 + 220 + 210 + 200 \\ \quad\; 19 \quad\; 36 \quad\; 52 \quad\; 67 \quad\; 80 \end{pmatrix} \cdot \underset{\text{interest}}{1000}$$

$$\sum i_{nop} = 1.604 \text{ mill. ÖS}$$

$$n = 1$$

$$\sum i = \sum i_{op} - \sum i_{nop}$$

$$= \mathit{0.556 \text{ mill. ÖS/patient}}$$

Table 4. Cost (c) of an operated and a nonoperated patient

$$\sum c = c_o + c_i + c_2 + c_3 + c_4 + c_5 \qquad (2)$$

$\sum$ operated patients ($\sum c_o$)

$$= \begin{pmatrix} 120 + 50 + 40 + 20 + 20 + 20 \\ \quad\; 4 \quad\; 6 \quad\; 5 \quad\; 6 \quad\; 8 \end{pmatrix} \cdot \underset{\text{interest}}{1000}$$

$$\sum c_o = 270\,000 \text{ ÖS}$$

$$n = 1$$

$\sum$ nonoperated patients ($\sum c_{nop}$)

$$= \begin{pmatrix} 50 + 60 + 70 + 80 + 90 + 100 \\ \quad\; 5 \quad\; 11 \quad\; 19 \quad\; 28 \quad\; 40 \end{pmatrix} \cdot \underset{\text{interest}}{1000}$$

$$\sum c_{nop} = 450\,000 \text{ ÖS}$$

$$n = 1$$

Table 5. Cost of a nonoperated patient with a myocardial infarction

$$\sum c_{nop} = \begin{pmatrix} 100 + 50 + 40 + 30 + 20 + 20 \\ \quad\; 4 \quad\; 6 \quad\; 5 \quad\; 6 \quad\; 8 \end{pmatrix} \cdot \underset{\text{interest}}{1000}$$

$$\sum c_{nop} = 917\,000 \text{ ÖS}$$

$$n = 1$$

$$\sum c = \sum c_{nop} - \sum c_{op} = 180\,000 \text{ ÖS} \quad \text{(Var. I)}$$

$$= 647\,000 \text{ ÖS} \quad \text{(Var. II)}$$

$$n = 1$$

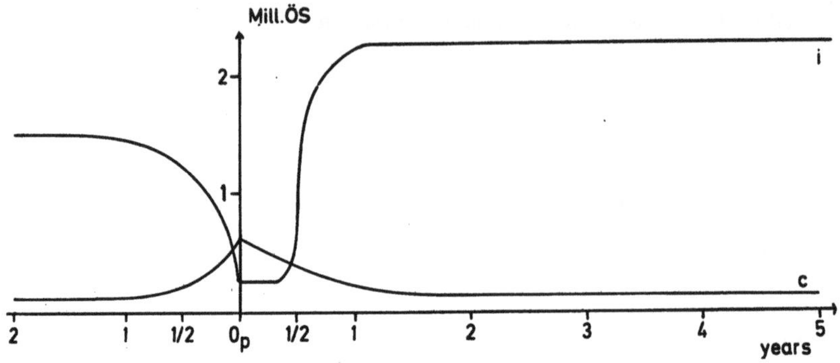

Fig. 4. Cost *(c)* and income *(i)* curves for an entrepreneur with optimal outcome after coronary artery bypass surgery

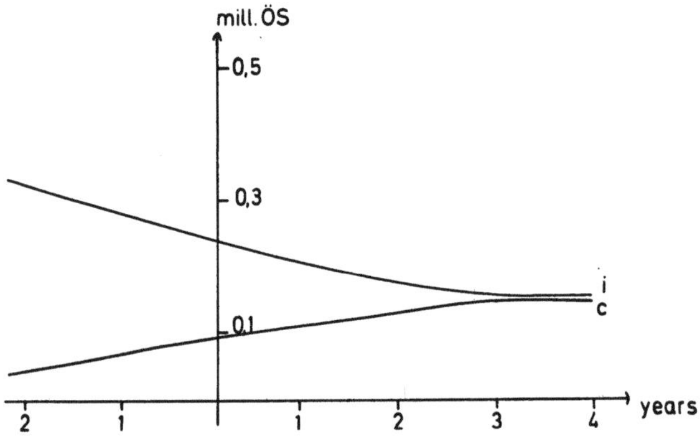

Fig. 5. Cost *(c)* and income *(i)* curves for a nonoperated employed patient

It is easier to calculate cost-effectiveness on 300 operated patients and 300 nonoperated patients (Fig. 6). Two years preoperatively the income will be ÖS 90 millions for the 300 operated patients; it falls to 60 millions at the time of operation and will recover to 90 millions 6 months postoperatively. The total costs are ÖS 20 millions for the operation, and they later costs fall to ÖS 6 millions per year.

In nonoperated patients, the income drops from ÖS 90 millions to ÖS 60 millions, while the costs rise to ÖS 100 millions.

Now we have to calculate the total income. This is done according to formula (1) in Table 3. Adding the annual income for the first five postoperative years and allowing for an 8% interest rate over this period, the total income for the 300 operated patients is ÖS 648 millions while for the nonoperated patients it is ÖS 481 millions. According to this calculation, the effective difference in income will be ÖS 167 millions.

In the group of 300 operated patients there are total costs of ÖS 81 millions. In the 300 nonoperated patients there are two groups: one group costs ÖS 135

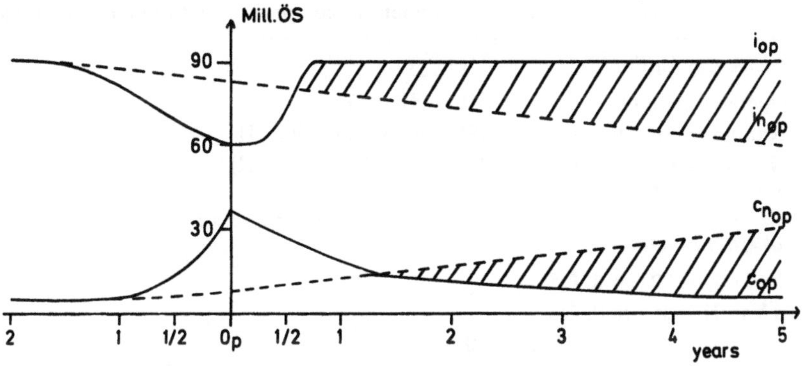

Fig. 6. Costs and income curves for 300 operated and 300 nonoperated patients

Table 6. Total income and costs in operated and nonoperated patients

	Operated patients ($n=300$)	Nonoperated patients ($n=300$)	$\Delta = \sum op - \sum nop$		
$\sum i =$	648	481	Δi	167	Mill. ÖS
$\sum c =$	81	135	Δc	54	Var. I
		275	Δc	194	Var. II
GNP					
$(\sum i - \sum c)$	567	346		*221*	Var. I
		206		*361*	Var. II

millions (Var. I), while the second group, comprising patients who have had a myocardial infarction, costs ÖS 275 millions (Table 6).

Conclusion

On the basis of the above data it can be demonstrated that the patients who are operated on produce less total costs than nonoperated patients. As a matter of principle everybody has the right to grow old in good health, and coronary artery surgery contributes to an improvement in this respect. Moreover an operated patient contributes actively toward the GNP.

The net benefit (income minus costs) is ÖS 567 millions in the operated group and ÖS 346 millions in the nonoperated group (Var. I). In the event of a myocardial infarction it will be ÖS 206 millions. The difference is ÖS 221 millions in Var. I and ÖS 361 millions in Var. II (Table 7). These sums of money will be lost in the case of the 300 patients who are not operated on.

The conclusion of this study is that the effectiveness of surgery can be expressed by quantifying of the costs which will be incurred if the patient is not

Table 7. Effectiveness of surgical treatment in comparison with medical therapy

Effectiveness (mill. ÖS)	$= \sum i - \sum c$	
Operated patients	$= 648 - 81 = 567$	
Nonoperated patients	$= 481 - 135 = 346$	(Var. I)
Nonoperated patients with myocardial infarction	$= 481 - 275 = 206$	(Var. II)
Real effectiveness		
Δ Var. I = 221 mill. ÖS		
Δ Var. II = 361 mill. ÖS		
	$n = 600$	

operated on. A single nonoperated patient produces costs which, according to this calculation, would cover 9–18 operations. Long-term studies show the benefits of coronary artery surgery, and from the viewpoint of the GNP, coronary artery surgery is superior to medical therapy.

Acknowledgment. This work was supported by the Austrian Research Council, Project No. P5186 (Principal Investigator F. Unger) and by the Austrian National Bank, Project No. 2341.

References

1. OECD (1973) List of social concerns common to most OECD countries. The OECD social indicator development program, Vol 1, Paris, p 14
2. WHO - Regional Office for Europe (1978) The long-term effects of coronary bypass surgery, Copenhagen 1978, ICP/CVD 003(8). World Health Organization (WHO), Geneva
3. Hesse H (1980) Nutzen-Kosten Analyse I: Theorie, Handwörterbuch der Wirtschaftswissenschaft (HdWW) Vol 5. Fischer, Stuttgart, p 361 (also published by J.C.B. Mohr (Paul Siebeck), Tübingen and Vandenhoeck & Ruprechts, Göttingen und Zürich)
4. Arnold V (1980) Nutzen-Kosten Analyse II: Anwendung, Handwörterbuch der Wirtschaftswissenschaft (HdWW) Vol 5. Fischer, Stuttgart, p 382
5. CASS (1983) Coronary Artery Study (CASS): A randomized trial of coronary artery bypass surgery: Survival data. Circulation 68:939
6. CASS (1983) Coronary Artery Study (CASS): A randomized trial of coronary artery bypass surgery: Quality of life in patients randomly assigned to treatment groups. Circulation 68:951
7. Chaitman BR et.al (1983) A life table and Cox regression analysis of patients with combined proximal left anterior descending and proximal left circumflex coronary artery disease: non left main equivalent lesions (CASS). Circulation 68:1163

The Contribution of Social Medicine to the Cost-Benefit Analysis of Coronary Bypass Surgery

H. Silomon

The tasks of medicine and of social insurance stand in a complementary relationship to one another. On the one hand, the benefits of medicine cannot be realized without taking appropriate legislative steps to make them available through social insurance. On the other hand, social insurance cannot keep the citizen in good health or restore his health without the help of medicine. This "steady-state" between medicine and social insurance is the result of a historical process, which has now entered a difficult phase.

The process of therapeutic and rehabilitative innovations in medicine has become so costly, due to the extensive involvement of technical resources and recruitment of manpower, that the financing of these innovations through social insurance will be problematic in the long run. The financial resources available are increasing in absolute terms, but declining in relation to the increasing demand.

At the same time, the capability of medicine to successfully master critical episodes in the clinical course of diseases, to provide relief for patients with chronic illnesses, and even to enable their rehabilitation has expanded on an unforeseeable scale. The labor market, however, is developing in the opposite direction: There is only demand for those who are not only fully and successfully rehabilitated in medical terms but who in addition are completely able-bodied and willing to work. The primary goal of rehabilitation is at least partly called into question by the fact that the employment market is not capable of absorbing the medically rehabilitated to the necessary degree [3, 5].

It is not surprising that at this point in time two instruments of measurement are becoming increasingly important: in medicine it is validity, in social insurance, cost-benefit analysis.

Even in the judgement of uncritical observers, the costs of medicine in relation to its benefits are too high. But luckily one could claim that for methodological reasons it is not possible to give a global estimation of its cost [9] and that its benefit can only be judged in part by means of so-called health indicators. On the other hand, it is possible in principle to make a critical analysis of single preventive, curative, and rehabilitative measures and strategies [6, 8] – for example, of rehabilitation after myocardial infarction.

From my understanding, the most important instruments on whose validity the success of coronary surgery as a part of the rehabilitation after myocardial infarction depends would be those which provide a basis for deciding whether or not the operation is indicated. The smaller the chances of an unsuccessful outcome, the greater the validity would be; in other words, the validity is governed by those cases that show too little improvement in regard to efficiency and by the rates of reinfarction and restenosis. Furthermore, it is those patients in whom an increase or decrease in productivity can be ascertained at the end of medical rehabilitation, on whom the success of social and economic rehabilitation depends.

It is self evident that the degree of validity of the individual methods will find its expression in the final result, which cost-benefit analysis shows. By cost-benefit analysis we mean investigations about the cost of a health measure in relation to its benefit [10]. Such calculations are difficult (a) because the total estimation of cost is not possible owing to delimitation difficulties, (b) because apart from financial costs other resources have to be taken into account as well, (c) because parameters and indicators by which benefit can be estimated are problematic, and (d) last but not least, because a benefit can also be gained which is of an unsubstantial character and cannot be operationalized.

Below I briefly present and discuss some data, in view of their properties and suitability as factors in the evaluation of the efficiency of coronary bypass surgery. Their usefulness and predictive value are influenced by the quality and purpose of the documentation from which they are taken as well as by the regulations controlling access to information.

To anticipate possible objections: No normal values are known with which these data can be correlated; at best we have are actual norms. The criterion "improvement" will probably be assessed variously by different clinics, and most likely in a broad rather than a narrow sense. There remains a lot of doubt whether those patients who have been successfully treated have also been successfully rehabilitated professionally, i.e., that they have not only made an improvement and regained their earning capacity in abstract terms, but that they actually earn their own living. A factor which cannot be operationalized and taken into account in a cost-benefit analysis is the relief of physical complaints.

Nevertheless, political decisions in the field of health will depend on the results of cost-benefit analyses, which has to be made against the background of the oft-quoted paradigmatic change taking place in medicine, i.e., more prevention, less therapy, and less rehabilitation. One decision that will have to be made is whether to build more cardiac centers or to spend more money on research funds for the prevention of coronary heart disease [1, 2, 4, 7].

The results of cardiac rehabilitation are much better in white-collar workers than in blue-collar workers, because more white-collar workers are able to continue with their professional activities shortly after coronary surgery (Table 1). Promoting vocational rehabilitation measures proved more essential than providing further medical treatment, and more so for in blue-collar than for white-collar workers.

In summary, after coronary bypass surgery on white-collar workers good results in terms of rehabilitation are achieved in less time, with less effort, and at a lower cost. Perhaps nonsurgical factors are even more important in blue-collar workers than are surgical problems. This should be taken into consideration when considering surgical procedures.

Table 1

	1982 ($n = 1267$)		1983 ($n = 1709$)	
	Blue-collar workers	White-collar workers	Blue-collar workers	White-collar workers
	62.8%	37.2%	17.3%	82.7%
Continuiation of previous occupation	48.1%	77.3%	17.3%	63.8%
No earning capacity	14.8%	16.4%	12.1%	25.2%
Further medical rehabilitation	12.4%	6.0%	11.1%	6.1%
Promotion of vocational rehabilitation	24.7%	2.0%	36.5%	0.21%
Potentially employable	26.7%	41.7%	22.8%	31.5%
Disabled	73.3%	58.3%	77.2%	68.5%

Source: statistics of the *Verband Deutscher Versicherungsträger* (German Association of Pension Insurance Funds)

In the above discussion, I have been dealing with decisions in health policy. In democracies, decisions regarding the raising, allocation, and use of public monies as health care resources are made by political bodies. In this sense, these decisions are political; nevertheless, they should not be reached on the basis of political ideology but rather, by examining data and information gained through investigations in the field of social medicine, as outlined here. Such investigations can form a platform for rational and verifiable conclusions and decisions.

References

1. Mc Keown T (1982) Die Bedeutung der Medizin. Suhrkamp, Frankfurt
2. Kuhn TS (1981) Die strukturwissenschaftlichen Revolutionen, 5. Aufl. Suhrkamp, Frankfurt
3. Silomon H (ed) (1980) Herzinfarktrehabilitation - Licht und Schatten. Hippokrates, Stuttgart
4. Silomon H (1983) Ökonomischer Exkurs. In: Silomon H (ed) Technologie in der Medizin - Folgen und Probleme. Hippokrates, Stuttgart, pp 33-39
5. Silomon H (1984) Der medizinische Sachverständige in der Sozialversicherung. Med Sachverständige 80:9-11
6. Schach E (1983) Technologie im Gesundheitswesen - einige empirisch-ökonomische Überlegungen. In: Silomon H (ed) Technologie in der Medizin - Folgen und Probleme. Hippokrates, Stuttgart, pp 152-173
7. Schaefer H (1979) Plädoyer für eine neue Medizin. Piper, München
8. Weißenböck H (1979) Studien zur Effizienz von Gesundheitssystemen. Thieme, Stuttgart
9. Szameitat K (1970) „Was kostet die Gesundheit". Öff Gesundheitswes 32:672-690
10. Thome R, Spencer WA, Wagner G (1975) „Kosten - Nutzen - Analyse". In: Koller S, Wagner G (eds) Handbuch der medizinischen Dokumentation und Datenverarbeitung. Schattauer, Stuttgart, pp 942-952

Summary of the Discussion

W. B. Stason

I would like to summarize the main messages from the economic studies that have been presented here today. For me, the most important message of all is the fact that people, at long last, are measuring costs and are beginning to consider costs in relation to the benefits of various medical treatments. Costs have attracted sufficient attention for physicians, as well as administrators, to try to measure the true resource costs of the treatments that we offer. I want to reemphasize the importance of differentiating between resource costs and charges. In the United States, at least, any relationship between charges and costs may be purely coincidental.

The second message was exemplified beautifully by Dr. Smith in his discussion of PTCA. Namely, we cannot focus only on the cost of an expensive treatment, such as surgery or PTCA, but, rather, we have to look at the continuum of costs for a given patient over a period of time. It is the sum total of costs for health care over 1, 3, or 5 years that is the important quantity from an economic perspective.

Third, we need to distinguish between medical care costs, on the one hand, and economic costs, on the other. One reason to do this is that fact that different costs affect different decision-makers. Medical care costs are of interest primarily to those who either pay for medical care directly or pay for it through insurance. Economic costs, such as lost wages, have very different implications. Both are important.

The main differences between cost-effectiveness analysis, as I presented it today, and Dr. Unger's cost-benefit analysis is that his analysis converts health care benefits into dollars. Though possible, this is difficult. We find it preferable to leave health benefits in terms of years of life, or quality-adjusted years of life; measures with which physicians can more easily identify.

In my view, the cost-effectiveness of PTCA is still not known. One major issue is whether PTCA will substitute for coronary bypass surgery or will, in fact, extend the indications for intervention to patients who are less severely ill and are presently treated medically. The overall cost for care of coronary artery disease will almost certainly increase if the latter occurs. We will need to confront this question as we attempt to assess the cost-effectiveness of PTCA.

Finally, I would like to argue that a cost-effectiveness analysis is not really that different, in the message it conveys, from the risk-benefit analysis with which physicians are so familiar. In our study there is very strong parallelism between cost-effectiveness results and risk-benefit results. The advantages of taking costs into account are several, not the least of which is the increasing role that we, as physicians, will have to play in influencing policy-makers. Arguments in terms of cost, as well as human benefits, are much more likely to be influential than either alone.

Rehabilitation and Return to Work: Strategies for Improving the Work Status of Patients After Coronary Artery Bypass Surgery

Return to Work After Coronary Bypass Surgery: Problems and Prospects*

N. K. Wenger, D. Almeida, J. M. Bradford, S. B. King, and J. W. Hurst

Coronary bypass surgery relieves angina pectoris and improves function in many patients with atherosclerotic coronary heart disease. However, the correlation of symptomatic and functional improvement with the return to work and the resumption of preillness life-style is poor. Between 51% and 74% of patients who recover from coronary bypass surgery are reported to return to work postoperatively, but a significant number of patients are described to have an impaired psychosocial adjustment. Nonmedical as well as medical variables have been reported to be important determinants of whether or not patients return to work [2–4].

This study was designed to assess the return to work of 2284 patients who had coronary bypass surgery at Emory University Hospital between June 1977 and June 1980; these patients were either working at the time of surgery or had discontinued work because of cardiac symptoms. Demographic data, symptoms, work and income status before and after surgery, and so forth were assessed by a mail-in questionnaire. The responses were correlated with the patients' clinical and hemodynamic data as recorded in the Emory Cardiovascular Data Bank.

Seventy percent of the patients responded to the mail questionnaire with adequate usable information, and data on these 1602 patients provide the basis for this report. The patients ranged in age from 29 to 64 years, with a mean of 53 years; 90% of the patients were male, 83% were white, and 92% were married. Occupational characteristics are listed in Table 1.

Table 1. Demographic characteristics (no. of patients = 1602)

Characteristic	Percent
Occupational status	
Professional	19
Executive/administrative	29
Clerical/sales	14
Self-employed	16
Military	0.1
Civil servant	2
Skilled	10
Semiskilled	9

* Adapted with permission of the authors and the editors of Circulation

Of the patients, 46%, 42%, 9%, and 3% had, respectively no, one, two, or three or more prior myocardial infarctions (Table 2). 23%, 32%, 36%, and 10% of the patients respectively had significant single, double, triple, and left main coronary artery disease at coronary angiography. The myocardial contractility was assessed as normal in 63% (Table 3).

Table 2. Prior myocardial infarction, NYHA functional class, and history of congestive heart failure ($n = 1602$)

Characteristic	Percent
Prior myocardial infarction	
0	46
1	42
2	9
3 or more	3
NYHA functional class	
I	55
II	27
III	13
IV	5
History of congestive heart failure	
Yes	5
No	95

Table 3. Coronary artery disease, myocardial contractility, and ejection fraction ($n = 1602$)

Characteristic	Percent
Coronary artery disease	
Single	23
Double	32
Triple	36
Left main	10
Myocardial contractility	
Normal	63
Abnormal	37
Ejection fraction	
50% or less	31
>50%	69
35% or less	4
>35%	96

Myocardial revascularization was considered complete in 76%. 70% of patients described no chest pain at follow-up after surgery. Of the 30% who continued to have chest pain, 80% described symptomatic improvement (Table 4). 51% of the patients were taking propranolol at the time of follow-up. The duration of follow-up ranged from 10 to 56 months, with a mean of 32 months.

Table 4. Myocardial revascularization and chest pain at follow-up ($n = 1602$)

Characteristic	Percent
Myocardial revascularization	
Complete	76
Incomplete	24
Chest pain at follow-up	
None	70
Less pain	24
Same or more pain	6

Of the patients, 66% were working prior to surgery; 34% had stopped work because of cardiac symptoms. 66% of these patients returned to work following surgery, with 70% of those working postoperatively returning to the same job (Table 5). 92% of the patients returning to work held full-time jobs. 91%, 69%, and 62% of the patients respectively were working at 6, 24, and greater than 36 months of follow-up after surgery (Table 6). 58% of patients characterized their jobs as having minimal or light activity; 34% and 9% respectively described moderate and heavy work activities (Table 7). Thus, the majority of our patients returned to the same job and held full-time jobs; over more than half had jobs demanding only minimal or light physical work.

Table 5. Working status before and after surgery ($n = 1602$)

Characteristic	Percent
Working prior to surgery	
Yes	66
No	34
Return to work following surgery	
Yes	66
No	34
Return to same job	
Yes	70
No	30

Of the patients, 32%, 45%, and 23% respectively described their financial status as less, the same, or more satisfactory than preoperatively (Table 7).

The variables which influenced the postoperative return to work were, in order of importance: (1) absence of chest pain at follow-up, (2) working preoperatively, (3) younger age, (4) fewer jobs held before surgery, (5) higher educational level, (7) male sex, (7) completeness of myocardial revascularization, (8) not taking propranolol postoperatively, (9) normal myocardial contractility, and (10) no or fewer preoperative myocardial infarctions. The relative importance of each variable was determined by both discriminant analysis and contingency tables. All of these variables were statistically significant at the 0.05 level or less (Tables 8, 9).

Table 6. Work load and numbers working at follow-up ($n = 1602$)

Characteristic	Percent
Work load of patients working after surgery	
Full-time	92
Part-time	8
Return to same job by work load	
Full-time	70
Part-time	68
Working at time of follow-up after surgery	
6 months	91
24 months	69
>36 months	62

Table 7. Job activity level, job satisfaction, and financial status ($n = 1602$)

Characteristic	Percent
Job activity level	
Minimal or light	58
Moderate	34
Heavy	9
Job satisfaction at follow-up compared with before surgery	
Less	12
Same	54
More	33
Financial status at follow-up compared with before surgery	
Less	32
Same	45
More	23

Absence of chest pain at follow-up after surgery best predicted the return to work. 79% of patients without chest pain returned to work, compared with 36% with chest pain after surgery (Table 8).

The work status prior to surgery was the best nonmedical variable predicting return to work. 80% of patients working preoperatively returned to work, versus 44% who had stopped working preoperatively because of cardiac symp-

Table 8. Most important variables influencing return to work after coronary artery bypass surgery

Variable	Percent return to work	
Chest pain at follow-up		
Absent	79	$P<0.0001$
Present	36	
Work status before surgery		
Working until surgery	80	$P<0.0001$
Stopped working (cardiac symptoms)	44	
Age		
<50	80	$P<0.0001$
≥ 50	61	
Number of jobs before surgery		
One	75	$P<0.0001$
Multiple	60	
Educational level		
Elementary	40	$P<0.0001$
High school	62	
Technical school	66	
College	78	

Table 9. Other variables influencing return to work after coronary artery bypass surgery

Variable	Percent return to work	
Sex		
Male	69	$P<0.0001$
Female	41	
Degree of myocardial revascularization		
Complete	70	$P<0.01$
Incomplete	56	
Taking of propranolol postoperatively		
Yes	60	$P<0.05$
No	72	
Myocardial contractility		
Normal	70	$P<0.01$
Abnormal	59	
Number of prior myocardial infarctions		
None	75	$P<0.0001$
Multiple	59	

toms (Table 8). Patients not working preoperatively for reasons other than their cardiac symptoms were *not* included in this study.

Age was the next best nonmedical predictor, with 80% of patients 50 years or younger returning to work versus 61% of patients older than age 50. The number of jobs held preoperatively was influential; 75% of patients with only one job before surgery returned to work, versus 60% who had multiple jobs preoperatively. Educational level was also a predictor, with return rates of 78%

for college educated, 66% for technical school educated, 62% for high school educated, and 40% for elementary educated patients (Table 8). The patient's sex was also a predictor, with 69% of males and 41% of females returning to work after surgery (Table 9).

Completeness of myocardial revascularization was the second most important medical predictor, although five nonmedical predictors were more important. 70% of the patients with complete revascularization returned to work, as compared with 56% of patients with incomplete revascularization. Even though the taking of propranolol was related to chest pain, it remained a significant predictor of return to work by itself. 72% of patients not taking propranolol postoperatively returned to work, versus 60% of those taking propranolol (Table 9).

Normal myocardial contractility was another predictor, with 70% of patients with normal contractility returning to work, versus 59% without normal contractility. The number of preoperative myocardial infarctions significantly predicted returned to work; 75% of patients without prior infarction returned to work, versus 59% with one or more myocardial infarctions prior to surgery (Table 9).

Of 906 patients who did not consider themselves disabled preoperatively, 86% of the pain-free patients returned to work, versus 59% of those who continued to have chest pain at follow-up. In comparison, of the 640 patients who considered themselves disabled preoperatively, 65% of those subsequently pain-free returned to work, versus 20% of those with residual chest pain at follow-up. Those patients who stopped working preoperatively *because* of their cardiac symptoms returned to work when free of these symptoms, although not in as large a number as those who had not stopped work before surgery (Table 10). Type of work also significantly influenced return to work (Table 11).

Of patients not working postoperatively, 80% reported their income to be less than prior to surgery, whereas among patients working postoperatively

Table 10. Preoperative "disability" and return to work

Variable	Working at follow-up	
	"Disabled" preoperatively (640)	Not disabled preoperatively (906)
Chest pain at follow-up		
Absent	65	86[a]
Present	20	59[a]
Work status before surgery		
Working until surgery	62	82[a]
Stopped working (cardiac symptoms)	45	16[a]
Age		
<50	64	90[a]
≥50	40	76[a]

[a] $P<0.001$

Table 11. Type of work and return to work

Type of work	Percent return to work
Professional	81[a]
Executive/administrative	75[a]
Clerical/sales	61[a]
Self-employed	62[a]
Military	42[a]
Civil service	64[a]
Skilled	62[a]
Semiskilled	34[a]

[a] $P<0.0001$

Table 12. Income at follow-up: percent of patients[a]

	Patients not working postoperatively	Patients working postoperatively
Income at follow-up compared with before surgery		
Less	80	15
Same	15	41
More	6	44
Financial status at follow-up compared with before surgery		
Less	65	16
Same	26	54
More	9	30

[a] $P<0.0001$

only 15% reported that their income level was less than preoperatively. The patient's income and total financial status were comparable. So our patients did *not* appear to stop working because their income or financial status would remain comparable whether or not they worked (Table 12).

A total of 542 patients did not return to work after surgery. "Physician advice" was the most common reason cited. 92% of women and 95% of men who failed to return to work did so for this reason. 52% of patients not working postoperatively reported medical reasons for failure to return to work. No socioeconomic factor reached this level of importance in the patients' opinion. Of the 318 patients who reported being advised by their physician not to return to work, only one patient did not follow this advice and returned to work (Table 13).

Thus patients who failed to resume gainful employment had residual chest pain, a medical variable, as the major determinant of their failure to return to work. However, not working before surgery and older age, nonmedical factors,

Table 13. Reasons for failure to return to work (542 nonworking patients)[a]

Reason	Number of patients	Percent
Physician advice	317	59
Cardiac symptoms	284	52
Adequate pension	124	23
Personal decision	88	16
Work too hard	82	15
Employer would not rehire	28	5
Would lose disability benefits	24	4
Could not find work	15	3
Union problem	1	0.2
Other	124	23

[a] Not mutually exclusive reasons

Table 14. Variables influencing physician advice not to return to work

Characteristic	Percent
Prior myocardial infarction	
0	15%[a]
1	27%[a]
2	48%[a]
3 or more	57%[a]
Working prior to surgery	
Yes	10%[a]
No	36%[a]
Educational level	
Elementary	40%[a]
High school	23%[a]
Technical school	22%[a]
College	11%[a]
Number of jobs before surgery	
One	14%[a]
Multiple	24%[a]

[a] $P<0.0001$

were the second and third major determinants. The other variables predicting failure to return to work included, in order of importance, more jobs held before surgery, lower educational level, female sex, incomplete myocardial revascularization, the taking of propranolol after surgery, abnormal myocardial contractility, and a greater number of prior myocardial infarctions. These demographic features can help identify the patient groups requiring increased attention to rehabilitation [5–10].

The same variables that predicted the failure to return to work were all significant determinants of the physician's advice that the patient should not return to work (Table 14). Therefore, physician attitudes and their specific advice to patients, both preoperatively and postoperatively, regarding return to work at levels appropriate for their functional status, would appear likely to encourage a return to work [11, 12]. This thesis is enhanced by the knowledge that the income and financial status of patients not working after surgery were significantly less satisfactory than among patients who returned to work.

References

1. Almeida D, Bradford JM, Wenger NK, King SB, Hurst JW (1982) Return to work after coronary bypass surgery. Circulation [Suppl II] 66:220
2. Hurst JW, King SB III, Walter PF, Friesinger GC, Edwards JE (1982) Atherosclerotic coronary heart disease: Angina pectoris, myocardial infarction, and other manifestations of myocardial ischemia. In: Hurst JW (ed) The heart, 5th ed. McGraw-Hill, New York, pp 1009–1148
3. National Institutes of Health Consensus-Development Conference Statement (1981) Coronary-artery bypass surgery: Scientific and clinical aspects. N Engl J Med 304:680–684
4. Wenger NK, Hurst JW (1984) Coronary bypass surgery as a rehabilitative procedure. In: Wenger NK, Hellerstein HK (eds) Rehabilitation of the coronary patient, 2nd ed. Wiley, New York, pp 115–132
5. Benesch L, Neuhaus KL, Rivas-Martin J, Loogen F (1979) Clinical results and return to work after coronary heart surgery. In: Roskamm H, Schmuziger M (eds) Coronary heart surgery. Springer, Berlin Heidelberg New York, pp 379–384
6. Anderson AJ, Barboriak JJ, Hoffmann RG, Mullen DC (1980) Retention or resumption of employment after aortocoronary bypass operations. JAMA 243:543–545
7. David P (1979) Contributing factors preventing return to work of cardiac surgery patients. In: Roskamm H, Schmuziger M (eds) Coronary heart surgery. Springer, Berlin Heidelberg New York, pp 370–374
8. Blümchen G, Scharf-Bornhofen E, Brandt D, van den Bergh C, Bierk G (1979) Clinical results and social implications in patients after coronary bypass surgery. In: Roskamm H, Schmuziger M (eds) Coronary heart surgery. Springer, Berlin Heidelberg New York, pp 375–377
9. Johnson WD, Kayser KL, Pedraza PM, Shore RT (1982) Employment patterns in males before and after myocardial revascularization surgery. A study of 2229 consecutive male patients followed for as long as 10 years. Circulation 65:1086–1093
10. Smith HC, Hammes LN, Gupta S, Vlietstra RE, Elveback L (1982) Employment status after coronary artery bypass surgery. Circulation [Suppl II] 65:120–125
11. Oberman A, Wayne JB, Charles ED, Kouchoukos NT (1981) Which of your coronary bypass patients are likely to return to work? J Cardiovasc Med 6:1107–1114
12. Russell RO, Wayne JB, Oberman A, Charles ED, Kouchoukos NT (1981) Return to work after treatment for coronary artery disease: Role of the physician. Primary Cardiol 7:12–23

Can We Improve Work Status After Surgery?

F. Boulay, P. David, N. Danchin, and M. G. Bourassa

It has been shown quite conclusively that coronary artery bypass surgery decreases myocardial ischemia, improves the quality of life, and prolongs survival in selected subsets of patients (National Institutes of Health Consensus-Development Conference Statement 1981; CASS principal investigators and their associates 1983, p 939–950). Surprisingly however, bypass surgery has apparently not succeeded in returning more patients to gainful employment (Oberman et al. 1983; CASS principal investigators and their associates 1983, p 951–960). We investigated the work status of four subgroups of patients who underwent coronary surgery between September 1969 and March 1980. The objectives of these studies were: (1) to determine what percentage of patients return to work after operation; (2) to identify which patient characteristics appear to influence return to work, and (3) to compare the results obtained with and without a postoperative rehabilitation program. This information should enable us to develop policies to improve the percentage of patients returning to work after coronary bypass surgery.

Material and Methods

Follow-up Questionnaires

The pre- and postoperative work status of 1543 patients was investigated by review of their clinical data and follow-up questionnaires in 1973 and 1978. The first survey (David and Juneau 1975) included 326 consecutive male patients (mean age at surgery: 52.7 years) who were operated on between September 1969 and December 1972. The average duration of follow-up was 30 months. In this study, over half of the patients who were not working after surgery were 55 years of age or older. Age was thus considered a detrimental factor for those who were near the usual age of retirement. The second survey (Danchin et al. 1980) therefore included 1217 consecutive male patients, under age 60 at operation (meanage: 49.8 years), who underwent bypass surgery between January 1973 and June 1978. The mean duration of follow-up was 36 months.

Statistical Analyses

In the second series, the follow-up was complete in 96% of the cases. A detailed analysis of 30 clinical and socioeconomic variables was carried out. Nine variables were independently correlated with work status in the univariate analysis. These nine variables were ranked by their order of importance in a multivariate analysis.

Pilot Rehabilitation Program

A pilot rehabilitation program was initiated in 1978, in order to evaluate prospectively the role of psychological, economic, and social factors in influencing the work status of patients and the methods which could lead to their improvement after surgery. Between November 1978 and March 1980, 59 consecutive patients were included in the study prior to coronary bypass surgery. The patients were men, less than 60 years of age, French speaking, living in the greater Montreal area, and inactive for less than 1 year. They had chronic stable angina, underwent bypass grafting without associated surgical procedures, and were free of any condition which could limit or prevent physical rehabilitation.

The following pre- and postoperative evaluation was carried out. A clinical examination was performed preoperatively and 6 weeks, 5 months, and 1 year postoperatively. The functional capacity was evaluated following submaximal stress testing on a bicycle ergometer before and after participation in the physical reconditioning program following surgery. A battery of psychological tests was administered and evaluated by the same psychologist before operation and 5 months and 1 year after operation. A social worker completed structured interviews with the patient at the same time intervals. The anamnesis questionnaire was elaborated by our Social Work Department (Table 1).

On the basis of the preoperative evaluation, a global return to work prognosis was made by the rehabilitation team.

Table 1. Psychological and social evaluation

Psychological tests:

1. The French Canadian Adaptation of the McGill-Melzack Pain Questionnaire (Melzack 1975)
2. The IPAT Anxiety Scale (Cattell and Scheier 1964)
3. The Bortner Rating Scale (Bortner 1969)
4. The Self-Rating Depression Scale (Zung 1975)
5. The IE Scale (Rotter 1975)
6. The MMPI (Welsh and Dahlstrom 1956)
7. The 16 PF Questionnaire (Cattell and Eber 1964)
8. The Rod-and-Fram Test (Witkin 1973)
9. The Visual Retention Test (Benton 1965)

Social tests:

1. The Goldberg's Questionnaire (20 Item Version) (Goldberg 1972)
2. The Personality Self-Perception Questionnaire (Croog 1976)
3. The Social Adjustment Scale (Weissman 1975)
4. The Anamnesis Questionnaire

The rehabilitation program was a team effort. Two physiotherapists took charge of the patients. A schedule of daily exercises was initiated at home during convalescence, with weekly follow-up at the Institute during the first 5 weeks. The reconditioning program was carried out between the 6th and 22nd postoperative weeks in our exercise laboratory. The social follow-up consisted of daily visits during hospitalization and weekly contacts thereafter until the end of the reconditioning program. Then telephone communications were encouraged whenever the patient felt that he needed assistance. Whenever a medical or psychological problem was noted by a member of the team, two cardiologists and a psychologist were available for assistance.

Control Group

Sixty-four patients operated on during the period of our study served as a control group. They were evaluated by a follow-up questionnaire and were not submitted to any form of rehabilitation. These patients met all the criteria for admission to the pilot study but were not included because of lack of communication between the surgeon and the members of the team or because a short preoperative interval did not permit us to carry out the complete battery of psychological and social evaluation tests. The follow-up was complete 1 year after operation in 97% of the patients. Therefore 62 control patients were studied. There was no significant difference in the nine most predictive variables for work status at 1 year between the control group and the group in the pilot study except in the percentage of the work load of the patients, which was heavier in the control group (subjective evaluation by the patient) than in the pilot study (objective evaluation by the multidisciplinary team).

Results

Percentage of Patients Returning to Work After Surgery

The results of the surveys are summarized in Table 2. In the first study, 58% of the patients were working, 11% had worked and quit subsequently, and 31% had never returned to work. Thus 69% of the group had made an attempt to resume work. In the second survey, 66% of the patients were working at 1 year after surgery, 10% had worked and quit, and 24% had never returned to work. Therefore 76% had, at one time or another, returned to work. The yearly work status in the second series showed that 66% of the patients were working at 1 year, 67% at 2 years, 62% at 3 years, 56% at 4 years, and 53% at 5 years. On the other hand, 84% of the patients had been working 1 year before surgery.

Variables Predictive of Work Status After Surgery

In the univariate analysis, nine variables were independently correlated with the work status at 1 year after surgery: age, anginal class, duration of symp-

Table 2. Work status of male patients after coronary artery bypass surgery

	First survey Sept. 69– Dec. 72	Second survey Jan. 73– June 78	Rehabilitation program Nov. 78– March 80	Control group Nov. 78– March 80
Number of patients	326	1217 (under age 60)	59	62
Length of follow-up	Mean: 30 mo.	1 yr	1 yr	1 yr
Working	58%	66%	86%	82%
Worked and quit	11%	10%	6%	7%
Never worked	31%	24%	8%	11%
Percentage returning to work	69%	76%	92%	89%

toms, associated vascular disease, noncardiovascular illness, length of preoperative inactivity, level of education, type of occupation, and total annual income. Taking these variables into account, Table 3 shows the most favorable and unfavorable factors influencing return to work in a given patient. Of these nine independent variables, by far the most influential in the multivariate analysis was the length of preoperative inactivity ($F=166$). Occupational status ($F=52$), noncardiovascular illness ($F=16$), educational level ($F=12$), anginal class ($F=8$), and duration of symptoms ($F=6$) followed in that order.

Results of the Rehabilitation Program

The patients were satisfied with the program in a proportion of 93%. The attendance at the psychosocial sessions was very good. Many patients had to quit the reconditioning program especially when they returned to work. Therefore, the program was followed partially by 69% of the patients and completely by 51%. The results showed that 92% of these 59 patients did return to work and 86% were working 1 year after operation. The profile of the eight patients not working at the end of 1 year is summarized in Table 4. One patient had to quit work because of a medical complication (constrictive pericarditis). Seven of the eight other patients had one to three unfavorable factors for return to work after surgery and six of these seven patients (86%) could be classified as suffering from alcoholism (Feighner 1972) as compared to 24% of the patients who were working at 1 year. The correlation between work status at 1 year and the preoperative psychological and social evaluation was excellent. When one of the two evaluations was found to be excellent, 100% of the patients were working. When both evaluations were good or excellent, 100% of the patients were working at 1 year. The preoperative multidisciplinary team prognosis of return to work was also found to be a valuable element: when the prognosis was good or excellent, 94% were working 1 year after their operation.

Table 3. Variables independently influencing work status after surgery

Variable	Influence on work status					
	Favorable			Unfavorable		
	Factor	Patients *n*	Patients % working	Factor	Patients *n*	Patients % working
Length of preoperative inactivity	≤3 months	506	82	>1 year	173	28[a]
Total annual income	>20000 dollars	242	81	<10000 dollars	321	48[a]
Type of occupation	Light or moderate	608	78	Heavy	395	50[a]
Education level	≥7 years	639	76	≤6 years	350	52[a]
Age at surgery	≤49 years	470	73	55–59 years	287	59[a]
Duration of symptoms	<1 year	281	78	>1 year	768	62[c]
Anginal class	Class 1 and 2	448	75	Class 3	440	57[a]
Noncardiovascular illness	Absent	744	72	Present	230	55[b]
Associated vascular disease	Absent	930	68	Present	120	53[b]

[a] $P<0.001$; [b] $P<0.002$; [c] $P<0.05$

Table 4. Profile of patients not working at 1 year in the pilot rehabilitation program

Patient	Preoperative inactivity (months)	Type of work	Level of education	Total annual income	Alcoholism	Psychosocial factors
1	1	Moderate	Low[a]	10–20000	No	Hypochondria
2	2	Heavy[a]	Low[a]	<10000[a]	Yes	Psychopathic behavior
3	10[a]	Moderate	Intermediate	10–20000	Yes	Psychiatric history
4	0	Heavy[a]	Intermediate	10–20000	Yes	Social inadaptation
5	8[a]	Heavy[a]	Intermediate	10–20000	Yes	Chronic depression
6	0	Moderate	Intermediate	>20000	No	Medical complication
7	12[a]	Moderate	Low[a]	<10000[a]	Yes	Lack of motivation
8	2	Heavy[a]	Low[a]	10–20000	Yes	Hypochondria

[a] Unfavorable predictive factor

Comparison with the Control Group

In the control group, 89% of the patients returned to work and 82% were working at 1 year. These percentages were not different from those of patients in the pilot study. Of the 11 patients who were not working at 1 year in the control group, four had no unfavorable factors, two had one, two had two, and three had three unfavorable factors. One patient had to quit working following the discovery of cancer. Three patients attributed their inactivity to noncardiac illnesses. Four patients had obtained a medical certificate of invalidism. Three were unable to readapt to their previous occupation. It was quite clear that explanations for not working were different when evaluated objectively by the multidisciplinary team in the pilot project and subjectively by the patient in the control group.

Discussion

A wide variation (between 17% and 92%) in the percentage of patients who return to work after coronary artery bypass surgery has previously been reported (Gundle et al. 1980; Anderson et al. 1980; Oberman et al. 1983). These reports, however, may not be comparable since they frequently deal with different patient populations (in terms of age, sex, etc.), with different lengths of follow-up (from 1 to 5 years) or did not consider the importance of classification into subsets (with respect to the length of preoperative inactivity, social status, etc.). The purpose of this report is to compare the results of four patient subsets studied over the last decade. Our first study of 326 consecutive patients did not show the expected socioeconomic benefit of an increased return to work rate after coronary bypass surgery, while other reports (National Institutes of Health Consensus-Development Conference Statement 1981) had shown that this surgery could relieve angina pectoris, which in most cases was felt to be the reason for unemployment. To explain this paradoxical effect, we carried out two study designs: (1) the perioperative sociodemographic and medical variables most predictive of return to work were determined and (2) the psychological and social components of the return to work behavior in a given individual and the influence of a multidisciplinary rehabilitation program were explored.

Among 30 perioperative variables, the uni- and bivariate analysis found nine most predictive factors. All were preoperative variables, while postoperative relief or improvement of symptoms was found to be highly predictive by others (Niles et al. 1980; Smith et al. 1982; Almeida et al. 1983). In the multivariate analysis, the preoperative work status defined by the length of preoperative unemployment and the physical work load was by far the most important factor; in conjunction with the educational level this was more influential than the medical variables. The other published multivariate analysis (Hammermeister et al. 1979; Niles et al. 1980) are in agreement with these findings. In our study, age was less predictive than in previous reports (Hammermeister et al. 1979; Niles et al. 1980; Almeida et al. 1983), probably in part because of patient selection (our patients were less than 60 years of age). However, these preoperative objective factors cannot explain all the return to work situation, since the square of the canonical variable (proportion of variance explained by these variables) is only 51%, as noted in another report (Gutmann et al. 1982). The pilot study tried to investigate these other factors. Table 4 shows the frequency of psychological problems. Alcoholism (Feighner 1972) was found in most of our patients who were not working at 1 year. More studies are needed to determine whether alcoholism is an independent predictive factor or only correlated to the socioeconomic status. In our control group, some patients who did not work had obtained a certificate of permanent disability from their physicians. Such a document has serious long-term consequences and should be given only in well-documented cases. The exercise test for functional capacity can be utilized as a mean of identifying those who are functionally impaired and who may require disability benefits. A strategy should be developed to inform physicians in this respect. The negative attitude of employers toward cardiac patients must be modified.

Following our early observations and the reports of other workers (Barnes et al. 1977; Symnes et al. 1978; Hammermeister et al. 1979), the importance of reducing the length of preoperative unemployment was stressed to physicians in our community. The percentage of patients who underwent surgery following less than 3 months of preoperative inactivity has increased from 44% between 1969 and 1972, to 51% between 1973 and 1978, and finally 74% in 1979–1980. In a parallel direction, the percentage of our patients who have returned to work after surgery has increased progressively from 69% between 1969 and 1972, to 76% between 1973 and 1978, and finally 89% in 1979–1980. Although several other factors, such as more complete revascularization, better pain relief, and more enlightened attitudes toward employment after CABG, may have contributed to this improvement, this medical strategy may have increased the return to work rate by preventing unnecessary inactivity before coronary arteriography and coronary bypass surgery and in spite of increased unemployment due to economic recession.

Using nine predictive factors and a psychosocial evaluation, we are able to identify subsets of patients in whom unfavorable results can be expected. This ability to predict preoperatively the work status may be used to indicate individually the need for rehabilitation, so we can concentrate our rehabilitation resources on patients who have a poor return to work prognosis. In the pilot project and in the control group, the majority of patients (more than 80%) had a favorable preoperative prognosis of return to work in terms of age and preoperative length of inactivity (less than 1 year). The rehabilitation program could not demonstrate any significant improvement in such a small number of patients who really needed rehabilitation. More studies are needed to show the effectiveness of rehabilitation.

In the future, we plan to introduce, as part of the routine preoperative work-up, the most significant psychological and social evaluations, a detailed questionnaire on alcohol consumption, and a chart of the nine most predictive factors. With this information, the rehabilitation team will make a return to work prognosis and patients with a poor return to work prognosis will be screened and submitted to an individualized rehabilitation program as previously described (Danchin et al. 1982). Before and after surgery, such comprehensive rehabilitation programs will concentrate on strategies (1) to improve the work conditions of the patient and prevent premature retirement; (2) to solve, whenever possible, the psychological problems of the patient and improve his quality of life; (3) to decrease coronary risk factors following individual or group sessions of information. Many questions remain and will be the subjects of future research, e.g., "what is the influence of alcoholism?" and "How can we screen with the greatest accuracy the patient subsets where the rehabilitation can be cost-effective?" Other studies must also be designed to explore other rehabilitation benefits. If, for society, the return to work of one of its member is very important and cost-effective, for the patient himself it may be equally important to evaluate how the rehabilitation will improve his quality of life and survival and will contribute to the secondary prevention of coronary artery disease.

References

Almeida D, Bradford JM, Wenger NK, King SB, Hurst JW (1983) Return to work after coronary bypass surgery. Circulation [Suppl II] 68:II 205-II 213

Anderson AJ, Barboriak JJ, Hoffmann RG, Mullen DC (1980) Retention or resumption of employment after aortocoronary bypass operations. JAMA 243:543-545

Barnes GK, Ray MJ, Oberman A, Kouchoukos NT (1977) Changes in working status of patients following coronary bypass surgery. JAMA 238:1259-1262

Benton AL (ed) (1965) Manuel du test de rétention visuelle, applications cliniques et expérimentales. Centre de Psychologie Appliquée, Paris

Bortner RW (1969) A short rating scale as a potential measure of pattern a behavior. J Chronic Dis 22:87-91

CASS principal investigators and their associates (1983) Coronary artery surgery study (CASS): A randomized trial of coronary artery bypass surgery. Survival data. Circulation 68:939-960

Cattell RB, Scheier (eds) (1964) Handbook for the IPAT anxiety scale. Institute for Personality and Ability testing. Champaign

Cattell RB, Eber WE (eds) (1964) Handbook for the 16 personality factor questionnaire. The Institute for Personality and Ability Testing. Champaign

Croog S (1976) Personality self-perception of male heart patients and their wives: Issues of congruence and "coronary personality". Percept Mot Skills 43:927-938

Danchin N, David P, Robert P, Bourassa MG (1980) Evolution du statut de travail après pontage aorto-coronarien dans une population canadienne française. Arch Mal Coeur 73:585-592

Danchin N, David P, Robert P, Bourassa MG (1982) Return to work after coronary surgery: is there a need for a comprehensive rehabilitation program? In: Mathes P, Halhuber MJ (eds) Controversies in cardiac rehabilitation. Springer, Berlin Heidelberg New York Tokyo, pp 81-83

David H, Juneau M (1975) Le pontage aortocoronarien, étude socioeconomique. Actual Cardiovasc Medicochir 7:94-105

Feighner JP (1972) Diagnostic criteria for use in psychiatric research. Arch Gen Psychiatry 26:57-63

Goldberg DP (ed) (1972) The detection of psychiatric illness by questionnaire. Oxford University Press, London

Gundle MJ, Reeves BR, Tate S, Raft D, McLaurin LP (1980) Psychosocial outcome after coronary artery surgery. Am J Psychiatry 137:1591-1594

Gutmann MC, Knapp DN, Pollock ML, Schmidt DH, Simon K, Walcott G (1982) Coronary artery bypass patients and work status. Circulation [Suppl III] 66:III 33–III 42
Hammermeister KE, DeRouen TA, English MT, Dodge MT (1979) Effect of surgical versus medical therapy on return to work in patients with coronary artery disease. Am J Cardiol 44:105–111
Melzack R (1975) The McGill pain questionnaire, major properties and scoring method. Pain 1:277–299
National Institutes of Health Consensus-Development Conference Statement (1981) Coronary-artery bypass surgery. Scientific and clinical aspects. N Engl J Med 304:680–684
Niles NW, Vandersalm TJ, Cutler BS (1980) Return to work after coronary artery bypass operation. J Thorac Cardiovasc Surg 79:916–921
Oberman A, Wayne JB, Kouchoukos NT, Charles ED, Russel RO, Rogers WJ (1983) Employment status after coronary artery bypass surgery. Circulation [Suppl II] 65:II 115–II 119
Rotter JB (1975) Some problems and misconceptions related to the construct of Interval VS. External control of reinforcement. J Consult Clin Psychol 43:56–67
Smith HC, Hammes LN, Gupta S, Vlietstra RE, Elveback L (1982) Employment status after coronary artery bypass surgery. Circulation 65 [Suppl II] 65:II 120–II 125
Symmes JC, Lenkey SCM, Berman MD (1978) Influence of aortocoronary bypass surgery on employment. Can Med Assoc J 118:268–270
Weissman M (1975) The assessment of social adjustment: A review of techniques. Arch Gen Psychiatry 32:357–365
Welsch GS, Dahlstrom WG (eds) (1956) Basic readings on the MMPI. University of Minnesota Press, Minneapolis
Witkin HA (ed) (1974) Field dependence-independence and psychological differentiation. A bibliography through 1972 with index. Educational Testing Service, Princeton
Zung WWK (1965) A self-rating depression scale. Arch Gen Psychiatry 12:63–70

The Rehabilitation of Patients Following Coronary Revascularization Surgery: Social and Economic Aspects

H. V. Liddle, P. D. Jones, B. Gould, and P. D. Clayton

Coronary revascularization surgery remains controversial with respect to its enduring influence on patient survival, relief of symptoms, rehabilitation, and cost-benefit. Reports in the literature concerning initial postoperative rehabilitation vary considerably, and there is general consensus in America that coronary surgery patients have a poor initial rehabilitation experience and even if they do become rehabilitated, they do not tend to remain employed for long. The psychologic impact of the disease itself (Gundle et al. 1980) and physician attitudes (David 1978; Oberman et al. 1982) about postoperative management tend to discourage work rehabilitation. The purpose of this paper is to determine the rate of rehabilitation of coronary surgery patients and to determine the duration of rehabilitation. The study examines the survival curves of coronary surgical patients and the effects on rehabilitation of patient's age, education, type of preoperative employment, preoperative work status, preoperative disability, duration of disability, and the effects of early and late graft patency on both initial rehabilitation and duration of work. The cost-benefits of the operation are also examined.

Materials and Methods

The study is composed of two groups of patients: Those patients who had a single revascularization procedure and those patients who had two or more such procedures. Eligibility for inclusion in this study was determined postoperatively by patient survival for more than 6 months and by completion of a demographic questionnaire. Postoperative angiograms were done between the 4th and 19th months postoperatively (average 6.6 months) as part of a routine protocol and without regard to symptomatic status in all patients who were willing to undergo the examination. All patients were operated upon by the same surgeon using standardized surgical methods and were followed at intervals of 1, 6, and 12 months postoperatively and biannually thereafter. Patients agreed in advance of surgery to a protocol of 6-month, 5-year, and 10-year arteriograms as well as analysis of occupational status and were also advised in advance of surgery that disability claims would be supported only if revascularization failed.

Nine hundred and ninety-eight patients had a single operation and of these, 960 patients (96%) survived for 6 months or more. There were 792 patients

(83%), average age of 58 years, who completed demographic questionnaires (710 males and 82 females). Of the men who completed demographic questionnaires 612 patients underwent a postoperative angiogram at 6 months. Four patients were studied between the fourth and sixth postoperative month because of recurrent symptoms. Patients who refused postoperative angiograms did so because of dye reaction (1.5%), patient refusal (6%), at the instruction of the referring physician (2.5%), or had their first postoperative angiogram later than 19 months postoperatively (4%). One hundred and thirty-seven male patients who returned to work had late postoperative arteriograms. The high rate of voluntary compliance suggests the data are free of selection bias. Of the 82 females who were eligible for this study, only 36 had an occupational history of gainful employment. For this reason females will not generally be included in the subsequent analysis of rehabilitation. Patients who submitted no questionnaire or whose questionnaires were incomplete were discounted from the study. There were 40 patients who underwent two or more revascularization procedures. There were no operative and two late deaths in this group. Thirty-six of these patients completed the demographic questionnaire.

The single operation patients were classified according to occupational status (working, retired, disabled) before and after surgery. Using the chi-square test, the male patients were examined to see whether the preoperative work status influenced their return to work. The null hypothesis that the duration of preoperative disability, type of occupation, level of education, early graft patency, and age at surgery did not influence the rate of return to work after surgery was also tested. To determine the duration of rehabilitation, the number of months that the rehabilitated patients actually worked after surgery was plotted against the possible number of months that they could have worked to their appropriate retirement age, death, or completion of this study. The patients were then grouped as to whether they worked as expected to retirement or whether they worked beyond that age, or quit work early. The patients who had both early and late postoperative arteriograms were then tested to see whether early or late graft failure influenced the duration of postoperative employment. Late graft status was assessed between 48 and 84 months postoperatively. To assess whether the strong emphasis placed on rehabilitation of this patient population had a negative effect on survival, Kaplan Meier survival curves were plotted for the entire population as well as for groups of patients according to the number of grafts they had.

To assess the economic aspects of coronary surgery, the cost of surgical care was compared to the salary production of patients who returned to work after surgery. The cost of surgery is defined as the total of hospital charges, physician fees, and disability payments both before and after surgery. The salary production was calculated by multiplying the monthly salary by the months worked postoperatively. The salary was based on the initial dollar amount reported by the patients in the questionnaire and does not reflect fluctuations in compensation which may have occurred over the duration of employment. For the 40 patients with multiple coronary surgeries the pre- and postoperative occupational status and salary production were calculated. The duration of the symptom-free interval for single and multiple surgery patients was compared using the Kaplan-Meier method. Cox regression was used to test significance.

Results

Single Operation Patients

Education

Of the 710 male respondents, 15% had an elementary education, 61% had completed high school, 17% were college graduates, and 7% had attended graduate school. Work rehabilitation for the elementary school graduates was only 60% as compared to 76%, 79%, and 79% respectively for patients with a higher level of education. The difference in return to work for the elementary school educated patients was significantly different ($P < 0.002$) than the rate for those with more education. The less educated patients were also older, with a median age of 61.5 years as compared to 57.8, 56.3, and 56 years respectively for the more educated patients. However, the elementary school graduates had a lower rate of rehabilitation in all age groups. There were no significant differences in return to work among the patients with more than elementary education ($P = 0.66$).

Occupation

Of 710 male respondents, 627 patients specifically listed a preoperative occupation, even though 83 of them had already retired. Of those whose occupation is known, 18% were farmers or ranchers, 44% were blue-collar workers, 25% were white-collar workers, and 13% were professional people. The rates for return to work were 77% for farmers, 84% for blue-collar workers, 83% for white-collar workers, and 84% for professional people. There were no significant differences in the rate of return to work among these various occupational categories ($P = 0.25$).

Preoperative and Postoperative Work Status by Age

The occupational status of single surgery patients before and after surgery is shown in Tables 1–3. There were 558 men under age 65 at the time of their operation, of whom 275 men were working preoperatively, 221 men were disabled for more than 1 month preoperatively, and 62 men were retired. Of the 275 working men, 265 (96%) returned to work, 1 man retired, 2 became disabled, and 7 (2%) elected to quit work, though they were deemed able to work. Of the 221 men who were disabled preoperatively, 198 (90%) returned to work, 6 retired, 7 remained disabled, and 10 (4%) elected to quit. Of the 62 retired men, only 2 (3%) returned to work and the balance remained retired. Thirty-eight of these 62 patients who retired prior to the age of 65 were over the age of 60 at the time of their surgery. Preoperatively 275 of 558 patients (49%) who were under age 65 at the time of surgery were working, but postoperatively 465 (83%) of these men had returned to work ($P < 0.00001$).

Table 1. Rehabilitation to work: 558 men under 65

Preoperative work status	Postoperative work status			
	Working	Retired	Disabled	Quit
Working (*n* = 275)	265 (96%)	1 (0.4%)	2 (0.6%)	7 (3%)
Disabled (*n* = 221)	198 (90%)	6 (3%)	7 (3%)	10 (4%)
Retired (*n* = 62)	2 (3%)	60 (97%)	0	0
Total (*n* = 558)	465 (83%)	67 (12%)	9 (2%)	17 (3%)

Table 2. Rehabilitation to work: 152 men over 65

Postoperative work status	Postoperative work status			
	Working	Retired	Disabled	Quit
Working (*n* = 32)	27 (85%)	2 (6%)	1 (3%)	2 (6%)
Disabled (*n* = 31)	29 (94%)	2 (6%)	0	0
Retired (*n* = 89)	4 (4%)	85 (96%)	0	0
Total (*n* = 152)	60 (39%)	89 (58%)	1 (0.7%)	2 (1.3%)

Table 3. Rehabilitation to work: 82 women

Preoperative work status	Postoperative work status			
	Working	Retired	Disabled	Quit
Working (*n* = 12)	12 (100%)	0	0	0
Disabled (*n* = 24)	14 (59%)	3 (12%)	1 (4%)	6 (25%)
Retired (*n* = 46)	0	46 (100%)	0	0
Total (*n* = 82)	26 (32%)	49 (60%)	1 (1%)	6 (7%)

There were 152 men over age 64 at the time of surgery, of whom 32 men were working, 31 were disabled, and 89 were retired. Twenty-seven (85%) of the 32 working men returned to work, and 29 (94%) of the 31 disabled men did so, but only 4 (5%) of the 89 retired men returned to work. Preoperatively there were only 32 of these 152 (21%) men over age 64 years who were working but postoperatively 60 (39%) men were doing so ($P < 0.00001$).

Because the women often classified themselves as homemakers, it was more difficult to assess their state of rehabilitation. All of the females who said they were gainfully employed before surgery and 59% of those who were disabled preoperatively returned to work postoperatively. For the 792 patients who completed questionnaires, including patients of all ages and sex, the increase in the number working postoperatively (70%) compared to the number working preoperatively (40%) was significant ($P < 0.00001$).

Age

Among 240 male patients who were under the age of 55 years at the time of surgery, 224 (93%) returned to work, whereas only 241 of 318 (76%) patients between the ages of 55 and 64 years returned to work. Among patients over 65 years, 60 of 152 (39%) returned to work. The differences were highly significant ($P < 0.00001$).

Effect of Preoperative Disability

When all 792 eligible patients who had a single operation are considered, 304 of 319 (95%) of those working preoperatively returned to work, and of the 276 patients who were disabled preoperatively, 241 (87%) returned to work. This difference is significant ($P < 0.0008$).

Among the men under 65 years of age at the time of surgery, the rehabilitation of preoperative working patients (96%) and disabled patients (90%) was also significantly different ($P < 0.005$).

The duration of preoperative disability for all disabled men had no influence on postoperative working status ($P = 0.34$). Of 175 men disabled 1–6 months preoperatively, 155 (89%) returned to work. Of 37 who were disabled for 7–12 months, 34 (92%) returned to work, and of 40 patients who were disabled for more than 1 year, 38 patients (95%) returned to work. Nor was the duration of disability a significant factor when only males under age 65 years were examined.

The Effect of Graft Patency

Early graft patency (6 months) had no influence on the initial rate of return to work. Of 243 males with early arteriograms who were working before surgery, 8 were not working after surgery, and 2 of them had at least one graft fail, while 86 (37%) of the patients who returned to work after surgery had at least one graft fail. The difference was not significant ($P = 0.77$). Of the 196 patients who were disabled before surgery and who had an early arteriogram, there were 20 who were not working after surgery and 9 of these (45%) had at least one graft fail early. Fifty-nine of the 176 (34%) disabled patients who went to work after surgery had at least one graft fail. These differences were not significant ($P = 0.44$). Patients with one or more failed grafts had a similar initial rate of return to work as did those patients with all patent grafts.

Duration of Postoperative Rehabilitation

The duration of employment for male patients of all ages is shown in Figs. 1 and 2. The points along or above the line of identity represent patients who worked to or beyond the expected duration and the points below the line represent those patients who quit prematurely. The patients who legitimately retired between the ages of 60 and 65 years were considered to have worked to retirement and are plotted on the line of identity. There were 26 working and 22 disabled patients preoperatively who legitimately retired postoperatively between ages 60 and 65 years. Patients who died later than 6 months postoperatively, but who were working until the time of death, worked as long as possible and are therefore plotted on the line of identity. There were 292 men of all ages who were working at the time of surgery and who returned to work postoperatively. Of these, 194 (66%) patients worked the expected duration and an additional 47 patients (16%) worked up to 10 years beyond retirement. Seventeen percent of patients quit prematurely. Twenty of these 292 patients (8%) patients sought less strenuous jobs postoperatively. There were 227 men of all ages who were disabled preoperatively and who returned to work postoperatively. Of these men, 139 (61%) worked the expected duration and an additional 44 patients (19%) worked up to 10 years beyond retirement. Forty-four patients (19%) quit work prematurely. Of the disabled patients who were rehabilitated, 40 (20%) sought a less strenuous job. The percentages of men who worked longer than, shorter than, or as expected did not differ ($P=0.12$) among those who were working and those who were disabled preoperatively.

Influence of Early and Late Graft Failure on Duration of Work

Among men who worked before and after surgery and who had an early arteriogram, 15% who quit work early, 5% of those who worked to retirement, and 5% of those working beyond retirement had no grafts open early (Table 4). Conversely, 33%, 28%, and 35% respectively had some grafts open, and 52%, 67%, and 60% of men in these groups had all grafts open. These differences were not significant ($P=0.30$), indicating that duration of work was independent of graft patency. However, when patients with no grafts open early were compared to patients with some or all grafts open, there was a significant difference ($P<0.05$) wherein duration of work was improved by graft patency. Duration of work was also positively influenced ($P<0.003$) by continued late patency of some or all grafts. Patients with no grafts open at the late arteriogram were much more likely to quit early. The results among men who were disabled before but working after surgery showed that graft patency is independent of duration of work (Table 5). It did not matter what degree of graft patency existed either early ($P=0.30$) or late ($P=0.78$) nor whether patients with no patent grafts were compared to those with some or all grafts patent ($P=0.73$), duration of work was unaffected.

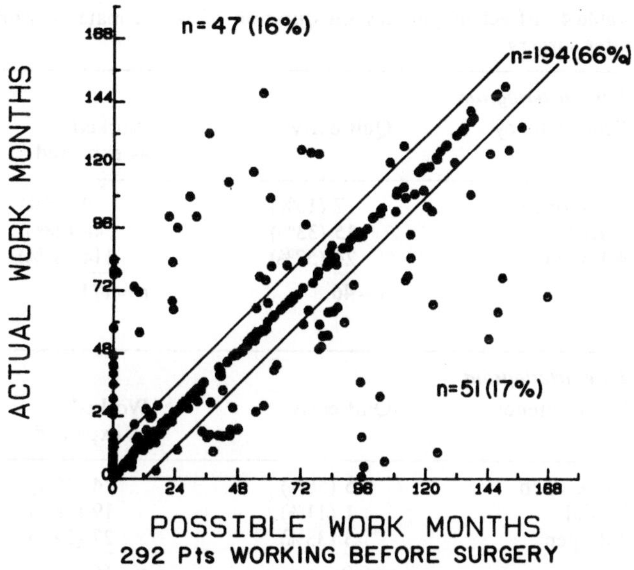

Fig. 1. Duration of postoperative work for 292 males working before and after surgery. The *horizontal axis* is the months the patient could work to retirement. The *vertical axis* is the actual months worked. Patients who actually worked as expected to retirement are plotted on the line of identity. Those who quit early are plotted below and those who worked beyond retirement are plotted above the line of identity

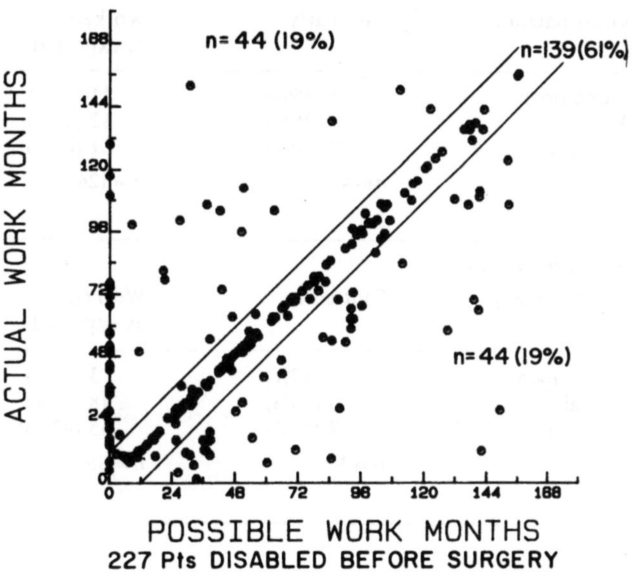

Fig. 2. Duration of postoperative work for 227 males disabled before but working after surgery. The *vertical axis* represents the actual months worked. Patients who actually worked as expected to retirement are plotted on the line of identity. Those who quit early are plotted below and those who worked beyond retirement are plotted above the line of identity

Table 4. Effect of patency on duration of work: males – working before surgery, working after surgery

Early arteriogram Graft patency	Quit early	Worked as expected	Worked extra
None open	7 (15%)	9 (5%)	2 (5%)
Partial	15 (33%)	48 (28%)	14 (35%)
All open	24 (52%)	114 (67%)	24 (60%)
	$n=46$	$n=171$	$n=40$
			$P=0.12$, NS
Late arteriogram Graft patency	Quit early	Worked as expected	Worked extra
None open	5 (56%)	4 (8%)	1 (7%)
Partial	1 (11%)	19 (38%)	6 (40%)
All open	3 (33%)	27 (54%)	8 (53%)
	$n=9$	$n=50$	$n=15$
			$P<0.003$

Table 5. Effect of patency on duration of work: males – disabled before surgery, working after surgery

Early arteriogram Graft patency	Quit early	Worked as expected	Worked extra
None open	2 (5%)	11 (9%)	3 (8%)
Partial	10 (25%)	32 (26%)	16 (42%)
All open	28 (70%)	81 (65%)	19 (50%)
	$n=40$	$n=124$	$n=38$
			$P=0.30$, NS
Late arteriogram Graft patency	Quit early	Worked as expected	Worked extra
None open	1 (7%)	3 (8%)	0 (0%)
Partial	6 (43%)	18 (50%)	8 (62%)
All open	7 (50%)	15 (42%)	5 (38%)
	$n=14$	$n=36$	$n=13$
			$P=0.78$, NS

Cost–Benefit Analysis

For the 792 patients who had a single revascularization operation, the surgical costs, including preoperative and postoperative disability payments, and the postoperative salary production for those patients who returned to work were analyzed. The total cost of medical care for the entire patient population was $ 12178071.00. The accumulated postoperative dollar production was $ 48002700.00. Postoperative earnings exceeded the cost of surgery by a factor of 4.

There were 247 patients who were either disabled or retired before surgery but who returned to work postoperatively. The salary production of this group of patients was $ 19422058.00, or 1.5 times the cost of medical care of the entire patient population (Table 6).

Table 6. Productivity of rehabilitated patients ($n = 247$)

Number	Sex	Age	Preop status	Postop status	Total earned income
11	F	<65	Disabled	Working	$ 653074.00
198	M	<65	Disabled	Working	17551783.00
2	M	<65	Retired	Working	10635.00
29	M	>64	Disabled	Working	1091390 00
4	M	>64	Retired	Working	73529.00
3	F	>64	Disabled	Working	41647.00
Total					19422058.00
Cost of surgical care of 792 patients					= 12178071.00
Excess of income of rehabilitated patients over total surgical cost					= 7243987.00

Life table analysis (Kaplan Meier) (Fig. 3) for the total population showed a 5-year survival of 93%, and the 10-year survival was 85%. When subdivided by the number of grafts done, single graft patients had a 10-year survival of 93%, while double and triple graft patients had 10-year survival of 83% and 78% respectively. The patients with four or more grafts had a 6-year survival of 87%, and there were no further deaths between the 6th and 10th years.

Multiple Operation Patients

Demographic data are available for 34 of 38 surviving male patients who underwent multiple revascularization procedures. These patients ranged in age from 36 to 68 years at the time of their first operation. Eight patients were over 65 years at the time of the second procedure. Of 14 patients who were working before the first procedure, 11 (79%) returned to work, one patient remained disabled, and two patients quit work, though they were considered fit to work. Of 16 patients who were disabled preoperatively, 14 patients (88%) returned to work and two patients quit. All four of the retired patients remained in retirement. At the time of the second procedure, 10 patients were working, 17 pa-

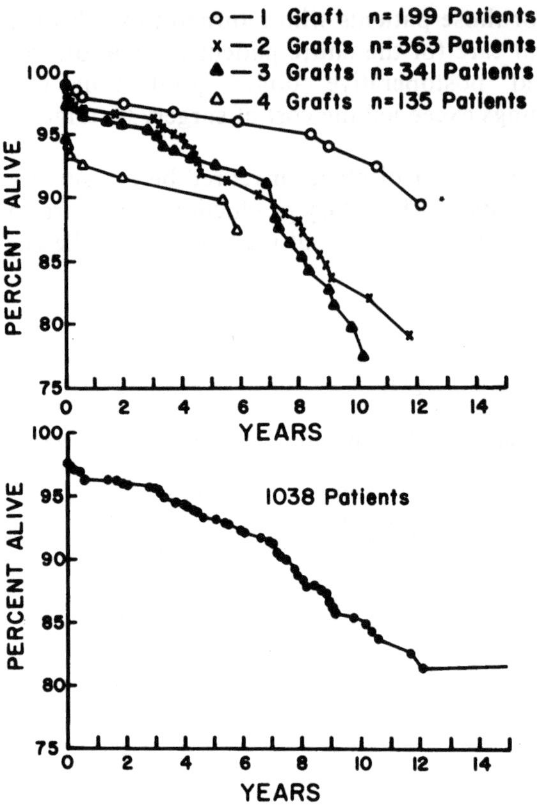

Fig. 3. Survival of operated patients. The *top panel* shows survival according to the number of grafts done. Each point on the curve is a coronary related death. For patients with four or more grafts the last death was at 6 years and in the subsequent 4 years no further deaths have occurred. The *bottom panel* shows survival for all patients. Five-year survival is 93% and 10-year survival is 85%

tients were disabled, and 7 had retired. Following the second surgery only 26 patients were still of working age and 18 (70%) of them returned to work. Fourteen patients were or became retired and 2 remained disabled. Additionally, the rate of return of symptoms postoperatively was no different ($P=0.10$) for the multiple operation patients than was the case for the patients who had a single operation (Fig. 4). At 5 years 75% of both groups were symptom free and at 10 years 50% were symptom free.

The total cost of medical care of these patients for all operative procedures was $ 1 208 370.00. The accumulated earned income of those patients who did return to work was $ 6 095 100.00, or five times greater the than cost of surgery.

Discussion

The studies which have been conducted in the United States and in Western Europe concerning rehabilitation following coronary surgery are at considerable variance. Most of the American studies (Oberman et al. 1982; Gutman et al. 1982; Rimm et al. 1976; Barnes et al. 1977) report disappointingly poor reha-

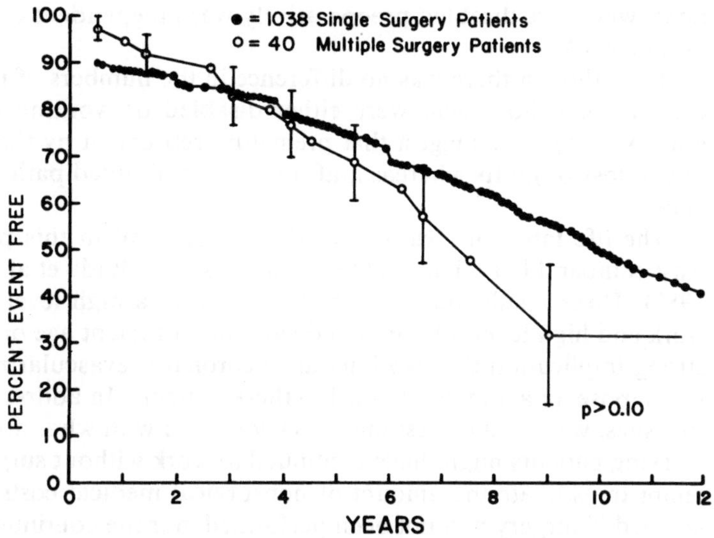

Fig. 4. Event curves demonstrate the rate of return of symptoms for single and multiple surgery patients. The differences between these curves was not significant ($P = 0.10$)

bilitation, whereas the European (Wallwork et al. 1978; Guvendik et al. 1982; Frick et al. 1979) results are more encouraging. The principal factors cited in the American literature which negatively influenced return to work are duration of preoperative disability, disability payments, age, educational status, occupation, and recurrence of symptoms. Our results and those cited previously by us (Liddle 1981; Liddle et al. 1982) agree that educational level is a significant factor ($P < 0.002$). The elementary educated patients had a lower rate of return to work in all age groups. On the other hand, occupation had no influence on return to work.

Age had a negative influence on rehabilitation. Patients under age 55 years at the time of surgery had a much higher rate of return to work than did the older patients. We found that preoperative disability also negatively influenced rehabilitation. Though the difference in return to work by men of all ages who were working (95%) and men who were disabled (87%) is significant, the rehabilitation in both groups was very high. In our experience the duration of preoperative disability had no effect on rehabilitation. Initial rehabilitation is the immediate goal of the operation but it is equally important that the patients remain productive to their retirement age. We have found that more than 80% of male patients who returned to work either worked to retirement or up to 10 years beyond retirement. We have previously shown that the rate of early graft patency did influence the duration of symptomatic relief (Jensen et al. 1982; Gould et al. 1984). When the effects of early graft patency and the subsequent loss of grafts during the first seven postoperative years was examined, there was a significant positive influence of graft patency on duration of work in men who were working preoperatively. Though a favorable influence of graft patency on duration of work was expected, the effect of graft patency in patients who were disabled preoperatively was independent of patency and duration of work.

Even though there was no difference in the numbers of men who quit work early among those who were either disabled or working preoperatively, the graft patency data suggest that premature retirement by the working men was due to loss of grafts whereas graft loss in the disabled patients made no difference.

The life table survival curves showed survival in this population to be at least comparable to that in other reported series (Buda et al. 1981; Lawrie et al. 1982). These results occurred in the setting of a high level of initial return to work and high levels of continued work to retirement age or beyond. There is a strong implication that working after coronary revascularization surgery does not impose an avoidable hazard to these patients. In addressing the cost-benefit issues, we could not estimate how long and with what dollar production the working patients might have continued to work without surgery. We did not attempt to estimate the amount of nonsurgical medical costs which might have accrued if surgery had not been performed, nor the continued cost of disability payments and loss of income production by disabled patients, nor the cots for patients in this study who died within the first 6 months after surgery. Based on the economic data we could measure, the productivity of the patients who returned to work far exceeds the surgical costs for the entire group. Of greater importance is the fact that the group of patients who were truly rehabilitated from retirement or disability to a productive capacity by the surgical intervention produced an accumulated postoperative income that was 1.5 times the cost of care for the entire patient population.

Our experience with reoperation for recurrent disease and/or graft failure is also favorable. After the second operation these patients had the same rate of freedom from symptoms as did the patients who had only one operative intervention. Their rate of return to work after the first surgery was slightly lower than was the case for the single surgery patients, but it still exceeded 70%. Their further attrition following the second operation was largely a result of age. Seventy percent of the eligible patients did return to work following the second operation.

It is difficult to explain why the rehabilitation results in this patient population are different than those cited in other reports. The pattern of follow-up is one of regular visits and the insistence on control of risk factors as well as return to work is firmly repeated. The patients knew in advance that rehabilitation was the goal of the surgery and that principle was frequently repeated. It may be that attitudes of physicians, families, and employers may be the critical factors in rehabilitation. This study suggests that effective rehabilitation depends on low operative mortality, on the determination of the patient to remain productive, and on reassurance to the patient that he is capable of being productive. This reassurance is justified by the evidence that return to work does not have a deleterious effect on survival.

Acknowledgment. This work was supported in part by the National Library of Medicine (LM 03688) and a grant from William R. Hewlett.

References

Barnes G, Ray M, Oberman A, Kouchoukos NT (1977) Changes in working status of patients following coronary bypass surgery. JAMA 238:1259–1262

Buda A, Macdonald I, Anderson M, Strauss H, David T, Berman N (1981) Long-term results following coronary bypass operation. J Thorac Cardiovasc Surg 82:383–390

David P (1978) Contributing factors preventing return to work of cardiac surgery patients. Cleve Clin Q 45:177–178

Frick M, Harjola P, Valle M (1979) Work status after coronary artery bypass surgery. A prospective randomized study with ergometric and angiographic correlations. Acta Med Scand 206:61–64

Gould B, Clayton P, Jensen R, Liddle HV (1984) Association between early graft patency and late outcome for patients undergoing artery bypass graft surgery. Circulation 69:569–575

Gundle M, Reeves B, Tate S, Raft D, McClaurin L (1980) Psycho-social outcome after coronary artery surgery. Am J Psychiatry 137:1591–94

Gutmann M, Knapp D, Pollock M, Schmidt D, Simon K, Walcott G (1982) Coronary artery bypass patients and work status. Circulation [Suppl III] 66:33–41

Guvendik L, Rahan M, Yacoub M (1982) Symptomatic status and pattern of employment during a five-year period following myocardial revascularization for angina. Ann Thorac Surg 34:383–387

Jensen R, Clayton P, Liddle HV (1982) Relationship between graft patency, postoperative work status, and symptomatic relief. J Thorac Cardiovasc Surg 83:503–511

Lawrie G, Morris G, Calhoon J, Safi H, Zamora J, Beltengady M, Baron A, Silvers A, Chapman D (1982) Clinical results of coronary bypass in 500 patients at least 10 years after operation. Circulation [Suppl I] 66:I-1–5

Liddle HV, Jensen R, Clayton P (1982) The rehabilitation of coronary surgical patients. Ann Thorac Surg 34:374–382

Liddle HV (1981) Perspectives in coronary artery surgery. J Thorac Cardiovasc Surg 81:1–10

Oberman A, Wayne JB, Kouchoukos NT, Charles E, Russell R, Rogers W (1982) Employment status after coronary artery bypass surgery. Circulation [Suppl II] 65:II-115–119

Rimm A, Barboriak JJ, Anderson AJ, Simon J (1976) Changes in occupation after aortocoronary vein-bypass operation. JAMA 236:361–364

Wallwork J, Potter B, Caves P (1978) Return to work after coronary artery surgery for angina. Br Med J 16:1680–81

The Significance of Radionuclide Ventriculography for the Prognosis and Social Fate of Heart Infarction Patients (With or Without Left Ventricular Aneurysm)

E. Grodzinski, T. Fentrop, T. Keller, G. Bierck, J. S. Borer, W. Schoop, and G. Blümchen

Introduction

The prognostic applicability of the left ventricular function and the morphology of the coronary arteries has been described in numerous studies. With radionuclide ventriculography (RNVA), we possess a method which enables us to recognize, noninvasively, hemodynamically, important coronary obstructions by analyzing the behavior of the ejection fraction. These parameters should be meaningful for the social medical evaluation of coronary patients as well. In this study, the early estimative ability of RNVA for the prognosis and social medical grouping of heart infarction patients will be demonstrated.

Patient Group

We examined 240 heart infarction patients, whose infarcts had occurred an average of 8 weeks earlier (217 men, 23 women). RNVA was also carried out on 188 of these patients during submaximal ergometry. 114 patients had suffered an anterior infarct and 126 a posterior infarct. 34 patients were shown, also using nuclear medical means, to have apical anterior aneurysms. The average age was 52±5 years (27–72 years). After an average of 2½ years, a survey was conducted, directed toward both the personal physician and the patient. One patient (a foreigner) could not be located (0.4%).

Methods

The technique of radionuclide ventriculography has been described in detail (Borer et al. 1976, 1977, 1979, 1980, 1981; Grodzinski et al. 1983 a, b). For technical reasons, the first 51 examinations were conducted only at rest.

The statistical calculations were carried out according to the chi-square test. The total probability of error should be less than 0.05%.

Results

For the examinations, 239 patients remained (126 posterior infarcts, 113 anterior infarcts). The average ejection fraction (EF) at rest was 52±11.4% (from

18% to 85%). The average rise or fall of the left ventricular function during exercise was $-1.6\% \pm 9.5\%$, i.e., on average, the ejection fraction fell 1.6%.

After 2½ years, 16 of 239 patients (6.7%) had died. One of these patients had had a second illness (carcinoma) and the cause of death could not with certainty be attributed to a cardiac problem.

In Fig. 1 one recognizes the high mortality for patients with a *resting* ejection fraction of under 30%, compared to the two other groups. In this group, three out of ten patients (30%) had died, whereas the mortality for the second group (EF at rest 30%–44%) was 3.4% and for the third group (EF at rest 45% or greater) 6.4%.

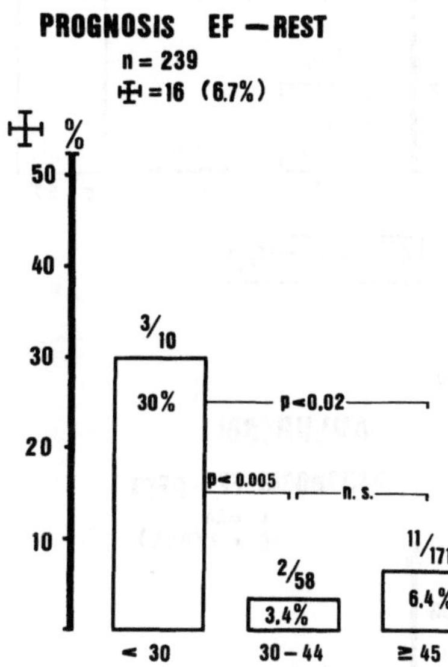

Fig. 1. The prognosis with regard to mortality for infarction patients (without aneurysm) with ejection fractions *at rest* of under 30%, between 30% and 44%, and greater than 44%. One recognizes that those patients with severely reduced ejection fractions of less than 30% demonstrate, after 2½ years observation, a distinctly poorer prognosis than those patients with larger resting ejection fractions

In Fig. 2 the heart infarction patients on whom RNVA *during exercise* was carried out are considered. In order to determine the prognostic usefulness of a decline in left ventricular function during exercise, patients with an ejection fraction of less than 30% at rest were excluded, as they are already recognized as high-risk patients. From the remaining 180 patients, eight patients (4.4%) had died within 2½ years. The mortality of the third group with a distinct decline of the ΔEF of 5% or more was significantly higher compared to the other two groups. Of 70 patients, seven (10%) had died, opposed to a mortality of 2% (one patient out of 49) in the first group with a distinct rise of the ΔEF of 5% or greater. In the second group (the so-called gray zone) there were no deaths.

Thirty-four of the anterior infarct patients had aneurysms. Three patients (8.8%) had died within the 2½ year period. The average resting ejection fraction in this group was $40.8\% \pm 10.6\%$, and the average decline in ejection fraction during exercise was 3.9%.

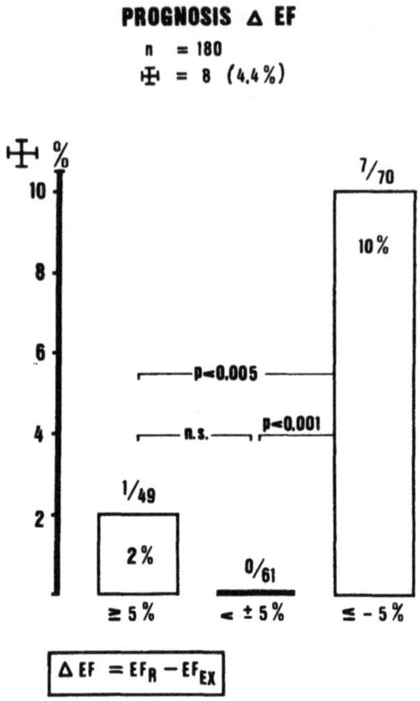

Fig. 2. Results in those infarction patients (without aneurysm) whose ejection fractions were determined both *at rest* and during *exercise*. These patients were categorized into three groups: increase (more than 5%), stable, and decrease (more than 5%). One sees that those patients who showed declines in ejection fraction have a distinctly poorer prognosis after 2½ years of observation than do the other two groups

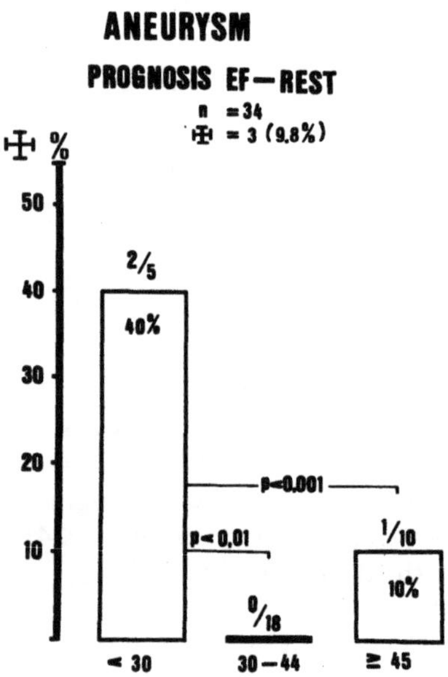

Fig. 3. Mortality of the 31 patients with anterior wall *aneurysms*. One sees that those patients having a distinctly reduced ventricular output at rest (<30%) demonstrate a poorer prognosis than do the other two groups

In Fig. 3 one sees that two of the five patients having a resting ejection fraction of under 30% had died, i. e., 40%, and one patient out of ten (10%) with an ejection fraction at rest of over 45%.

In Fig. 4 the changes in ejection fraction during *exercise* are shown in aneurysm patients. The expired patient in the third group with an ejection fraction of 48% at rest is depicted. A distinct fall in left ventricular function during exercise was observed. The ΔEF was minus 21%.

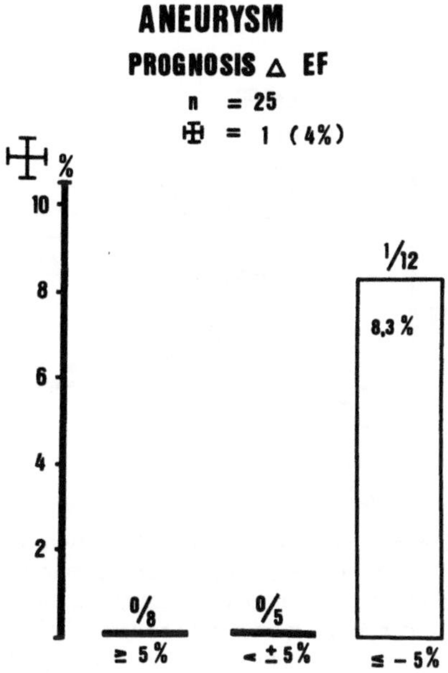

Fig. 4. Behavior of the *aneurysm* patients ($n = 25$) *during exercise.* Here again, one sees that a decline in ejection fraction during exercise indicates a poor prognosis

Figure 5 shows the social medical situation of 221 heart infarction patients correlated with left ventricular function *at rest.* Two patients had already received their pensions before the infarction for reasons of age. None of the group of five patients with resting ejection fractions of under 30% were able to return to work. All were given pensions. 102 out of 221 (46.2%) patients were able to return to work after heart infarction. 24 patients with ejection fractions ranging from 30% to 44% were again able to work, and in the third group with ejection fractions at rest of over 45%, 78 out of 160 (48.4%) went back to work. Correspondingly, the pension rate for these two groups was distinctly lower compared with the first group having resting ejection fractions of under 30%. 42.5% in the second group and 37.9% in the third group were given pensions. Only 28 out of 221 patients (12.7%) were unable to return to work. In the group having ejection fractions at rest of between 30% and 44%, 12.5% and in the third group with resting ejection fractions of more than 45%, 13.1% of the patients were pensioned.

Figure 6 shows the social medical situation of 172 patients correlated to the behavior of the left ventricular function *during exercise.* This number of patients results from the total number of patients who were ergometrically exercised, minus the patients with resting ejection fractions of less than 30%, who were all pensioned, and minus the eight patients who had expired. 50% of these

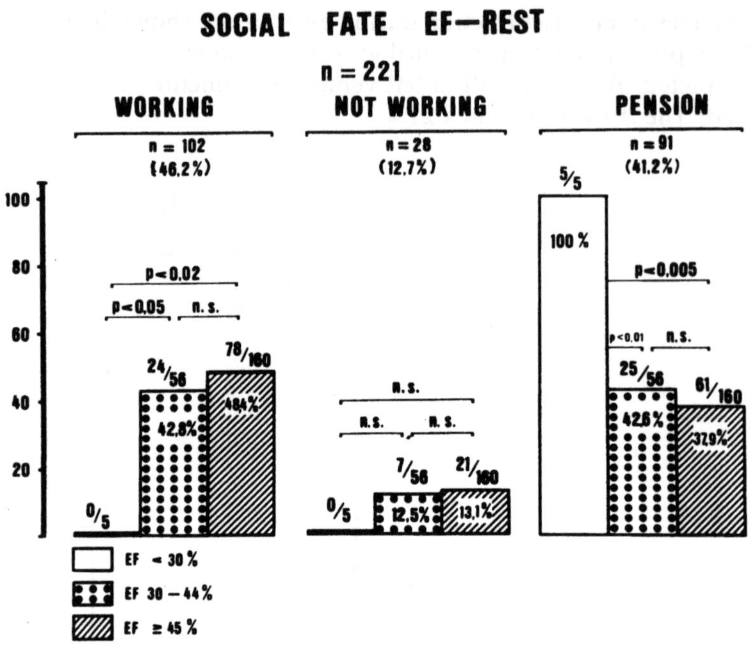

Fig. 5. Social medical data (ability to work, inability to work, pension) from the 221 heart infarction patients without aneurysms taken after a 2½ year observation period. The figure shows the social medical categorization of patients with distinctly restricted ejection fractions (under 30%), moderately restricted ejection fractions (30%–44%), and normal *resting* ejection fractions (over 45%). See text for explanation

patients were able to return to work (86 out of 172) after heart infarction. There were no major differences with regard to working ability in the separate groups having an increase or decrease in the ejection fraction during exercise. The pension rate was 37.3% (64 out of 172 patients). Those patients with a distinct decline of the ΔEF (26 out of 63 patients) are not pensioned with a significantly greater frequency, as 41.3% were given pensions. 12.8% were unable to work, i.e., 22 out of 172 patients. The patients who were most often given pensions, although the difference is not significant, were those having a distinct increase in ejection fraction during exercise. 17% received pensions.

Figure 7 shows the social fate of the 31 *aneurysm patients*. 31%, i.e., 9 out of 31 patients were able to return to work. Only those patients having a *resting* ventricular function of over 30% were allowed to work. The group with resting ejection fractions of between 30% and 44% had a higher return to work rate (39%) than the group which had resting ejection fractions of 45% or more. In this group, 22% were able to go back to work. 65.5% (16 out of 31) of the patients with aneurysm were given pensions. All patients having resting ejection fractions of less than 30% were pensioned (4%). This pension rate was significantly higher compared to the other two groups. The second group, all having ejection fractions at rest ranging from 30% to 44%, had a pension rate of 55%. The third group, all having resting ejection fractions of 45% or more, had a

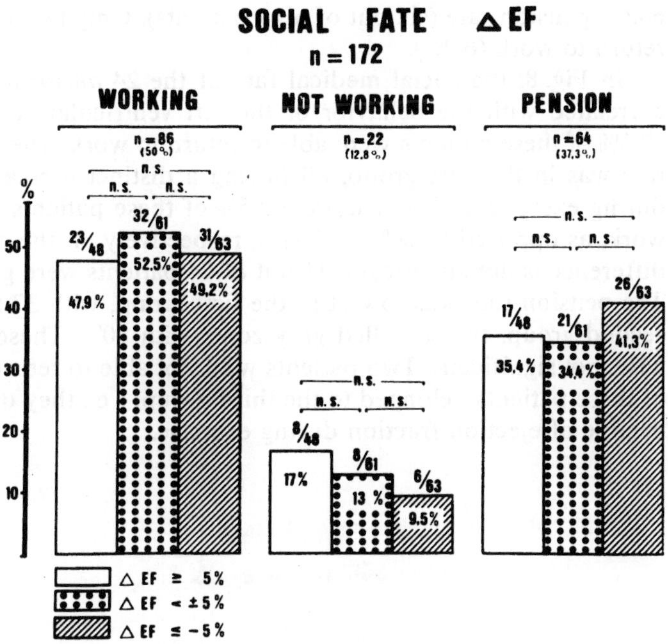

Fig. 6. Social medical situation of 172 heart infarction patients without aneurysms whose ejection fractions were determined both *at rest* and during *exercise*. See text for explanation

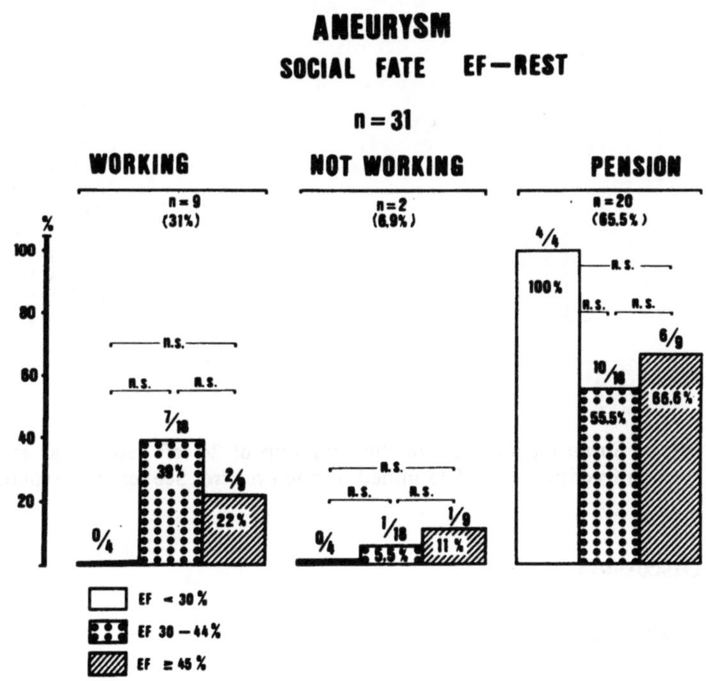

Fig. 7. Social medical fate of the subgroup of 31 left ventricular anterior wall aneurysm patients according to the EF at rest. See text for explanation

66.6% pension rate (six out of nine patients). Only two patients were unable to return to work (6.9%).

In Fig. 8, the social medical fate of the 24 *aneurysm* patients is depicted, correlated with the behavior of the left ventricular function *during exercise.* 37.5% of these patients were able to return to work. The highest return to work rate was in the first group, all having a distinct increase in ejection fraction during exercise of 5% or more. 62.5% of these patients were able to return to work, as opposed to 20% and 27%, respectively, in the other two groups. This difference is not significant. 13 out of 24 patients were given pensions (54.2%). The pension rate was lowest in the first group, with 37.5%, and highest in the second group, the so-called gray zone, with 80%. These differences are, likewise, not significant. Two patients were not able to return to work (8.3%). Both of these patients belonged to the third group, i.e., they demonstrated a distinct decline of ejection fraction during exercise.

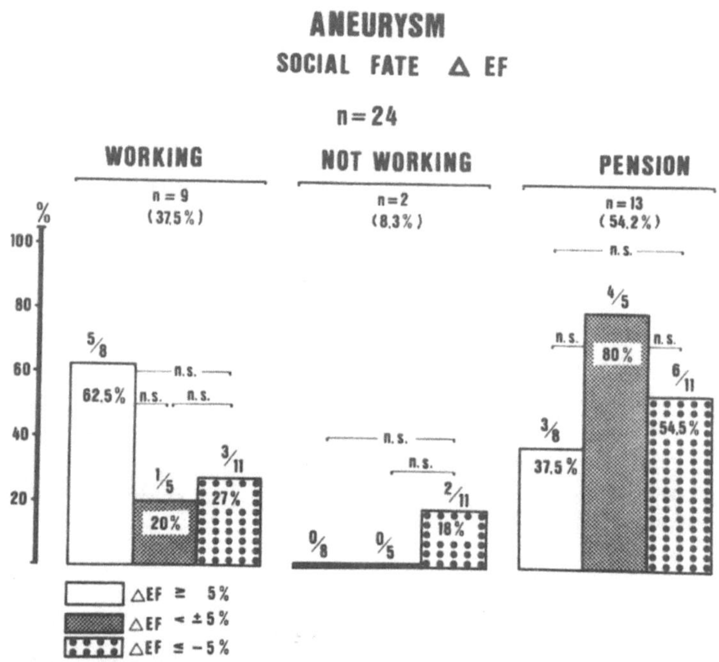

Fig. 8. *Social medical fate* of the subgroup of 24 left ventricular aneurysm patients whose ejection fractions were determined during *exercise.* See text for explanation

Discussion

Prognosis

Approximately 14 days after heart infarction, left ventricular function will no longer show any noteworthy changes (Wallis et al. 1983). For this reason, the prognosis for heart infarction patients can be determined in the first few weeks after infarction. Using RNVA, the ejection fraction at rest and during exercise can be determined noninvasively. For the patient, the examination is relatively safe and stressless. Aside from the determination of the left ventricular function, one can detect the existence of hemodynamically important coronary obstructions early, making proper diagnostics and therapy easier.

As was the case in other studies, we found a distinctly higher mortality in patients with markedly restricted left ventricular function of under 30% after 2½ years of follow-up. The mortality for these patients is 30%. By contrast, patients having slightly restricted or normal left ventricular ejection fractions at rest demonstrated lower mortality rates of 3% to 6%. The prognosis for patients with a left ventricular function of over 30% is more accurately determined by calculating the ejection fraction during exercise. Patients having a decline of left ventricular function during exercise of more than 5% demonstrate a higher mortality, namely 10%, than patients whose ejection fractions climb during exercise. Our results are in agreement with studies by Wallis et al. (1983). One of our patients, in spite of a distinct climb in left ventricular function during exercise, expired. This patients was suffering from serious rhythm disturbances of Lown classification IVa.

A prognostic prediction with regard to the invasively examined patients is, at this time, not practical. Only 4 of these 75 patients have expired. The trend shows, however, that the mortality for patients with three-vessel disease is higher than that for patients who underwent bypass surgery. Borer and his group were able to confirm this with a larger patient group (600 patients).

The mortality for *aneurysm patients* after 2½ years of follow-up is, at 8%, somewhat higher than the 6.7% rate for the heart infarction patients without aneurysm. This difference is, however, not significant. This has already been reported by our study group (Grodzinski et al. 1983b). Nevertheless, the question remains as to whether or not the aneurysm patients were properly categorized and perhaps incorrectly recommended for aneurysmectomy. As in the case of the heart infarction patients without aneurysm, the mortality for aneurysm patients having a resting ejection fraction of less than 30% is distinctly higher. Aneurysmectomy seems to be a positive factor for the prognosis for these patients, as long as the remaining myocardium continues to demonstrate good function. One of the deceased aneurysm patients was examined during exercise using RNVA. He demonstrated a decline in ejection fraction from 48% to 27%. The patient was not invasively diagnosed, as he achieved an 80 W exercise level without showing any signs of symptoms. A decline of the ejection fraction is probably caused by increasing myocardial insufficiency during exercise, meaning that the determination of the left ventricular function at rest alone does not suffice. Using this example, one recognizes that interpretation of the decline in the ejection fraction is sometimes difficult. As in the case of a pathologic increase in pulmonary artery pressure, an exercise ejection fraction decrease can be of myocardial scar or ischemic origin. Differentiation is only possible through clinical means.

Social Fate

The social fate of heart infarction patients is closely related to the left ventricular function, though it is also related to other factors (Wenger 1984). In fact, all patients with a resting ejection fraction of under 30% were pensioned. The significance of the left ventricular function is then correctly recognized by social medical evaluators. A return to work rate of 46% after a 2½ year postinfarct period is, without noteworthy discrepancy, the general rule for patients with resting ejection fractions over 30%. Nevertheless, 13% of these cases are, after 2½ years, not yet clear. The patients are not able to work and are considered by evaluators to be disabled. For these patients and for those pensioned patients with ejection fractions at rest of over 30%, the behavior of the ejection fraction during exercise may be the key to their social medical outcome. Patients with a decline of the ΔEF would be categorized as high-risk patients, and further diagnostics and therapy should be conducted. This would make a removal of a patient from the working world understandable. However, the significance of the left ventricular function during exercise is apparently not well understood by German social medical evaluators. Independent of the behavior of the ΔEF, heart infarction patients are either classified as being capable of work or are given pensions. Only 41% of those patients with resting ejection fractions of more than 30% were correctly pensioned, as they showed a 5% decline of the ejection fraction during exercise. 49% of those patients classified as capable of work had in fact demonstrated a similar decline of 5% or more, and thus a poor prognosis as well. This is, in part, caused by patients themselves who wish to continue working. Disabled patients applied for pensions from the National Health Fund during the 2½ year observation period. In 9.5% of these patients, the unclear social medical situation is solely caused by the improper classification of these patients on the part of the evaluators.

Those patients with a subnormal climb or small decline (EF $\leqq \pm 5\%$) of the ejection fraction during exercise (so-called gray zone), could neither be put into the first group of patients with a normal rise (over 5%) nor into the third group having a distinct decline of the ejection fraction during exercise (over 5%). This is due to the methodological margin of error involved. This group is medically difficult to classify. For these patients, depending upon the clinical picture involved, further diagnostics should be carried out.

Aneurysm patients show a similar, parallel development with regard to the social situation. The pension rate is, at 65.5%, higher than among the remaining heart infarction patients without aneurysm. Here as well, all patients with a left ventricular function at rest of less than 30% were pensioned. There is no significant difference in pension rate for those patients with a resting ejection fraction greater than 30%. Approximately 55% of these patients demonstrate a distinct decline of the ejection fraction during exercise and are, in spite of good ventriculare function, categorized as having a poorer prognosis. 31% of the aneurysm patients were able to return to work. All of these patients had resting ejection fractions of more than 30%. However, 27% of these patients are, due to the decline of the ΔEF, high-risk patients. Only two patients were, after 2½ years, still incapable of working, and both showed distinct declines of

ΔEF. These patients should be pensioned. The social medical evaluation of aneurysm patients shows a cautious trend and a higher pension rate compared to the remaining heart infarction patients. Here as well, the uncertainty on the part of the evaluators as to the significance of the exercise ejection fraction can be seen.

According to our experiences, the prognosis for heart infarction patients can, using radionuclide ventriculography, be recognized early: Patients with resting ejection fractions of less than 30% (without aneurysm) should not return to work. Expensive rehabilitation does not seem to be useful for these patients. The existence of an aneurysm should be dealt with in relation to the ΔEF and the function of the remaining myocardium, and further diagnostics leading to possible operative procedures may be necessary. Myocardial infarction patients without aneurysm and with resting ejection fractions of 30% or more have a good prognosis and should undergo in-patient rehabilitation. If a distinct decline of left ventricular function during exercise is discovered, further diagnostics are indicated, along with consideration of bypass surgery.

Summary

Two hundred and thirty-nine patients were examined using radionuclide ventriculography (RNVA) at rest average of 8 weeks following heart infarction. In the cases of 188 patients, the ejection fraction was also determined during exercise. After an average of 2½ years, 16 patients (6.7%) had died. For patients with a left ventricular function at rest of under 30% the mortality was 30%, and therefore significantly higher than for patients whose ejection fractions at rest were over 30%. Patients with a decline in ejection fraction during exercise of 5% or more demonstrated a mortality of 10%, likewise significantly higher. Out of 34 aneurysm patients, three died (8.8%), two of whom had an ejection fraction at rest of less than 30%, while the one remaining patient showed a decline in ejection fraction during exercise of over 5%.

The social medical evaluation often considers the left ventricular function solely at rest. All patients with an ejection fraction at rest of under 30% were pensioned. The question of working ability was only considered in patients with a resting ejection fraction of over 30%. 46% of these patients were able to return to work. The significance of the behavior of the ejection fraction during exercise (ΔEF) is not known to social medical evaluators. Independent of the behavior of the ΔEF, patients were either classified as capable of work or given pensions. Aneurysm patients have a higher pension rate, but the tendency is comparable to the evaluation of heart infarction patients without aneurysms.

References

Borer JS, Bacharach SL, Green MV, Kent KM, Epstein SE, Johnston GS (1976) Rapid evaluation of left ventricular function during exercise in patients with coronary artery disease. Circulation [Suppl II] 54

Borer JS, Bacharach SL, Green MV, Kent KM, Epstein SE, Johnston GS (1977) Realtime radionuclide cineangiography in the noninvasive evaluation of global and regional left ventricular function at rest and during exercise in patients with coronary artery disease. N Engl J Med 296:839

Borer JS, Kent KM, Bacharach SL, Green MV, Rosing DR, Seides SF, Epstein SE, Johnston GS (1979) Sensitivity, specificity, and predictive accurary of radionuclide cineangiography during exercise in patients with coronary artery disease: comparison with exercise electrography. Circulation 60:572

Borer JS, Rosing DR, Miller RH, Stark RM, Kent KM, Bacharach SL, Green MV, Lake CR, Cohen H, Holmes D, Donohuc D, Baker W, Epstein SE (1980) Natural of history of left ventricular function during one year after acute myocardial infarction: Comparison with clinical, electrocardiographic and biochemical determinations. Am J Cardiol 46:1

Borer JS, Blümchen G, Bacharach SL, Green MV (1981) Application of radionuclide-based methods in exercise rehabilitation therapy: An overview and preliminary data. Echocardiography and radionuclid methodes lifelong rehabilitation in phase III. International Society and Federation of Cardiology, Munich

Grodzinski E, Kreutz F, Blümchen G, Borer JS (1983a) Über das Verhalten der Ruhe- und Belastungs-Auswurffraktion (EF) bei Herzinfarktpatienten vor und nach vierwöchigem Training. Vergleich zu einer Kontrollgruppe. Z Kardiol 72:105–118

Grodzinski E, Fentrop T, Koanantakul B, Bierck G, Minning E, Rücker H, Borer J, Schoop W, Blümchen G (1983b) Die Bedeutung der Radionuklidventrikulographie (RNV) für die sozialmedizinische Begutachtung von Herzinfarktpatienten. Öff Gesundheitswes 45:620–626

Wallis J, Borer JS, Moses JW, et al (1983) Radionuclide cineangiography during exercise: Prognostic importance in coronary artery disease (Abstr). J Am Coll Cardiol 1:733

Wenger NK (1984) Return to work or active life-style in patients with atherosclerotic coronary heart disease: Rehabilitation of the coronary patient. In: Hurst JW (ed) Clinical Essays on the heart, vol 2. McGraw-Hill, New York, p 319

Comparison of Active Participation in the Rotterdam Outpatient Cardiac Rehabilitation Program and Home Rehabilitation: A 5-Year Follow-up of a Controlled Clinical Trial on Psychological Well-Being: A Presentation on Behalf of CAPRI

R. A. M. Erdman and P. G. Hugenholtz

Material and Methods

The Rotterdam rehabilitation-program is named CAPRI, which stands for *Car*diopulmonary *R*esearch *I*nstitute and is an adaptation of the CAPRI program from Seattle [1]. It is an interactional rehabilitation program consisting of two sessions of 2 h training a week in a conventional gymnasium, supervised by a multidisciplinary team including a cardiologist, a psychologist, two physiotherapists, a social worker, and a nurse. Each training session consists of a period of warming up, jogging, gymnastics, volleyball, soccer or hockey, and relaxation exercises. Training is done under cardiologic supervision and resuscitation equipment is available. The entire program takes 6 months. The main goals of the CAPRI program are to restore physical capacity, to reduce fear and anxiety, and to enhance self-esteem [2, 3, 4]. Within the context of this rehabilitation program we were able to investigate changes in psychic functioning, work resumption, smoking habits, and the taking up of gymnastics as a habit, over a period of approximately 5 years.

During 1½ years 328 cardiac patients were referred to the CAPRI program and of these 80 conformed to the selection criteria of this study. Only male and married patients with a myocardial infarction which had occurred not longer than 6 months before the first psychological investigation were considered for the trial. Furthermore, they had to be younger than 65 years and mentally and physically fit to take part in the program. The 80 patients were randomly allocated either to participation in the CAPRI program or to physician-encouraged home rehabilitation. The patients of the home rehabilitation group (our control group) received a brochure with guidelines and advice for physical fitness training and jogging. All patients received the usual outpatient cardiological care. The dropout rate was 20% in both groups at the end of a rehabilitation period. Eight patients quit the CAPRI group earlier than planned: two died, two had a reinfarction, two had cardiac interventions, and two failed to attend. In the home group, 6 patients were removed from the study since they were no longer motivated to participate in the psychological tests, and two sets data were incomplete. Thus each group consisted of 32 patients after 6 months. Five years later the groups were reduced to 27 and 30 patients.

In the CAPRI group, two patients died, two were not longer motivated to participate in the study, and one was lost to follow-up. In the home group, two patients were eliminated: one got a reinfarction and participated in the CAPRI program, and one was treated in hospital for cancer. Both groups were examined three times by means of a structured interview and one psychological questionnaire entitled: Medical Psychological Questionnaire for Cardiac Patients [5]. This measures the four psychological concepts: WELL-BEING, FEELING OF BEING DISABLED, DISPLEASURE, and SOCIAL INHIBITION. The test was validated on a large reference group consisting of 1649 cardiac patients in the Netherlands. The interview gave information about cardiac events, smoking habits, sporting activities, work resumption, and life events.

Results

The 32 CAPRI patients who completed the study attended on average 75% of the training sessions offered. The two groups were comparable as to the incidence of life events, age, occupational level, and the incidence of cardiac events. At intake, the mean age of all 80 patients was 51 years (range 35–60 years).

Smoking Habits. After 6 months, within the CAPRI group only 28% reported they were smokers vs 47% in the home group ($P<0.01$). Five years later however, the results had changed completely; the CAPRI group included 52% smokers, while in the home group 36% reported they were smokers.

Gymnastics. As could be expected, after 6 months in the CAPRI group 87% participated in doing active sports vs only 50% in the home group ($P<0.01$). Five years later, this favourable results is continued. The majority of the CAPRI group (67%) has taken up gymnastics as a habit vs 45% in the home group. This result, however, was not statistically significant.

Work Resumption. It was striking that in the CAPRI group, after a follow-up period of 5 years 44% had resumed their work activities full-time, vs only 27% in the home group. The greater part of those who resumed their work activities part-time after 5 years were rehabilitated in the home group: 23% vs 11%. None of these findings were statistically significant.

Psychological Measurement. Figure 1 illustrates the data on the scales of the Medical Psychological Questionnaire for Cardiac Patients. The horizontal axis shows the three measurements over about 5 years, and on the vertical axis the test score is represented. Each mark in the graph represents the mean test score on the appropriate scale. In the case of well-being, the better the feeling, the higher the score.

During the second measurement, i. e., just after the end of the rehabilitation program, the difference in feelings of well-being is at the largest, in favour of the CAPRI group. Thus one can state: CAPRI has a favourable short-term affect on WELL-BEING, but these findings are reversed 5 years later. On the other three

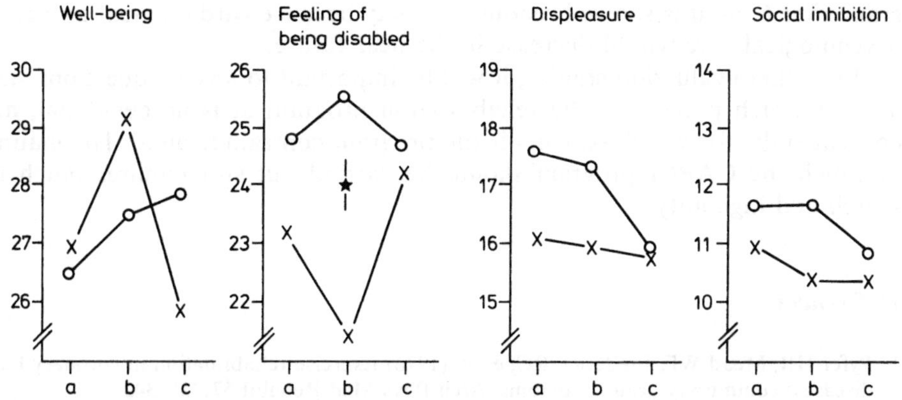

Fig. 1. Psychic functioning in both study groups: ×——×, CAPRI group; o——o, control group. ★, Mann-Whitney test, $P<0.05$, two-tailed. *a*, intake; *b*, 6 months; *c*, 5 years

graphs, the higher score means an unfavourable result. The only statistically significant result is in FEELINGS OF BEING DISABLED. After 6 months the rehabilitated group feels statistically significant less disabled than the control group. After 5 years this effect has practically disappeared. This tendency repeats itself in the remaining two items, DISPLEASURE and SOCIAL INHIBITION. After 6 months there exists a difference between the groups in favour of the CAPRI group. However, these results are not statistically significant, and after 5 years these findings have faded away.

Conclusions

1. Participation in the CAPRI program has a short-term favourable effect on smoking habits; this result is abolished 5 years later.
2. After 5 years, 67% of the rehabilitated group continued with sporting activities versus only 45% in the home group.
3. Participation in the CAPRI program has a long-term favourable effect on full-time work resumption.
4. Group rehabilitation on an outpatient basis enhances feelings of well-being and diminishes feelings of being disabled, displeasure, and social inhibition after 6 months. This effect disappeared almost completely after 5 years.

Discussion

Due to the small sample size, the results of this study are tentative and as yet not generalizable. Perhaps our patient groups were too small or the attendance rate within the rehabilitation group was not sufficient. Another explanation for our results could be that those patients who had to leave the rehabilitation program after 6 months showed rebound anxiety because cardiological as well as psychological care would decrease in the near future.

In further evaluation studies, it will be important to answer questions such as: For which patients is the rehabilitation program at issue beneficial, and consequently, for which patients is the program contraindicated? The manner in which the CAPRI program should be carried out still requires much research and ingenuity.

References

1. Pyfer HR, Mead WF, Frederick RC, et al (1976) Exercise rehabilitation in coronary heart diseases: community group programs. Arch Phys Med Rehabil 57:335–342
2. Bruce RA, Kusumi F, Bruce EM, et al (1977) Cardiovascular and psychological adaptations to prolonged physical training of coronary patients. Cardiology 62:83–84
3. Croog SH, Levine S, Lurie Z (1968) The heart patient and the recovery process. Soc Sci Med (1970) 2:111–164
4. Mulcahy R, Hickey N (1970) The rehabilitation of patients with coronary heart disease. Scand J Rehabil Med 2:108
5. Erdman RAM (1982) M.P.V.H.: Medisch Psychologische Vragenlijst voor Hartpatiënten. Swets & Zeitlinger, Lisse

Medical Problems and Hemodynamic Responses of Myocardial Revascularization Surgery Patients to Early Cardiac Rehabilitation

W. F. Dion, M. L. Pollock, C. Foster, P. Grevenow, S. Sennett, and D. H. Schmidt

In response to the development of alternative modes of treatment for individuals with coronary artery disease (CAD), formal cardiac rehabilitation programs have evolved. Most research concerning medical problems, functional capacity, and hemodynamic response to exercise prior to 1977 was conducted on myocardial infarction (MI) patients [10]. With the onset of 170000 coronary artery bypass surgery (CABS) procedures performed last year [2], documentation of responses to exercise with postsurgery patients was needed to help establish guidelines for exercise and a timetable for return to normal activity, such as gainful employment. Our experience with postsurgery patients spans 7 years of in-patient and out-patient cardiac rehabilitation (a combined total of 3500 patients). This text will summarize several studies conducted at this institution concerning the medical problems, heart rate (HR) and hemodynamic responses, electrocardiographic (ECG) changes, and level of functional capacity of CABS patients involved in a cardiac rehabilitation program.

In-Patient Cardiac Rehabilitation

Rehabilitative Exercise

Two studies have documented the effects of early exercise following CABS [5, 17]. Initially, 521 consecutive patients who had undergone CABS and entered an in-patient cardiac rehabilitation program were studied. Patients averaged 56 years of age and 86% were men. The average number of bypass grafts was four per patient and 12% had previously undergone CABS. Perioperative infarcts were found in 8% of those studied.

Patients were usually treated twice daily. The program began in the intensive care unit with range of motion (ROM) exercises and ambulation as tolerated. Exercise continued on the intermediate ward with ambulation increased by 100 ft (30.5 m) daily, and increased repetitions of the ROM exercises. When patients could perform a series of these exercises and ambulate 400 ft (121.9 m), rehabilitation sessions were conducted in the In-patient Exercise Center. These sessions consisted of a warm-up (ROM exercise), an aerobic period (treadmill ambulation or stationary cycling), stair-climbing, and a cooldown period.

Bedside ROM exercise and ambulation began 12–24 h after surgery for 65% of patients. Symptoms occurring most frequently were incisional discomfort (sternal, arm, or leg) (14%) and light-headedness (14%), with the incidence of angina pectoris and claudication low (4% and 3%, respectively). In the United States there are cardiac rehabilitation programs which prohibit CABS patients from performing upper extremity stretching until the sternum is healed (6–8 weeks); however, our experience with this type of activity has been successful in maintaining preoperative ROM and preventing surgery-related limitations. ROM exercises are especially important during this stage of recovery to help decrease postsurgical stiffness, to prevent chest wall adhesions and muscle shortening, and to maintain muscle tone. The appearance of sternal "clicking" or movement and wound infection would be an indication to stop the exercises until symptoms abate. Less than 5% of patients had sternal complications that precluded performing ROM exercise.

Ventricular dysrhythmias were the most frequently occurring medical problem (44%), with 22% of these dysrhythmias first detected during monitored cardiac rehabilitation. Hypotension was common in CABS patients and included orthostatic and exertional types (8%). Hypotension was defined as a standing resting systolic blood pressure (SBP) below 90 mmHg or an orthostatic decrease in SBP of 20 mmHg or more. A decrease in SBP of 10 mmHg with symptoms was a reason to terminate the exercise session.

In the Exercise Center (5–6 days postsurgery), treadmill exercise began at 2.0 METs for 8.6 min, with 61% of patients able to walk 10 min or more on their first day. HR increased by an average of 11.6 beats/min from standing rest, and SBP rose by 14.5 mmHg. At hospital discharge (11 days postsurgery), patients performed at 2.3 METs for 22.5 min. Forty-one percent of patients walked for 30 min at 2.0–2.5 mph (3.2–4 kph). HR increased by an average of 13.6 beats/min, and SBP rose by 16.3 mmHg. Patients tolerated this increase without persistent or increasing fatigue or significant morbidity.

ECG changes were manifested primarily by the incidence of ventricular dysrhythmias. Significant ventricular ectopy occurred in 37% of those studied and included frequent unifocal premature ventricular contractions (PVCs) (15%), multifocal PVCs (48%), ventricular couplets (32%), and nonsustained ventricular tachycardia (VT) (5%). The occurrence of VT resulted in additional drug manipulation, with follow-up holter monitoring prior to hospital discharge. Supraventricular dysrhythmias (atrial fibrillation, atrial flutter, and PAT) occurred in 17% of patients. Eight patients (2%) displayed significant ST-segment changes from baseline. Of the total medical problems seen in this study, 29% were first detected by the rehabilitation team, thus showing the importance of the cardiac rehabilitation program. This type of surveillance is thought to improve patient management. During 7 years of in-patient cardiac rehabilitation no cardiac arrest or mortality has been associated with this program.

Discharge Exercise Testing

Four studies have documented the safety of graded exercise testing (GXT) prior to discharge [6, 7, 13, 15], two of which conducted tests to symptom-limited maximum [6, 15]. Data from GXTs performed to symptom-limited maximum revealed an average functional capacity of 4.5 METs (range 2–9 METs), with 33 of the 86 patients in one study (38%) able to perform ≥6 METs at 11 days postsurgery. It was concluded that predischarge GXT was both safe and feasible for uncomplicated CABS patients prior to hospital discharge.

Out-Patient Cardiac Rehabilitation

Rehabilitative Exercise

Patients began the out-patient program within 1 week of hospital discharge. Exercise sessions were conducted three times per week for 45–75 min/session for up to 12 weeks. Telemetric monitoring was utilized during exercise for many, while others regulated exercise intensity by HR palpation. The initial 10–15 min were utilized as a warm-up and for muscle conditioning, and included both flexibility and strength exercises. During the first 8 weeks after surgery, patients used light dumbbells weighing 1–5 lbs (0.5–2.3 kg). Heavier weights [up to 17.5 lbs (8 kg)] were used later, as well as arm ergometry and combination arm-leg stationary cycling. More recently, Nautilus strength training equipment has been integrated into the out-patient program. The issue of weight training with cardiac patients is discussed in greater depth by Pollock et al. [12, 14]. The rationale for strength training will be addressed later in this paper.

The aerobic phase began at 20 min and increased to 45 min as adaptation took place. Those patients in need of weight reduction exercised up to 60 min. A variety of equipment was utilized, including treadmill, stationary cycle (traditional or arm-leg type), rowing machine, and arm ergometer. The exercise session concluded with a 5–10 min cool-down consisting of slow walking or free pedalling, stretching, and relaxation exercise. Intensity of training was kept low (20 beats/min above standing rest or 60%–70% of maximum HR range) until 30–45 min of aerobic exercise was well tolerated. After 8 weeks postsurgery, a symptom-limited GXT was performed and exercise intensity adjusted to 70%–85% of maximum HR range. The adjustment of training intensity after the 8-week GXT usually resulted in an increase in training HR of 10 beats/min.

Medical problems of 365 medical and surgical patients during a 12-week out-patient cardiac rehabilitation program were studied [16]. The average patient age was 57 years. MI and *CABS* patients differed significantly in medical problems for the following: angina 34 vs *19%*, hypotension 9 vs *4%*, and low-back discomfort 13 vs *6%*. Other problems prevalent but statistically nonsignificant between groups included ST-segment changes 14 vs *9%*, hypertension 6 vs *5%*, dyspnea and light-headedness 22 vs *22%*, orthopedic problems 7 vs *10%*, and claudication 6 vs *5%*. Sternal movement was reported by 3% of the postsurgical group. Patients who exhibited evidence of sternal instability or "clicking" were restriced from ROM and upper body strengthening exercises. These activities were later resumed with permission from the surgeon or primary physician.

The most predominant ECG change was dysrhythmia. Complex ventricular dysrhythmias occurred in 30% of those studied and supraventricular dysrhythmias occurred in 19%. The frequency and type of dysrhythmias occurred fairly equally in the medical and surgical groups, with the exception of VT. The higher percentage of VT in the surgical group (4 vs 12%) was also associated with greater drug manipulation and need for electrophysiology follow-up. In general, medical problems were prevalent but not life threatening. No cardiac arrest or mortality has occurred in the out-patient program.

The results of an exercise program on CABS patients were evaluated [6]. The overall MET level of the experimental group increased from 3.9 METs to 7.3 METs with exercise training, as compared to the increase of 3.7 METs to 5.7 METs for the control group. The randomized study clearly showed that an aggressive 24-week aerobic training program increased functional capacity at a faster rate than just ROM exercise and relaxation.

In the out-patient study of 365 patients, training MET levels for surgical patients were 2.8, 3.7, and 5.0 METs for the 1st, 2nd, and 3rd months, respectively [16]. Thus, the data suggest that by 8 weeks postsurgery, most uncomplicated CABS patients are physically capable of returning to work. Patients whose occupational or leisure time activity requires heavy arm work or moderate to heavy energy requirements may need a longer rehabilitation program.

As stated previously, strength training is thought to enhance recovery from CABS. More recently, Nautilus strength training equipment has been integrated into the out-patient program. The equipment includes machines designed to develop chest, shoulder, abdomen, low back, and trunk rotation muscles. Nautilus equipment is variable resistant and uses several different means to alter the mechanical advantage of the lever arm. This results in altered resistance to the patient through range of motion even though the weight on the weight stack is constant. The equipment is also designed to avoid hand gripping and may help minimize significant blood pressure increases with low to moderate lifting. The Nautilus strength training program is experimental at this time and CABS patients must meet the following criteria to participate: 6 weeks postsurgery, no sternal instability or infection, controlled hypertension, and normal left ventricular function (EF 50%). The extent of a strength training program is dependent upon medical status and patient need and desire. As an essential part of a rehabilitation program, it potentially can help prepare individuals for return to work and leisure time activity. A strength training program with selected cardiac patients appears safe since rhythmical arm activity at HRs (rate pressure products) similar to those with leg work has not been associated with increased dysrhythmia, ischemia, or incidence of cardiac events [4].

Major cardiovascular complications in cardiac rehabilitation programs have been infrequent [8, 9]. Early GXT has shown angina pectoris, significant dysrhythmias, significant ST-segment depression, poor blood pressure response, and poor exercise tolerance (≤ 3 METs) to be associated with increased risk of fatal and nonfatal events during the first year of recovery from an MI [1, 3, 11, 18]. Also, individuals with significant dysrhythmias and severe left ventricular dysfunction carry a much higher risk for sudden death [19]. These high-risk patients should be treated aggressively and followed carefully in cardiac rehabilitation programs. Hossack and Hartwig [9] demonstrated the need for closely monitoring exercise intensity to help prevent complications during training sessions. Individuals exhibiting cardiac arrest were found to exceed their upper limit training HR 56% of the time as compared to 24% for the controls. They were also above average in fitness and exercised with significant ST-segment depression. Thus, these data show that exercise in the range of 60%–85% of HR max reserve can be safe for most patients.

In summary, participation in a structured cardiac rehabilitation program soon after CABS is safe, hastens the overall recovery process, and provides additional surveillance resulting in better patient management. The frequency of dysrhythmias found during cardiac rehabilitation further documents the importance of monitoring and supervision during recovery after CABS. Program results seem to indicate that most patients are physiologically ready to return to work by 8 weeks after MI or surgery.

References

1. Bigger JT, Fleiss J, Kleiger R, Miller JP, Rolnitzky LM and the multicenter post-infarction research group (1984) The relationship among ventricular arrhythmias, left ventricular dysfunction, and mortality in the 2 years after myocardial infarction. Circulation 69(2):250–258
2. Braunwald E (1983) Effects of coronary artery bypass grafting on survival: Implications of the randomized coronary artery surgery study. N Engl J Med 309(19):1181–1184
3. Davidson DM, DeBusk RF (1980) Prognostic value of a single exercise test 3 weeks after uncomplicated myocardial infarction. Circulation 61:236–242
4. DeBusk RF, Valdez R, Houston N, Haskell W (1978) Cardiovascular reponses to dynamic and static effort soon after myocardial infarction. Application to occupational work assessment. Circulation 58:368–375
5. Dion W, Grevenow P, Pollock ML, Squires R, Foster C, Johnson WD, Schmidt DH (1982) Supervised inpatient cardiac rehabilitation: the patient after coronary artery bypass grafting. Heart Lung 11(3):248–255
6. Foster C, Pollock ML, Anholm J, Squires R, Ward A, Dymond D, Rod J, Saichek R, Schmidt DH (1984) Work capacity and left ventricular function during rehabilitation after myocardial revascularization surgery. Circulation 69(4):748–755
7. Gutmann MC, Squires RW, Pollock ML, Foster C, Anholm J (1981) Perceived exertion-heart rate relationship during exercise testing and training in cardiac patients. J Cardiac Rehabil 1:52–59
8. Haskell WL (1974) Cardiovascular complications during training of cardiac patients. Circulation 57:920–924
9. Hossack K, Hartwig R (1982) Cardiac arrest associated with supervised cardiac rehabilitation. J Cardiac Rehabil 2:402–408
10. Naughton JP, Hellerstein HK, Mohler LC (eds) (1973) Exercise testing and exercise training in coronary heart disease. Academic Press, New York
11. McNeer JF, Margolis JR, Lee KL, Kisslo JA, Peter RH, Kong Y (1978) The role of the exercise test in the evaluation of patients for ischemic heart disease. Circulation 57:64–70
12. Pollock ML (1984) Exercise regimens after myocardial revascularization (and other cardiac surgery): rationale and results. In: Wenger NK, Brest AN (eds) Exercise and the heart, 2nd ed. Davis, Philadelphia

13. Pollock ML, Foster C, Anholm J, Rod JL, Wolf FG, Akhtar M, Al-Nouri MB, Schmidt DH (1982) Diagnostic capabilities of exercise testing soon after myocardial revascularization surgery. Cardiology 69:358–365
14. Pollock ML, Wilmore J, Fox S (1984) Exercise in health and disease: Evaluation and prescription for prevention and rehabilitation. Saunders, Philadelphia
15. Rod J, Squires R, Pollock ML, Foster C, Schmidt DH (1982) Symptom-limited graded exercise testing soon after myocardial revascularization surgery. J Cardiac Rehabil 2:199–205
16. Sennett S, Pollock ML, Pels A, Foster C, Dolatowski R, Patel S (1984) Medical problems of cardiac patients in an outpatient cardiac rehabilitation program. Med Sci Sports Exerc 16(2):149
17. Silvidi GE, Squires RW, Pollock ML, Foster C (1982) Hemodynamic responses and medical problems associated with early exercise and ambulation in coronary artery bypass graft surgery patients. J Cardiac Rehabil 2(5):355–362
18. Theroux P, Waters DD, Halphen C, Debaisieux JD, Mizgala HF (1979) Prognostic value of exercise testing soon after myocardial infarction. N Engl J Med 301:341–345
19. Wolf FG, Akhtar M (1979) Sudden cardiac death. In: Pollock ML, Schmidt DH (eds) Heart disease and rehabilitation. Wiley, New York

Inability to Work After Myocardial Infarction: A 5-Year Follow-up Study

G. Stein, H. Jungmann, E. O. Krasemann, and M. Zothner

The rates of a return to work after myocardial infarction are still, even today, unsatisfactory. The factors which lead to a late return to work are well known. Apart from medical reasons it is above all the far-reaching sociological changes in the attitude to work and the declining job market which affect return to work after cardiac infarction. On account of these changes the positive effects of the follow-up therapeutic treatment and comprehensive rehabilitation are weakened. In a prospective study of 1019 random patients in Hamburg it emerged that only 53% of those under 60 were again employed 18 months after a first cardiac infarction from which they had recovered (Weiß 1983). In our experience the same well-known factors which impede reintegration into working life apply to patients after bypass operations.

Two questions were to be answered by our investigations:

1. Can early return to work after MI be improved by better collaboration between cardiologists, rehabilitation physicians, general practitioners, and patients?
2. Will the prognosis after *early* return to work be negatively influenced?

In 1976, in a retrospective study of 153 infarction patients, we had established that the date of return to work, fixed by the doctors of the rehabilitation clinic in conjunction with the patients, was only adhered to in 22% of cases. 73% of the patients had become fit for work at a later date than that previously expected by the rehabilitation clinic (Krasemann und Jungmann 1979). Therefore a prospective study was set up in the same rehabilitation clinic. The groups of patients in the study were similar in age, diagnosis, sex, and social background. In the second study only the style of the discharge discussion in the rehabilitation clinic and the cooperation with the G.P. was altered (Stein und Krasemann 1981).

The methodologies of the first (retrospective) and the second (prospective) studies are summarized in Tables 1 and 2. The results of both studies are summarized in Tables 3 and 4.

Table 1. Methodology of the first, retrospective study (patients aged 35–55 years, $n = 153$)

1. Agreement between rehabilitation physicians and each patient about return to work
2. Result of the discussion was noted in the report to the G.P.
3. In the discharge report a recommendation was made as to the duration of incapacity

Table 2. Methodology of the second, prospective study (patients aged 35–55 years, $n = 124$)

1. Agreement between rehabilitation physicians and each patient about return to work (corresponding to the first study)
2. Results of the discussion were noted in the report to the G.P. (corresponding to the first study)
3. Dialogue between the rehabilitation physician and patient about *date* of return to work
4. Cooperation between the rehabilitation physician and the G.P.
   a) Contact regarding the time of recommended return to work
   b) Discussion with the G.P. about reasons for patient's ability or inability to work

Table 3. Result of first study

Validity of prognosis	
1. Correct prognosis	$n = 32$ (22%)
2. Incorrect prognosis	
= later return to work	$n = 112$ (73%)
3. Retired	$n = 8$ (5%)

Table 4. Results of second study

Validity of prognosis	
1. Correct prognosis	
= fitness for work	
at recommended time	$n = 93$ (75%)
2. Incorrect prognosis	$n = 31$
a) Later return to work	$n = 25$ (20%)
b) Retired/deaths	$n = 6$ (5%)

By means of improved cooperation between the doctors of the rehabilitation clinic and the G.P., the period of incapacity for work after discharge from the rehabilitation clinic could be reduced from 4.3 months to 7 weeks.

The duration of incapacity for work, including the stay in intensive care, totalled 21 weeks (Fig. 1). According to the results of our investigations, neither the extent of the vascular disorder nor the degree of left ventricular damage nor the physical stress in the profession was a decisive criterion for the date of resumption of the profession (Table 5). Factors which negatively influenced early return to work are shown in Table 6.

Table 5. Factors which did *not* influence early return to work

1. Physical capacity (ergometry)
2. Symptoms of angina or dyspnea
3. ST-segment depression
4. Heart volume
5. Arrhythmias

Table 6. Factors which negatively influenced early return to work

1.	Insufficient cooperation between clinical/rehabilitation physicians and G.P.s
2.	Anxiety of the patient and members of his family
3.	Unsatisfactory knowledge of the work load entailed by the job
4.	Socioeconomic and organizational factors

In our experience the G.P. is often overtaxed with regard to the question of fitness for work, and, on account of insufficient data and misinterpretation of symptoms, tends to warn patients against a return to work. In the closing medical report, therefore, in a concluding assessment, the following are imperative: information about the job and circumstances of the job, a statement on the quantitative and qualitative performance capabilities, and an individual sociomedical assessment of the particular case. Moreover a recommendation by doctors from the rehabilitation clinic regarding the precise date of renewed fitness for work is of major importance. From our investigations the key position of the G.P. administering further treatment becomes clear. While in our previous investigations only 22% of petients became fit for work on the recommended date, this percentage was increased to 75% by additional contact with the G.P.

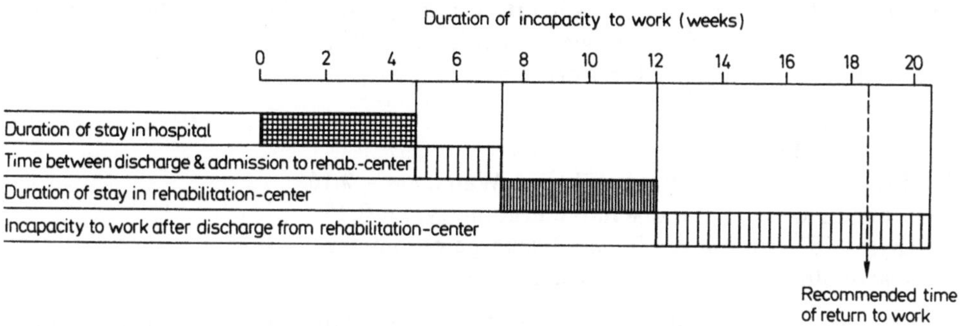

Fig. 1. Duration of incapacity (mean value, weeks) from admission to return to work ($n = 118$)

It was the object of a further investigation to establish whether a premature return to work negatively influences the course of coronary heart disease. Catamnestic surveys of the 124 patients of the second prospective study were conducted over 5 years. The results are summarized in Table 7.

In the course of the 5 years, ten patients (8.1%) died for cardiac reasons and one patient (0.8%) due to a stroke. Thirteen patients (10.5%) suffered a reinfarction and in the case of 25 patients (20%) a new incapacity for work temporarily occurred on account of coronary heart disease. During the period of observation only 13 patients (10%) were retired; 100 patients (80.7%) were fully fit for work even after 5 years.

Table 7. Does *early* return to work negatively influence coronary heart disease? Results in 124 patients, followed up by questionnaires for about 5 years

Mortality (cardiac death)		1.6% per year
Reinfarction (survived)		2.8% per year
Intermittent incapacity	$n = 25$	20.0%
Retired	$n = 8$	10.5%
Continued to work	$n = 100$	80.7%

The most deaths occurred in the third year after cardiac infarction; almost two-thirds of the survived reinfarctions occurred in the fourth and fifth years. In the case of workers and skilled workers retirement and cardiac deaths were somewhat, but not significantly, more frequent than in other professional categories.

In answer to the question of which factors led to a renewed incapacity for work due to coronary heart disease, a correlation analysis was conducted. This investigated the following variables: the connection between the duration of renewed incapacity for work due to coronary heart disease and social status, age, the highest Watt level reached at the time of discharge from the rehabilitation clinic, the absence or incidence of ischemia signs, the absence or incidence of rhythmic disturbances, as well as heart-volume in ml/kg body weight. The following correlation coefficients were calculated (Zothner 1983):

Duration of incapacity for work and

a) Social status, $r = 0.15$
b) Age, $r = 0.09$
c) Physical performance capability in Watts, $r = -0.16$
d) Ischemia signs in the discharge ergometry, $r = 0.26$
e) Rhythmic disturbances in the discharge ergometry, $r = 0.15$
f) Heart-volume (ml/kg body weight), $r = 0.18$

Nowhere in the results of the correlation calculation is a proven relation apparent between the duration of incapacity for work and the somatic or sociodemographic data listed.

Our investigations permit no direct comparison with other statistics on account of the positive selection of infarction patients. However, there are no indications in our investigations that, even 5 years after cardiac infarction, early reintegration into working life presents a particular threat.

In summary, our investigations permit the following conclusions:

1. Early return to work after MI should be improved by (a) motivation of, and provision of comprehensive information to patients, and (b) better cooperation between cardiologists, rehabilitation physicians, family doctors, and occupational physicians.
2. Coronary heart disease does not seem to be negatively influenced by early return to work.

References

Krasemann EO, Jungmann H (1979) Return to work after myocardial infarction. Cardiology 64:190

Stein G, Krasemann EO (1981) Prospektive Untersuchungen zur Dauer der Arbeitsunfähigkeit nach Herzinfarkt. Herz/Kreisl 11:526–532

Weiß B (1983) Wiederaufnahme der Arbeit nach erstem Herzinfarkt. Ergebnisse der Hamburger Infarkt-Nachsorge-Studie. Dtsch Med Wochenschr 108:1872–1875

Zothner M (1983) Katamnestische Untersuchungen über 5 Jahre bei Infarktpatienten, denen bei der Entlassung zur Wiederaufnahme der Arbeit innerhalb von 10 Wochen geraten worden war. Inaugural Dissertation, Hamburg

Postoperative Work Rehabilitation

B. Rigler, F. Iberer, J. Kraft-Kinz, and W. Klein

Successful coronary artery bypass (ACBG) surgery can favorably influence the postoperative work rehabilitation of patients as well as improve their symptomatic status and functional capacity. However, varying proportions of patients working postoperatively have been reported from country to country. For that reason a study was initiated to evaluate and compare effectively rehabilitated patients and nonworking patients in respect of a number of medical and socioeconomic factors which have been identified as predictive of return to work after ACBG surgery.

Patients and Methods

Three hundred and thirty unselected patients operated upon between 1974 and 1982 were analyzed retrospectively with regard to the incidence of myocardial infarctions (MIs), coexisting disorders, and the year and kind of surgical therapy (isolated or combined procedures). From January 1984 to March 1984 the patients were contacted either personally or by mailed questionnaires; complete information was available for 248. The patients' symptomatic status (at mild and moderate exertion), their present medications, worsening of symptoms, and frequency of postoperative MIs were compared. Furthermore, a set of characteristics like education, preoperative employment status, job classification, and income was taken into consideration as well as the influence of waiting periods and patients' participation in rehabilitation measures (Fig. 1).

Among the 248 patients who were included in the study there were 25 female and 223 male patients. At the time of surgery 15% (37) of the patients were less than 45 years old. The age of 38% ranged from 46 to 55 years. 47.2% (117) were older than 56 years, and 4% (10) were over the age of 65 years.

Preoperatively 74.6% of the patients had a history of one or more MIs. Of these patients, 16% were diabetic and 21.3% required antihypertensive treatment. 225 (91%) had undergone isolated ACBG surgery. 23 (9%) had concomitant resection of left ventricular aneurysms (LVA). Postoperatively, 65.4% of the patients presented free of angina pectoris (AP) at moderate exertion (the patients were requested to test their physical capacity by climbing one or two floors) (Fig. 2). During a follow-up period of 1–9 years documented MIs occurred in 8.8% (22) of the entire series. 31 (12.5%) developed mild to moderate heart failure and were treated by digitalis and diuretics. 41 (16.5%) patients had been restudied angiographically, mainly due to worsening of anginal symp-

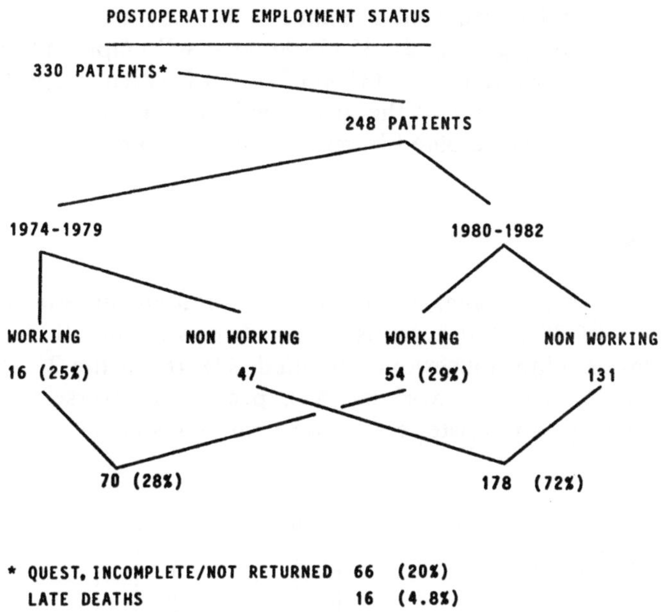

Fig. 1. Composition of the study

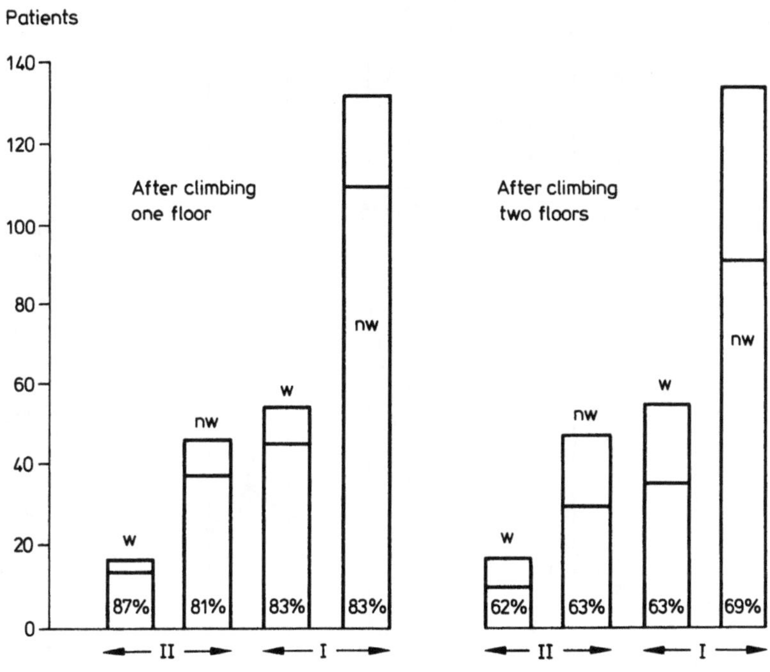

Fig. 2. Exertional pattern of angina pectoris in working *(W)* and nonworking patients *(NW)* with follow-up periods of 1–3 years *(I)* or 4–9 years *(II)*. (% – free of angina pectoris)

toms, and five required a second ACBG operation. 37 (15%) were college and/or university graduates, 45 (18%) were self-employed, and 79 (31.8%) had retired preoperatively. 77 (31%) of the 248 patients reported a major loss of annual income. 9.4% of the group waited more than 1 month for the operation and 85.4% participated in rehabilitation programs.

Results

Irrespective of age, sex, preoperative retirement, and duration of follow-up a total of 70 (28%) patients returned to work and 178 (72%) remained unemployed. With housework excluded, 32% (8) of the 25 women and 62 (27%) of the 223 men were working. As expected, an inverse relation was observed between age and postoperative occupational status (Fig. 3). After isolated ACBG

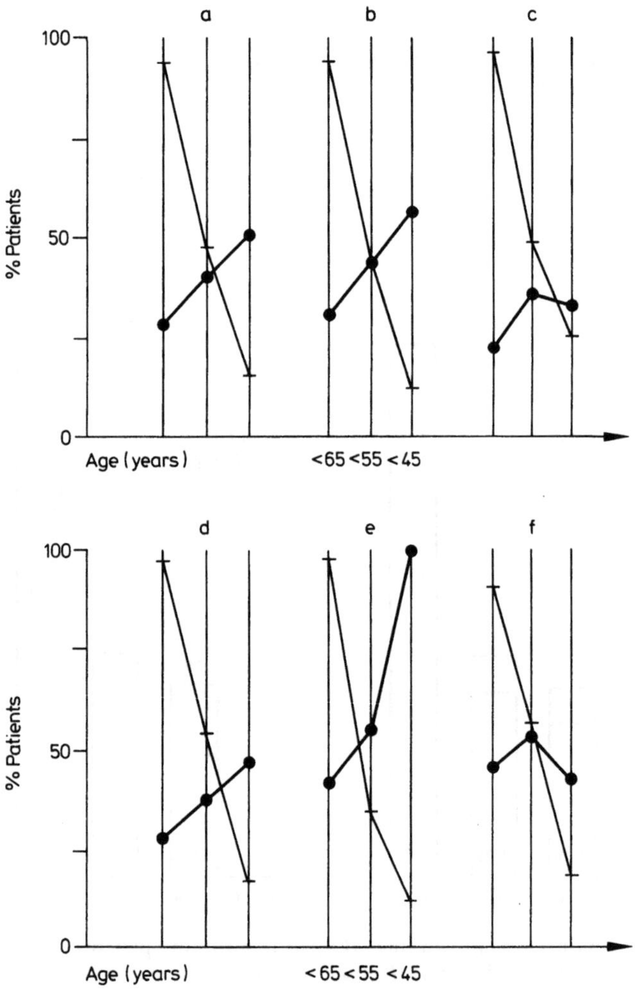

Fig. 3a–f. The influence on postoperative work rehabilitation of different factors is shown in relation to patients' age: *a* Entire series of 248 patients; *b* 225 patients with isolated ACBG surgery; *c* 23 patients with concomitant resection of left ventricular aneurysms; *d* 223 men; *e* 25 women; *f* 37 college and/or university graduates. +, percentage of patients operated upon; •, percentage of patients working postoperatively

surgery the percentage of working subjects decreased from 55% among patients less than 45 years old to 41% in patients less than 55 years old and 30% among patients aged less than 65 years (Fig. 3 B). With combined procedures the proportion of working patients of corresponding age groups was 33%, 35%, and 22% respectively (Fig. 3 C). The postoperative employment status was not affected by the history of myocardial infarction and diabetes. However, only 22.6% of hypertensive patients worked postoperatively, whereas 46.4% of normotensive patients did so. 40.5% of college and/or university graduates were employed, while 26% of those who had completed elementary and high school returned to work. Little difference in postoperative occupational status was seen with self-employed and salaried people (35.5% versus 27%). 35.5% of 107 white-collar workers and 23% of 141 blue-collar workers and professionals returned to work. Those patients who classified their jobs as executive were more likely to return to work (35% versus 23% nonexecutive). Out of 169 patients disabled or working at the time of surgery, 35.5% were working, and 12% of 79 patients who had retired preoperatively were found to be employed.

With regard to the waiting list, no difference could be found according to whether waiting periods were less or more than 1 month, since the corresponding working rates were 29% and 28%. 30% of the patients who participated in rehabilitation programs were employed. Among 36 subjects who did not participate in a rehabilitation program, only 19% worked postoperatively. A rather small improvement in postoperative work status was observed among patients operated on more recently (1980–1982 versus 1974–1979), since the percentages of employed patients were 29.2% and 25.4% respectively (Fig. 4). Within both groups (working and nonworking) of patients the incidences of MI (pre- and postoperatively) and diabetes were nearly identical: 64.3% of the working patients presented free of AP and 7% (5) suffered postoperative MIs, while the corresponding figures for the nonworking cohort were 65.7% and 9.5%. 11% of the employed patients and 13% of the nonworking group required digitalis and diuretics due to heart failure. In the two groups angiographic restudies were performed in 16% and 17% respectively (Table 1). 26% of the working subjects and 33% of the nonworking patients reported a major loss of income. Only five patients who worked postoperatively changed their occupational status, and 24 were periodically unemployed.

Comment

Postoperative work rehabilitation of working age patients is considered to be an important objective of ACBG surgery. In contrast to recent papers, in our series the proportion of patients successfully rehabilitated was rather small. The rate of postoperative employment did not increase significantly during the 9-year period despite more complete revascularization in recent years. Motivation to return to work was clearly influenced by age, educational level, and preoperative employment status Patients who participated in postoperative rehabilitation programs were more likely to return to work. Within a broad range the occupational status after ACBG surgery seemed to be unrelated to the

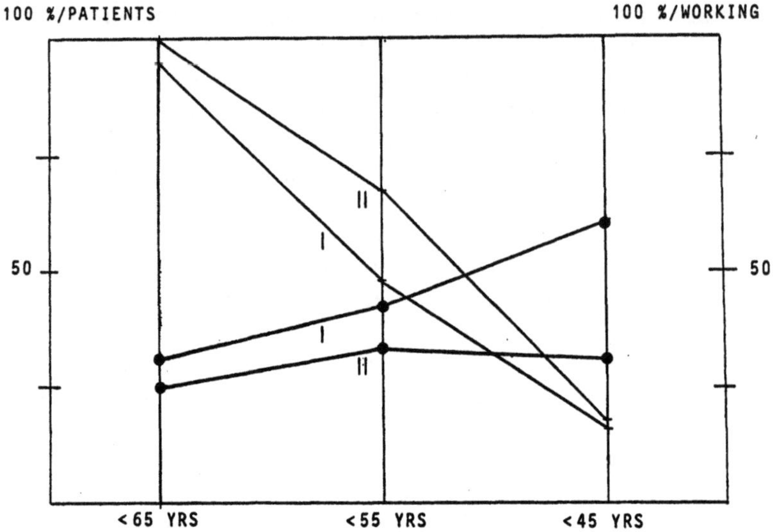

Fig. 4. Relation between age and postoperative work rehabilitation of two cohorts of patients with follow-up periods of 1–3 years (*I*, 185) or 4–9 years (*II*, 63). +, percentage of patients operated upon; •, percentage of patients working postoperatively

Table 1. Myocardial infarctions, coexisting disorders, and patients' present symptomatic status in relation to the postoperative occupational status. (% – percentage of the entire number of working/nonworking patients)

	Working	Nonworking
History of MI	50 (71%)	135 (76%)
Diabetes	10 (14%)	30 (17%)
Hypertension	12 (17%)	41 (23%)
Angina free postop.	45 (64%)	117 (66%)
MI during follow-up[a]	5 (7%)	17 (9.5%)
Digitalis and diuretics	8 (11%)	23 (13%)
Angiographic restudy	11 (16%)	30 (17%)
ACBG reoperation	1	4

[a] Follow-up, 1–9 years

symptomatic pattern of anginal symptoms, coexisting disorders, and the frequency of pre- and postoperative myocardial infarctions.

According to our national health care and insurance systems, major loss of income – probably one of the most important factors – was reported by only 32% of the unemployed patients, underlining the importance of better psychological preparation of patients, their families, and physicians.

References

1. Guvendik G, Rahan M, Yacoub M (1982) Symptomatic status and pattern of employment during a five-year period following myocardial revascularisation for angina. Ann Thorac Surg 34/4:383–389
2. Liddle HV, Jensen R, Clayton PD (1982) The rehabilitation of coronary surgical patients. Ann Thorac Surg 34/4:374–382

Survival After Return to Work

C. Seidel, U. Stocksmeier, and R. Wegscheider

Introduction

From a prospective study of male patients in rehabilitation after myocardial infarction, 57 persons from the Upper Bavarian Myocardial Infarction Study who underwent coronary arteriography and aortocoronary bypass graft surgery are analyzed, comparing those patients who returned to work after their infarction and were still working according to our last information with those patients who stopped working during observation. Further comparison was made between the men alive at the time of the last observation and the late postoperative deaths. The participants in the study went to rehabilitation to the Klinik Höhenried after their myocardial infarction and were examined twice a year until death or drop-out.

Material and Methods

The mean observation time after operation was 72.9 ± 38.6 months. The mean age was 49.2 ± 8.0 years. Two early postoperative deaths and six late deaths were observed. The following variables were analyzed, using either corrected chi-square or Student's *t*-test:

- Number and localization of preoperative MI
- Number and localization of bypass graft anastomosis
- Long-term medication during observation, diagnosis, risk factors, ECG changes, mean and highest exercise test work load of all examinations before and after the first coronary arteriography, number of diseased vessels (1–3), ventricular function (1–5), and coronary score (1–5).

Results

Workers vs Nonworkers

Observations comparing workers and nonworkers are shown in Table 1.

The number of diseased vessels, coronary score, ventricular function, number of bypassed vessels, and number of preoperative MIs did not differ significantly. The time of postoperative observations was longer for the worker group.

Table 1. Workers vs nonworkers

Variable	Workers ($n=28$)	Miss-ing	Nonworkers ($n=29$)	Miss-ing	Test
No. of diseased vessels	2.07 ± 0.87	1	2.22 ± 0.80	2	NS
Coronary score	3.70 ± 0.87	1	3.74 ± 0.86	2	NS
Ventricular function	2.56 ± 1.05	1	2.30 ± 0.37	2	NS
No. of bypassed vessels	1.79 ± 1.10		1.97 ± 1.09		NS
No. of preop. MIs	1.32		1.31		NS
Months of postop. observ.	77.6 ± 43.4		68.5 ± 33.5		NS
Year of operation	74.7 ± 2.5		76.0 ± 2.2		$P<0.05$
Age at operation	45.3 ± 8.4		52.8 ± 5.8		$P<0.001$
Lipid-lowering drugs	8 ≙ 29%		2 ≙ 7%		$P<0.1$
Digitalis	9 ≙ 32%		16 ≙ 55%		NS
Exercise, mean working load - before	80.3 ± 25.7	6	75.7 ± 16.8	6	NS
	↑		↑		
	$P<0.05$		NS		
	↓		↓		
- after	96.2 ± 29.6	3	67.6 ± 26.2	3	$P<0.001$
Exercise, max. working load - before	96.6 ± 34.8	6	94.6 ± 24.9	6	NS
	↑		↑		
	$P<0.005$		NS		
	↓		↓		
- after	125.0 ± 35.4	3	84.6 ± 28.4	3	$P<0.001$
Bypass LAD	20 ≙ 71%		26 ≙ 90%		NS
Death rate	6 ≙ 23%	($n=26$)	0		$P<0.05$

The workers were operated on at an earlier time ($P=0.05$), which is partially responsible for the longer observation time. They were far younger than the nonworkers ($P=0.001$) and were more frequently using lipid-lowering drugs ($P=0.1$) and less digitalis (NS). The exercise testing before and after the first arteriography showed a significant increase in physical capacity for the workers, whereas the nonworkers showed an even lower capacity, so that after arteriography the workers had significantly higher levels ($P=0.001$).

It was remarkable but not significant that the nonworker group had more frequently had the LAD bypassed.

Excluding the early postoperative mortality, the death rate was 23% for workers and 0 for nonworkers ($P=0.05$).

Survivors vs Nonsurvivors

Comparing the patients who died late ($n=6$) with all survivors ($n=49$), there was a significantly higher number of preoperative MIs in the dead group (1.67 ± 0.75 vs. 1.29 ± 0.50; $P=0.05$). The localization of the first MI was anterior for 5 (83%) of the dead and for 18 (37%) of the survivors, showing a difference on the $P=0.1$ level.

Three (50%) of the dead had ventricular conduction defects in the ECG compared to seven (14%) of the living ($P=0.1$; one-tailed probability). A myocardial aneurysm was found in three (50%) of the dead and in seven survivors (14%) ($P=0.1$; one-tailed probability).

Excluding the early and the late deaths produced no change in the comparison of workers and nonworkers, except for the difference in lipid-lowering drugs, which was no longer significant, and the observation time, which now differed significantly (workers $n=20$, 92.9±35.4; nonworkers $n=29$, 68.5±33.5; $P=0.01$). This difference could cause a disturbance, especially affecting the death rates. Therefore, observation time was limited to a level which half of the living patients exceeded. About half (25 of 49) of the survivors had more than 6 years of observation time. Thus excluding early deaths, the death rate for the workers fell to 5 (19%), which was still significant in comparison to the nonworkers ($P=0.05$). The cut observation time for workers was now 59.8±16.95, and that for nonworkers, 52.5±18.0 months (NS).

Due to the low number of cases in the late death group, only their worse ventricular function and the lower percentage of bypass grafts on the LAD were statistically different from findings in the survivors (Table 2). It is remarkable that the late deaths tended to be younger and to have a higher working capacity than the survivors.

Table 2. Survivors vs late deaths

Variable	Late deaths ($n=5$)	Missing	Survivors ($n=50$)	Missing	Test
No. of diseased vessels	2.0 ±1.15	1	2.15±0.12	2	NS
Coronary score	4.0 ±1.16	1	3.70±0.85	2	NS
Ventricular function	3.25±0.96	1	2.33±0.93	2	$P<0.1$
No. of bypassed vessels	1.40±0.55		1.88±1.10		NS
Age at operation	43.40±11.0		49.7 ±7.6		NS
Lipid-lowering drugs	2≙40%		6≙12%		NS
Exercise mean after	101±29.9	0	79.5±30.9	5	NS
Exercise max. after	116.7±30.3	0	103.4±38.7	5	NS
Bypass LAD	2≙40%		42≙84%		$P<0.1$

Discussion

It is a surprising result of our study that CABG patients who returned to work after MI seemed more likely to die, though they were younger than men who stopped working and had a significantly better operation result concerning their physical working capacity. We do not think that this increased mortality can be explained by the fact that the workers were operated on about 1.3 years earlier and did not profit from the advances in surgical technique. Also, the more frequent use of lipid-lowering substances seemed to be no definite reason. It may be that psychosocial variables strongly determine the return to work. It also may be that maximum work in exercise testing is influenced by the patient's wish to go to work or not. This could perhaps explain the higher death rate in a seemingly healthier collective that is exposed to remaining stress.

Survival was also negatively influenced by an anterior localization of a previous MI, the presence of myocardial aneurysm, and a deterioration in left ventricular function.

Cardiac Rehabilitation: Influence on Work Resumption

A. Vermeulen, J. J. Koolen, A. C. Moulijn, and N. Slangen-Schotermann

Introduction

Cardiac rehabilitation has been advocated as a measure to ameliorate the psychological and physical condition of the patient with myocardial infarction [1-3]. The study of Sanne [4] was the first controlled study, but the follow-up period was too short to show a definite effect on the prognosis. The study which was undertaken in our center was the first that showed a positive effect on prognosis by a reduction of 50% in coronary events in the 5 years after a first myocardial infarction (Fig. 1) [5]. As we in that study could not find any effect of cardiac rehabilitation [6] and angina pectoris proved to be the major determinant in return to work after myocardial infarction (Table 1), we decided to evaluate the effect of coronary artery surgery on work resumption.

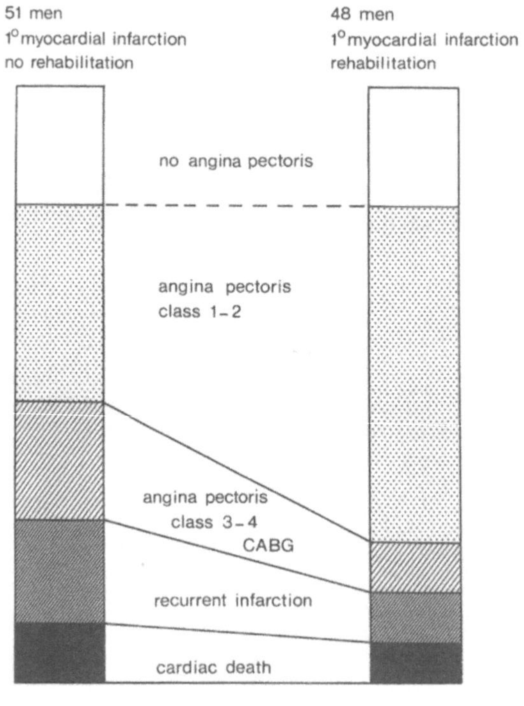

Fig. 1. Effect of rehabilitation on angina pectoris, recurrent infarction, and cardiac death in the 5 years after a first myocardial infarction

Table 1. The influence of angina pectoris on return to work after a first myocardial infarction in 77 men aged 40–55 years who were fully employed at the time of myocardial infarction and were still alive 5 years afterwards[a]

		Still at work 1 year after MI	Still at work 5 years after MI
Angina pectoris	38	25 (12)	13 (5)
No angina pectoris	39	34 (26)	27 (21)

[a] The figures in parenthesis give the number of patients working full-time

Patient Material and Methods

A retrospective study was undertaken on (a) the 100 consecutive patients who underwent coronary artery bypass surgery in our center during the period January 1972 till October 1976 and (b) the 27 patients who were referred to the rehabilitation institute for rehabilitation after coronary bypass surgery during the months January–October 1983. Referral was based on the indication of poor progression of the physical and/or psychological condition of the patients. A symptom-limited exercise test was performed using a bicycle ergometer starting with load of 30 W, with increases of 30 W every 3 min.

Results

Part I. At the moment of the study 6 of the 100 had died, of whom 4 suffered a cardiac death. Three patients were lost to follow-up. Of the remaining 91 still alive, 34 had no complaints, 28 were in class II/IV (New York Heart Association), 13 in class III/IV, and 16 in class IV/IV (Table 2). Only 33% of the patients alive were still at work 7–10 years after coronary artery bypass surgery.

Table 2. Functional status 7–10 years after coronary artery bypass surgery ($n=91$)

No complaints	34
II/IV (NYHA)	28
III/IV	13
IV/IV	16

Part II. Of the 27 patients 12 had either a sickness payment (9) or were retired (3), nine worked full-time, and six part-time. None of the patients retired or on sickness payment returned to work. At 6 months after coronary artery bypass surgery 12 of the 15 patients working before their hospitalization returned to work, mostly part-time with the intention of returning to full-time work. There was no difference in exercise tolerance between the patients who returned to work and those who did not (Table 3).

Table 3. Influence of work status and cardiac rehabilitation on exercise tolerance after coronary bypass surgery (expressed as a percentage of the expected exercise tolerance)

	Before rehabilitation	After rehabilitation
Returned to work	76 ± 12 ($n=12$)	84 ± 14 ($n=11$)
Did not return to work	73 ± 13 ($n=15$)	84 ± 16 ($n=13$)

Table 4. Angina pectoris after coronary artery bypass surgery and return to work in 27 patients referred for cardiac rehabilitation

	Returned to work	Did not return to work
Angina pectoris + ($n=11$)	4	7
Angina pectoris – ($n=16$)	7	9

Sixteen patients reported total relief of anginal complaints, but there was no relation between the existence of angina pectoris after coronary artery bypass surgery and return to work (Table 4).

Discussion

As angina pectoris was one of the major factors in determining return to work, one would expect that a therapy that relieves this symptom will reduce its influence. According to Westaby et al. [7] coronary artery bypass surgery led to an appreciable reduction of symptoms in 90% of the patients, clearing the way for work resumption, irrespective of the type of job. Russell et al. [8] likewise reported a decrease of symptoms, but also a substantial drop in income due to a very low degree of return of work (44.7%). In the Netherlands, employees on sick leave currently receive 80%–100% of their salary for 1 year and after that 70%–75% until retirement age. It is probably this type of social security and the bad status of the labor market that leads to the failure of surgery to improve the rate of return to work. The incapacity of the patients returning to work 3–6 months after surgery ranged from −28% to +11% with a mean of −16%. It is therefore remarkable that these patients did resume their work, and there must be psychological factors which determine this behavior. A lot of studies have stressed these factors as important for return to work after myocardial infarction, but it is not definitely known whether these factors are equally important after coronary artery bypass surgery. A controlled study of cardiac rehabilitation after coronary artery bypass surgery will hopefully answer these questions.

Conclusion

In a retrospective study a low rate of return to work was found in a group of Dutch patients, and there was no indication that cardiac rehabilitation improved the work status. Previous employment before surgery proved to be the main determinant of work, and the influence of cardiac rehabilitation may be counteracted by the relatively high disability benefits in the Netherlands.

References

1. Wenger NK (1969) The use of exercise in the rehabilitation of patients after myocardial infarction. JSC Med Assoc [Suppl I] 65:66–68
2. Hellerstein HK (1968) Exercise therapy in coronary disease. Bull NY Acad Med 44:1028–1047
3. Gottheiner V (1968) Long range strenuous sports training for cardiac reconditioning and rehabilitation. Am J Cardiol 22:426–435
4. Sanne H (1973) Exercise tolerance and physical training of nonselected patients after myocardial infarction. Acta Med Scand [Suppl] 551
5. Vermeulen A, Lie KI, Durrer D (1983) Effects of cardiac rehabilitation after myocardial infarction: changes in coronary risk factors and long-term prognosis. Am Heart J 105:798–801
6. Vermeulen A, Lie KI, Durrer D (1981) De invloed van revalidatie na een eerste hartinfarct bij mannen van middelbare leeftijd op de werkhervatting na 3–5 jaar. Ned Tijdschr Geneesk 125:1921–1924
7. Westaby S, Sapsford R, Bentall HH (1979) Return to work and quality of life after surgery for coronary artery disease. Br Med J 2:1028–1031
8. Russell RO, Wayne JB, Kronenfield J et al (1980) Surgical versus medical therapy for treatment of unstable angina. Am J Cardiol 45:134–140

Summary of the Discussion

N. K. Wenger

Wenger: I only regret that we did not have adequate time to discuss the last four papers (Dion, Stein, Seidel, Vermeulen, Rigler) because they are most interesting. Prof. Walter tells me that in the interest of rehabilitating the audience he will not schedule the concluding panel that is on your program.

You are free to discuss any of the issues with the individuals involved. He has asked me to summarize this session for you, realizing that perhaps some of our discussions will have to be deferred to a subsequent meeting on this topic.

I expect what we all have encountered is that although coronary bypass surgery decreases symptoms and improves function, there is considerable question as to its effect on return to work. The other issue of importance is whether return to work is a complete assessment of quality of life and we seem to think that it is not. Nevertheless, it is an important component in the assessment of patients simply because of the finite quantity of health dollars and the realization that return to work is an important component to be considered by physicians as well as by economists.

In terms of the strategy of encouraging return to work we have only preliminary descriptive information rather than data from randomized interventions in most of the studies. Much of the emphasis seems to be on what one of the authors in a recent *New England Journal of Medicine* article has called "compression of morbidity." Essentially, this "compression of morbidity" involves earlier definitive diagnosis of patients with chest pain, earlier decision about angiography, and earlier surgery in an attempt to improve return to work. This is because the duration of preoperative disability has been shown, in a number of studies, to influence the ultimate return to work; return to work is far less likely for patients unemployed for more than 6 months.

Therefore the physician has a major role not only in raising the issue of return to work, but in initiating a prompt diagnostic and then therapeutic approach for these patients. The physicians' specific recommendations about the ability of the patient to return to work and recommendations for the time of this return seem important.

However, the physician can be saddled with neither the total blame nor the total responsibility for the lack of return to work of patients after coronary bypass surgery. There is a major role of the patient and of the family in terms of their philosophy of return to work, of the employer, and indeed of the society, part of which relates to the government because regulatory and legislative aspects are often deciding features affecting return to work.

One area that must be investigated is the role of rehabilitation - structured or unstructured, formal or informal, exercise and/or education and counselling - in influencing the return to work.

These are the questions that have been raised; they must all be evaluated critically by prospective studies. That perhaps is the major task for many of the people in attendance at this meeting. Before returning the microphone to Prof. Walter, who will close the conference, I know you will want to join me in thanking him and the organizing committee for a program that has been scientifically superior, has enabled the formation of many friendships medically and socially, but most importantly has brought together a group of individuals in a multidisciplinary approach that unquestionably will have a favorable effect on the care of patients with coronary disease who undergo coronary bypass surgery. Please join me in thanking Dr. Walter.

Walter: Thank you, Dr. Wenger. Thank you all. I must confess it was a great pleasure for me to have organized this symposium, to listen to your papers, to participate in the discussions, and to hear your views. I would like to express my gratitude to the Pharma Schwarz Company in Monheim, represented by Mr. Gücker, whose mediation I gratefully acknowledge. The coordination and smooth running of this congress were only possible thanks to the enormous talents and energy of Mrs. Kratzenberg. Without her tremendous behind-the-scenes activity, the meeting could not have taken place. Please accept my greatest thanks, Mrs. Kratzenberg. I also want to thank the host, the *Herz- und Kreislaufzentrum*, and all others who helped in any capacity whatsoever.

MIX
Papier aus verantwortungsvollen Quellen
Paper from responsible sources
FSC® C105338

If you have any concerns about our products,
you can contact us on
ProductSafety@springernature.com

In case Publisher is established outside the EU,
the EU authorized representative is:
Springer Nature Customer Service Center GmbH
Europaplatz 3, 69115 Heidelberg, Germany

Printed by Libri Plureos GmbH
in Hamburg, Germany